Clinical Management and Challenges in Polytrauma

Clinical Management and Challenges in Polytrauma

Editor

Roman Pfeifer

MDPI • Basel • Beijing • Wuhan • Barcelona • Belgrade • Manchester • Tokyo • Cluj • Tianjin

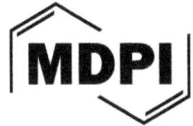

Editor
Roman Pfeifer
Universitats Spital Zurich
Switzerland

Editorial Office
MDPI
St. Alban-Anlage 66
4052 Basel, Switzerland

This is a reprint of articles from the Special Issue published online in the open access journal *Journal of Clinical Medicine* (ISSN 2077-0383) (available at: https://www.mdpi.com/journal/jcm/special_issues/Clinical_Polytrauma).

For citation purposes, cite each article independently as indicated on the article page online and as indicated below:

LastName, A.A.; LastName, B.B.; LastName, C.C. Article Title. *Journal Name* **Year**, *Volume Number*, Page Range.

ISBN 978-3-0365-5139-5 (Hbk)
ISBN 978-3-0365-5140-1 (PDF)

© 2022 by the authors. Articles in this book are Open Access and distributed under the Creative Commons Attribution (CC BY) license, which allows users to download, copy and build upon published articles, as long as the author and publisher are properly credited, which ensures maximum dissemination and a wider impact of our publications.

The book as a whole is distributed by MDPI under the terms and conditions of the Creative Commons license CC BY-NC-ND.

Contents

About the Editor vii

Jan Gewiess, Christoph Emanuel Albers, Hans-Christoph Pape, Hannes Bangerter, Wolf-Dieter Zech, Marius Johann Baptist Keel and Johannes Dominik Bastian
Characteristics of Prehospital Death in Trauma Victims
Reprinted from: *J. Clin. Med.* **2021**, *10*, 4765, doi:10.3390/jcm10204765 1

Daniel Schmitt, Sascha Halvachizadeh, Robin Steinemann, Kai Oliver Jensen, Till Berk, Valentin Neuhaus, Ladislav Mica, Roman Pfeifer, Hans Christoph Pape and Kai Sprengel
Trauma Team Activation: Which Surgical Capability Is Immediately Required in Polytrauma? A Retrospective, Monocentric Analysis of Emergency Procedures Performed on 751 Severely Injured Patients
Reprinted from: *J. Clin. Med.* **2021**, *10*, 4335, doi:10.3390/jcm10194335 11

Emilian Spörri, Sascha Halvachizadeh, Jamison G. Gamble, Till Berk, Florin Allemann, Hans-Christoph Pape and Thomas Rauer
Comparison of Injury Patterns between Electric Bicycle, Bicycle and Motorcycle Accidents
Reprinted from: *J. Clin. Med.* **2021**, *10*, 3359, doi:10.3390/jcm10153359 21

Julian Scherer, Yannik Kalbas, Franziska Ziegenhain, Valentin Neuhaus, Rolf Lefering, Michel Teuben, Kai Sprengel, Hans-Christoph Pape and Kai Oliver Jensen
The GERtality Score: The Development of a Simple Tool to Help Predict in-Hospital Mortality in Geriatric Trauma Patients
Reprinted from: *J. Clin. Med.* **2021**, *10*, 1362, doi:10.3390/jcm10071362 29

Alison Fecher, Anthony Stimpson, Lisa Ferrigno and Timothy H. Pohlman
The Pathophysiology and Management of Hemorrhagic Shock in the Polytrauma Patient
Reprinted from: *J. Clin. Med.* **2021**, *10*, 4793, doi:10.3390/jcm10204793 39

Valerie Kuner, Nicole van Veelen, Stephanie Studer, Bryan Van de Wall, Jürgen Fornaro, Michael Stickel, Matthias Knobe, Reto Babst, Frank J.P. Beeres and Björn-Christian Link
Application of Pelvic Circumferential Compression Devices in Pelvic Ring Fractures—Are Guidelines Followed in Daily Practice?
Reprinted from: *J. Clin. Med.* **2021**, *10*, 1297, doi:10.3390/jcm10061297 67

Christian Kleber, Mirja Haussmann, Michael Hetz, Michael Tsokos and Claas T. Buschmann
Epidemiologic, Postmortem Computed Tomography-Morphologic and Biomechanical Analysis of the Effects of Non-Invasive External Pelvic Stabilizers in Genuine Unstable Pelvic Injuries
Reprinted from: *J. Clin. Med.* **2021**, *10*, 4348, doi:10.3390/jcm10194348 81

Andrea Janicova, Nils Becker, Baolin Xu, Marija Simic, Laurens Noack, Nils Wagner, Andreas J. Müller, Jessica Bertrand, Ingo Marzi and Borna Relja
Severe Traumatic Injury Induces Phenotypic and Functional Changes of Neutrophils and Monocytes
Reprinted from: *J. Clin. Med.* **2021**, *10*, 4139, doi:10.3390/jcm10184139 97

Jan Tilmann Vollrath, Felix Klingebiel, Felix Bläsius, Johannes Greven, Eftychios Bolierakis, Aleksander J. Nowak, Marija Simic, Frank Hildebrand, Ingo Marzi and Borna Relja
I-FABP as a Potential Marker for Intestinal Barrier Loss in Porcine Polytrauma
Reprinted from: *J. Clin. Med.* **2022**, *11*, 4599, doi:10.3390/jcm11154599 117

Frederik Greve, Olivia Mair, Ina Aulbach, Peter Biberthaler and Marc Hanschen
Correlation between Platelet Count and Lung Dysfunction in Multiple Trauma Patients—A Retrospective Cohort Analysis
Reprinted from: *J. Clin. Med.* **2022**, *11*, 1400, doi:10.3390/jcm11051400 . . . . **129**

Jordan E. Handcox, Jose M. Gutierrez-Naranjo, Luis M. Salazar, Travis S. Bullock, Leah P. Griffin and Boris A. Zelle
Nutrition and Vitamin Deficiencies Are Common in Orthopaedic Trauma Patients
Reprinted from: *J. Clin. Med.* **2021**, *10*, 5012, doi:10.3390/jcm10215012 . . . . **143**

About the Editor

Roman Pfeifer

Roman Pfeifer is a consultant of Trauma Surgery at the Department of Traumatology, University Hospital Zurich, Switzerland. He studied medicine at Hanover Medical School (MHH), Germany, and performed a scholarship (supported by German Academic Exchange Service, DAAD) at the University of Pittsburgh Medical Center, Department of Orthopedics, Pittsburgh, USA. He was a resident at the Department of Orthopedic Surgery, University of Aachen Medical Center, Germany, and is a board-certified trauma surgeon (2017). He is also a Fellow of the European Board of Surgeons (FEBS, EBSQ exam). Since 2017, he has been working at the Department of Traumatology, University Hospital Zurich, Switzerland. He is a member of several surgical societies (ESTES, DGU, SICOT, AO etc.) and of TREAT (Translational Large Animal Research Network), performing translational projects in orthopedics and traumatology. Since 2022, he has been a Professor for Translational Research in Polytrauma at the University of Zurich.

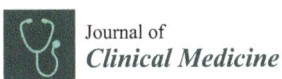

Article

Characteristics of Prehospital Death in Trauma Victims

Jan Gewiess [1,*], Christoph Emanuel Albers [1], Hans-Christoph Pape [2], Hannes Bangerter [1], Wolf-Dieter Zech [3], Marius Johann Baptist Keel [1] and Johannes Dominik Bastian [1]

- [1] Department of Orthopaedic Surgery and Traumatology, Inselspital, Bern University Hospital, University of Bern, 3010 Bern, Switzerland; christoph.albers@insel.ch (C.E.A.); hannes.bangerter@outlook.com (H.B.); marius.keel@insel.ch (M.J.B.K.); johannes.bastian@insel.ch (J.D.B.)
- [2] Department of Trauma, University Hospital of Zurich, 8091 Zurich, Switzerland; hans-christoph.pape@usz.ch
- [3] Institute of Forensic Medicine Bern, University of Bern, 3012 Bern, Switzerland; Wolf-Dieter.Zech@irm.unibe.ch
- * Correspondence: jan.gewiess@insel.ch; Tel.: +41-31-664-04-40

Abstract: Background: Using Injury Severity Score (ISS) data, this study aimed to give an overview of trauma mechanisms, causes of death, injury patterns, and potential survivability in prehospital trauma victims. Methods: Age, gender, trauma mechanism, cause of death, and ISS data were recorded regarding forensic autopsies and whole-body postmortem CT. Characteristics were analyzed for injuries considered potentially survivable at cutoffs of (I) ISS $\leq$ 75 vs. ISS = 75, (II) ISS $\leq$ 49 vs. ISS $\geq$ 50, and (III) ISS < lethal dose 50% (LD50) vs. ISS > LD50 according to Bull's probit model. Results: In $n = 130$ prehospital trauma victims (45.3 ± 19.5 years), median ISS was 66. Severity of injuries to the head/neck and chest was greater compared to other regions ($p < 0.001$). 52% died from central nervous system (CNS) injury. Increasing injury severity in head/neck region was associated with CNS-injury related death (odds ratio (OR) 2.7, confidence interval (CI) 1.8–4.4). Potentially survivable trauma was identified in (I) 56%, (II) 22%, and (III) 9%. Victims with ISS $\leq$ 75, ISS $\leq$ 49, and ISS < LD50 had lower injury severity across most ISS body regions compared to their respective counterparts ($p < 0.05$). Conclusion: In prehospital trauma victims, injury severity is high. Lethal injuries predominate in the head/neck and chest regions and are associated with CNS-related death. The appreciable amount (9–56%) of victims dying at presumably survivable injury severity encourages perpetual efforts for improvement in the rescue of highly traumatized patients.

Keywords: polytrauma; trauma victims; prehospital death; Injury Severity Score (ISS)

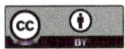

1. Introduction

The term 'polytrauma' has been widely established for patients suffering simultaneous injuries to multiple body regions or organ systems, in which the single injury or its combination is potentially life-threatening (Deutsche Gesellschaft für Unfallchirurgie (DGU)). More recent definitions include a priori assumptions of mortality rates >30% factoring the Injury Severity Score (ISS) and physiological parameters such as hypotension, unconsciousness, acidosis, coagulopathy, and age [1]. Prehospital mortality rates have been reported to reach >50% in polytraumatized patients [2,3]. Recent literature elaborating on epidemiology and specific injury patterns related to mortality in trauma victims focused primarily on in-hospital deaths and deaths during transport of trauma patients [4–6]. However, this study aimed to identify the most prevalent causes of death and potentially survivable constellations regarding trauma severity in prehospital trauma victims in order to uncover the quality and evolutional potential of trauma rescue.

According to the World Health Organization (WHO), the three leading causes of death from trauma are road-traffic injuries, self-inflicted violence, and homicide (WHO, 2021). A high number of traumatic prehospital deaths results from fatal trauma implying lethal injury with greatest possible severity across multiple body regions [7]. The ISS first described by Baker et al. in 1974 is commonly used to quantify overall trauma severity [8].

An ISS > 15 is usually adopted to characterize major trauma [9]. Patients with an ISS > 24 are considered to be critically injured [10].

Most deaths in trauma victims are reportedly secondary to central nervous system (CNS) injury, uncontrolled bleeding, airway insufficiency, or multiple organ failure (MOF) [11,12]. Establishing the most probable cause of death in dependency of quickly accessible data (trauma mechanism, injury pattern and injury severity) might give direction to possible treatment strategies even before complete Advanced Trauma Life Support (ATLS) assessment is performed.

Using ISS data obtained from autopsy reports and postmortem CT scan data of trauma victims, this study aimed to give an overview of:

- trauma mechanisms,
- causes of death,
- injury patterns,
- influence of regional trauma severity on causes of death,
- trauma mechanisms, causes of death, and injury patterns in potentially survivable injuries.

2. Materials and Methods

2.1. Patients and Parameters

Between 01/2005 and 12/2013, forensic autopsies and whole body postmortem CT scans prior to autopsy were undertaken for all trauma-related deaths in the canton Bern, Switzerland at the Institute of Forensic Medicine at the University of Bern (n = 489). Victims underwent forensic evaluation ordered by local prosecutors due to suspected non-natural cause of death. Within this 9-year period, 130 patients suffered prehospital death. Forensic examinations and postmortem reports were conducted by board certified forensic pathologists. From CT scans and records, an independent investigator assessed each patient's age, gender, trauma mechanism, cause of death, and injury severity. Victims were included with trauma mechanisms such as motor vehicle accidents (MVA), suicides, workspace accidents, sports accidents, and agriculture accidents. Among those committing suicide, only victims being run over by a train or falling/jumping from height were included. Other suicides, such as hanging, shooting, burning, and stabbing were excluded. Injury severity was assessed using total ISS, Copes' ISS intervals (proposed for mitigation of heterogeneity with the rationale of the most severe injury/combination included (ISS 16–24, 25–40, 41–49, 50–66, and 75)) [10], and the Abbreviated Injury Score (AIS98) for the respective ISS body region.

Regional injury severity was represented by the AIS98 categories (0 = none, 1 = minor, 2 = moderate, 3 = serious, 4 = severe, 5 = critical, 6 = maximum/currently untreatable). Calculation of the ISS is based on the sum of squares of the most severely injured three of six different body regions (face, head and neck, chest and thoracic spine, abdomen and lumbar spine, pelvis and extremities, external). External injuries included injuries such as abrasions, lacerations, burns, hypothermia, and electrical injury. The ISS ranges from 3–75. In the case of a category 6 trauma to any body region, the ISS is set to 75.

Injury characteristics of trauma victims sustaining potentially survivable injury were compared to those with unsurvivable injury. The respective graduation of lesser traumatization or potentially survivable injury was performed for (I) salvageable submaximal trauma (ISS < 75) according to Chiara et al. [13], (II) an ISS < 49, as proposed by Sampalis et al. [14] and (III) using Bull's probit model for the derivation of a lethal dose of 50% (LD50) [15]. Using the formula '$42 - 0.004167 \times age^2$', potential survivability was considered if the patient's probability of survival is >50%.

2.2. Statistical Analysis

Statistical analysis was performed using R (R Foundation for Statistical Computing, Version 4.1.0 (2021), Vienna, Austria). Data description is performed using the median and interquartile range (Q1–Q3) and absolute and relative frequencies, respectively. Frequencies were compared using Chi^2-tests and Fisher's exact test in the case of an expected frequency < 5. Normal distribution was tested using the Shapiro–Wilk test. Pairwise comparisons were performed using *t*-tests for parametric and Mann-Whitney-*U*-tests for non-parametric continuous data. Multivariable analyses were performed using logistic regression. Results are reported as Odds ratios (OR) and corresponding 95% confidence intervals.

3. Results

3.1. Overview of Trauma Mechanisms and Causes of Death

Within a 9-year period, $n = 130$ trauma victims died before arriving at the emergency department (mean age 45.3 ± 19.5 years; range 16–92). Seventy four percent victims were of male gender. The most common trauma mechanism was MVA (54%), followed by suicide (18%), industrial/workspace accidents (9%), sports accidents (7%), and agriculture accidents (2%). Among sports accidents, paragliding, parachuting, and base-jumping were most common followed by skiing/snowboarding or hiking and sledding or climbing. The most frequently coded cause of death was CNS injury (52%), followed by uncontrolled bleeding (42%), airway compromise (32%) and MOF (29%). A single cause of death was found in $n = 78$ (60%), a combination of 2 in $n = 37$ (29%), a combination of 3 in $n = 12$ (9%), and a combination of four in $n = 3$ (2%) patients. Numerical summaries of demographic data, trauma mechanisms, and causes of death are given in Table 1.

Table 1. Frequencies and numerical summaries of demographic data, trauma mechanisms, and causes of death.

	n	Mean Age (SD, IQR)	n f/m (%)	Median ISS (Q1, Q3)	n CNS Injury (%)	n Exsanguination (%)	n Airway Compromise (%)	n MOF (%)
Overall	130	45.3 (19.49, 32.75)	34/96 (26.15/73.85)	66 (50, 75)	67 (51.54)	54 (41.54)	41 (31.54)	38 (29.23)
MVA	70	48.48 (20.4, 32.00)	16/54 (22.9/77.1)	66 (54.75, 75)	36 (51.4)	32 (45.7)	20 (28.6)	22 (31.4)
Suicide	23	40.48 (17.06, 23.5)	11/12 (47.8/52.2)	75 (62.5, 75)	12 (52.2)	10 (43.5)	10 (43.5)	6 (26.1)
Industrial/ workspace	12	42.25 (14.06, 22.25)	0/12 (0/100)	62.5 (47.75, 75)	10 (83.3)	4 (33.3)	4 (33.3)	4 (33.3)
Sports	9	36.11 (15.99, 27)	3/6 (33.3/66.7)	50 (43, 66)	1 (11.1)	4 (44.4)	2 (22.2)	5 (55.6)
Agriculture	3	64 (17.78, 17)	1/2 (33.3/66.7)	57 (53.5, 66)	1 (33.3)	1 (33.3)	1 (33.3)	1 (33.3)

SD, Standard deviation; IQR, interquartile range; f/m, female to male ratio; ISS, Injury Severity Score; CNS, central nervous system; MOF, multiple organ failure; MVA, motor vehicle accident.

Median ISS was 66 in 130 deceased. According to causes of death, median total ISS was highest in (combined) CNS injuries (65) and lowest in (combined) MOF (56). Compared to victims of CNS injuries, total ISS was significantly lower in those dying of airway compromise ($p = 0.019$) or those dying of MOF ($p = 0.036$). According to trauma mechanism, median ISS was highest in suicides (66) and lowest in sports accidents (50). Differences were not significant ($p > 0.16$). Descriptive statistics of ISS distributions are shown in Table 2.

Table 2. Median (Q1, Q3) total ISS and severity in respective ISS body regions according to trauma mechanisms and causes of death.

	n (%)	Median Total ISS (Q1, Q3)	Median ISS Head/Neck (Q1, Q3)	Median ISS face (Q1, Q3)	Median ISS Chest (Q1, Q3)	Median ISS Abdomen (Q1, Q3)	Median ISS Pelvis/Extremities (Q1, Q3)	Median ISS External (Q1, Q3)
Overall	130	66 (50, 75)	5 (3.25, 6)	1 (0, 3)	5 (4, 5)	4 (0, 5)	3 (2, 4)	2 (2, 2)
MVA	70 (54)	66 (54.75, 75)	4 (4, 6)	2 (0, 3.75)	5 (4, 6)	4 (0, 5)	3 (2, 4)	2 (2, 2)
Suicide	23 (18)	75 (62.5, 75)	6 (3.5, 6)	2 (0, 4)	5 (4, 5)	5 (3, 5)	3 (3, 4)	2 (2, 2)
Workspace	12 (9)	62.5 (47.75, 75)	5 (3, 6)	0 (0, 2.25)	5 (3.75, 5)	5 (4.25, 5)	3 (0, 4)	2 (2, 2)
Sports	9 (7)	50 (43, 66)	4 (3, 5)	1 (0, 3)	5 (4, 5)	0 (0, 5)	3 (2, 3)	2 (2, 2)
Agriculture	3 (2)	57 (53.5, 66)	3 (1.5, 4.5)	0 (0, 0.5)	5 (5, 5)	4 (3, 4.5)	4 (3.5, 4)	2 (2, 2)
CNS injury	67 (52)	75 (57, 75)	6 (5, 6)	2 (0, 4)	5 (4, 5)	5 (1, 5)	3 (2, 4)	2 (2, 2)
Exsanguination	54 (42)	66 (57, 75)	4 (3, 5)	0 (0, 2.75)	5 (5, 6)	4 (3, 5)	3 (3, 4)	2 (2, 2)
Airway compromise	41 (32)	59 (50, 66)	4 (3, 5)	0 (0, 2)	5 (5, 5)	4 (3, 5)	3 (2, 4)	2 (2, 2)
MOF	38 (29)	61.5 (43, 75)	4 (3, 5)	0 (0, 2)	5 (4, 5)	3 (0.5, 5)	3 (2, 4)	2 (2, 2)

Q1, First quartile; Q3, third quartile; ISS, Injury Severity Score; CNS, central nervous system; MOF, multiple organ failure; MVA, motor vehicle accident.

3.2. Overview of Injury Patterns

No patient had injuries to only one body region. Two body regions were injured in $n = 3$ (2%), three in $n = 14$ (11%), four in $n = 18$ (14%), five in $n = 50$ (39%), and six in $n = 45$ (35%) patients. Face trauma was present in $n = 70$ (54%), head and neck trauma in $n = 117$ (90%), thoracic trauma in $n = 122$ (94%), abdominal trauma in $n = 96$ (74%), pelvic and extremity trauma in $n = 108$ (83%), and external injury in $n = 127$ (98%). Depending on the number of injury combinations, different body regions were predominantly injured (Figure 1). For example, abdominal injuries were rather infrequent when there were ≤ 3 different body regions affected (14%) compared to when ≤ 5 regions were affected (78%). The frequency of face or external injury was comparable, regardless of the number of injured body regions.

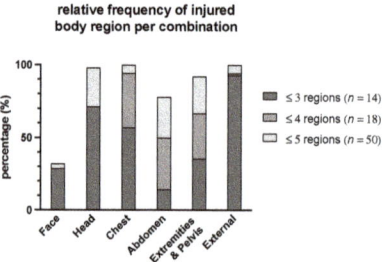

Figure 1. Relative distribution of injured body regions according to ISS per injury combination in prehospital trauma-related deaths.

3.3. Overview of Injury Severity

According to Copes' ISS intervals, $n = 6$ (5%) presented with an ISS of 1–24, $n = 22$ (17%) with an ISS of 24–49, $n = 45$ (35%) with an ISS of 50–74, and $n = 57$ (44%) with an ISS of 75. According to the ISS body regions, severity was critical (median = 5, Q1 = 3.25, Q3 = 6) in head/neck injuries, minor (median = 1, Q1 = 0, Q3 = 3) in face injuries, critical (median = 5, Q1 = 4, Q3 = 5) in chest injuries, severe (median = 4, Q1 = 0, Q3 = 5) in abdomen injuries, serious (median = 3, Q1 = 2, Q3 = 4) in pelvis/extremity injuries, and moderate (median = 2, Q1 = 2, Q3 = 2) in external injuries.

Face injuries were significantly less severe compared to injuries across all other body regions except for external ($p < 0.001$, Figure 2). Median head and neck injury and chest injury both were significantly more severe than injuries to abdomen, extremities, and external ($p < 0.001$). Abdominal injuries were significantly more severe compared to external injuries ($p < 0.001$). Extremity injuries were significantly more severe compared to external injuries ($p < 0.002$). Descriptive statistics of injury severity in respective ISS body regions are provided in Table 2 and Figure 2.

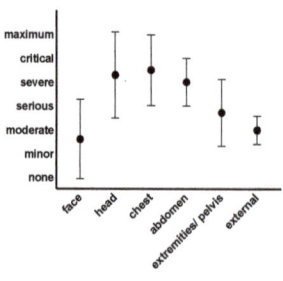

Figure 2. Median and 95% CI of injury severity across ISS body regions. Symbol: median, whiskers: 95% CI.

3.4. Influence of Regional Trauma Severity on Causes of Death

Relative risk (OR) of succumbing a specific cause of death relative to an increasing trauma severity to the respective ISS body region is shown in Figure 3. Among these, the clearest indicator for an increased OR for a specific cause of death is an increased trauma severity in the head/neck region for the CNS-injury related death (OR 2.7, CI 1.8–4.4). For the remaining causes of death, a clear monodirectional relation to regional injury severity could not be established.

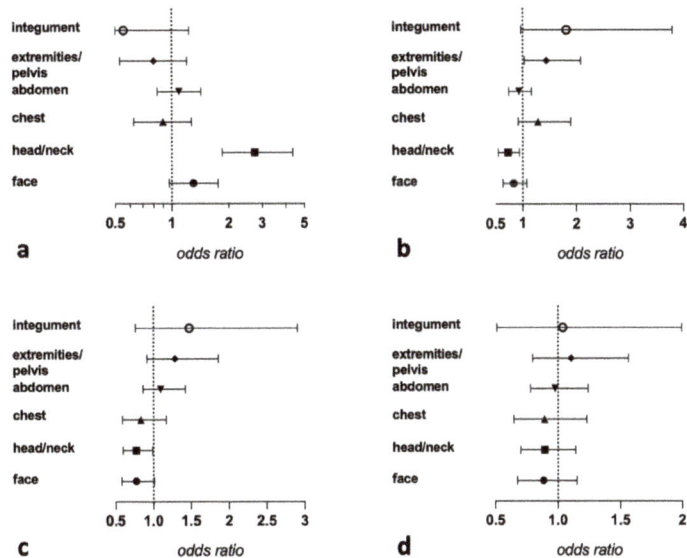

Figure 3. Coefplots (Odds ratios with 95% Wald confidence limits) for (**a**) CNS injury, (**b**) exsanguination, (**c**) airway compromise, (**d**) MOF. Most CI indicate no clear monodirectional relation between an increasing regional injury severity and a specific reason of death.

3.5. Comparison of Trauma Victims with Potentially Survivable Injuries versus Trauma Victims with Non-Survivable Injuries

N = 73 (56.2%) victims died with an ISS < 75 and n = 57 (43.8%) died with an ISS of 75. N = 28 (22%) victims sustained potentially survivable trauma characterized by an ISS < 49. According to Bull's model, n = 11 (9%) patients sustained potentially survivable trauma (Figure 4). Median ISS was 54 in the case of submaximal trauma, 37 for victims with an ISS < 49, and 24 for victims with an ISS < LD50. Age and gender of victims were comparable among respective groups for all three approaches (p > 0.4). Regarding trauma mechanisms, there were no significant differences between victims of maximal/submaximal or unsurvivable/potentially survivable trauma (Table 3). However, people committing suicide more frequently sustained maximal injuries compared to other trauma mechanisms (p < 0.07). People dying in sports accidents rather sustained submaximal (p < 0.08) or potentially survivable injuries (p < 0.17).

Relative frequencies of causes of death varied when comparing maximal to submaximal and unsurvivable to potentially survivable trauma. In the case of the respective higher suspected traumatization (maximal and unsurvivable injury), CNS injury was the most common cause of death (>52%), followed by exsanguination (>40%). For the suspected lesser traumatization (submaximal and potentially survivable injuries), frequencies of airway compromise and MOF were generally increased (up to 80%). A comparison of causes of death for the three approaches is presented in Figure 5.

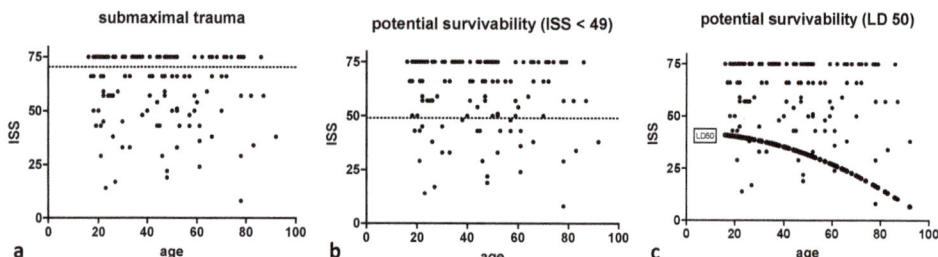

Figure 4. Age versus Injury Severity Score (ISS) for trauma victims with submaximal trauma/ISS < 75 (**a**), potentially survivable injuries/ISS < 49 (**b**), and age versus Injury Severity Score (ISS) and LD50 derived from Bull's probit analysis (**c**). Submaximal trauma was present in 56% and potentially survivable trauma in 22% and 9%, respectively.

Table 3. Absolute (relative) frequencies and comparison of demographic data, trauma mechanisms, and causes of death for trauma victims with submaximal trauma/ISS < 75, potentially survivable injuries/ISS < 49, and potentially survivable (ISS < LD50 as derived from Bull's probit analysis). N (ISS < 75) = 73, n (ISS < 49) = 28, n (ISS < LD50) = 11.

	Overall (%)	ISS < 75	ISS 75	p-Value	ISS < 49	ISS > 49	p-Value	ISS < LD50	ISS > LD50	p-Value
Median ISS	66	54	75		37	75		24	66	
Mean age	46	47	44	0.664	47	45.5	0.626	33	47	0.403
n female/male (%)	34/96 (26.15/73.85)	21/52 (28.8/71.2)	13/44 (22.8/77.2)	0.443	9/19 (32.1/67.9)	25/77 (24.5/76)	0.568	4/7 (36.4/63.6)	30/89 (25.2/75)	0.477
n MVA (%)	70 (54)	38 (52.1)	32 (56.1)	0.643	13 (46.4)	57 (55.9)	0.374	4 (36.4)	66 (55.5)	0.224
n suicide (%)	23 (18)	9 (12.3)	14 (24.6)	0.07	3 (10.7)	20 (19.6)	0.403	1 (9.1)	22 (18.5)	0.435
n workspace (%)	12 (9)	8 (11)	4 (7)	0.441	3 (10.7)	9 (8.8)	0.721	1 (9.1)	11 (9.2)	1
n sports (%)	9 (7)	8 (11)	1 (1.8)	0.077	4 (14.3)	5 (4.9)	0.1	2 (18.2)	7 (5.9)	0.169
n agriculture (%)	3 (2)	2 (2.7)	1 (1.8)	1	0 (0)	3 (2.9)	1	0	3 (2.5)	1
n CNS injury (%)	67 (52)	27 (37)	40 (70.2)	<0.001	10 (35.7)	57 (55.9)	0.059	5 (45.5)	62 (52.1)	0.673
n exsanguination (%)	54 (42)	32 (43.8)	22 (38.6)	0.548	9 (32.1)	45 (44.1)	0.255	3 (27.3)	51 (42.9)	0.36
n airway compromise (%)	41 (32)	33 (45.2)	8 (14)	<0.001	9 (32.1)	32 (31.4)	0.938	5 (45.5)	36 (30.3)	0.321
n MOF (%)	38 (29)	26 (35.6)	12 (21.1)	0.07	14 (50)	24 (23.5)	0.007	3 (27.3)	35 (29.4)	1

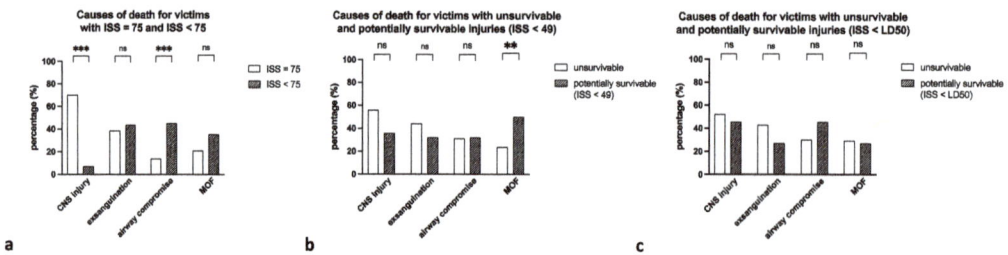

Figure 5. Relative frequencies of causes of death for (**a**) maximal (clear) vs. submaximal (patterned) trauma, (**b**) unsurvivable (ISS > 49, clear) vs. potentially survivable (ISS < 49, patterned) trauma, and (**c**) unsurvivable (ISS > LD50, clear) vs. potentially survivable (ISS < LD50, patterned) trauma. Relative frequency of CNS injury was always higher in the suspected higher traumatized group but reached significance only in the comparison of maximal to submaximal trauma (**a**). In turn, airway compromise was more frequently observed in victims sustaining potentially survivable injury with significance only when comparing maximal to submaximal trauma (**a**). Similarly, MOF was more frequent in submaximal (**a**) and potentially survivable (**b**,**c**) trauma. *** $p < 0.001$, ** $p < 0.01$, ns: not significant.

Overall, injury severity of specific body regions was lower in the suspected lesser traumatization (submaximal and potentially survivable injuries. Table 4 and Figure 6). There were significant differences for all body regions, except for the external. Especially, injury severity to the chest and abdomen was significantly lower in submaximal and potentially survivable injuries ($p < 0.001$).

Table 4. Means (SD, IQR) of total ISS and of injury severity to the respective body region.

	Overall	ISS < 75	ISS 75	p-Value	ISS < 49	ISS > 49	p-Value	ISS < LD50	ISS > LD50	p-Value
Face	1 (0, 3)	0 (0, 2)	3 (0, 4)	<0.001	0 (0, 2)	2 (0, 4)	0.03	0 (0, 1.5)	2 (0, 4)	0.148
Head/neck	5 (3.25, 6)	4 (3, 5)	6 (6, 6)	<0.001	4 (3, 5)	5 (4, 6)	<0.001	3 (3, 5)	5 (4, 6)	0.024
Chest	5 (4, 5)	5 (4, 5)	5 (5, 6)	<0.001	3 (2, 4.5)	5 (5, 5)	<0.001	2 (0, 2.5)	5 (5, 5)	<0.001
Abdomen	4 (0, 5)	3 (0, 5)	5 (4, 5)	<0.001	0 (0, 2)	5 (3, 5)	<0.001	0 (0, 0)	5 (3, 5)	<0.001
Pelvis and extremities	3 (2, 4)	3 (2, 4)	3 (3, 4)	0.022	1 (0, 3)	3 (3, 4)	<0.001	0 (0, 2)	3 (3, 4)	<0.001
External	2 (2, 2)	2 (2, 2)	2 (2, 2)	0.155	2 (2, 2)	2 (2, 2)	0.962	2 (2, 2)	2 (2, 2)	0.122

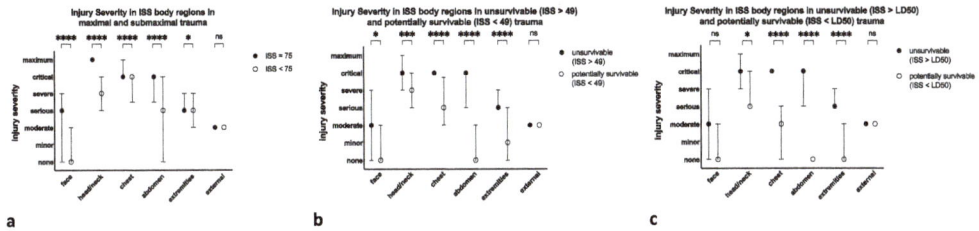

Figure 6. Median and IQR of injury severities according to the AIS-98 within the respective ISS body regions for prehospital deaths and submaximal (ISS < 75) injury (**a**), unsurvivable (ISS > 49) and potentially survivable (ISS < 49) injury (**b**), and unsurvivable (ISS > LD50) and potentially survivable (ISS < LD50) injury (**c**). There were significant differences in all body regions except for the external. **** $p < 0.0001$, *** $p < 0.001$, * $p < 0.5$, ns not significant. Symbol: median, whiskers: IQR.

4. Discussion

Means to identify injury patterns and causes of death in deceased patients are autopsy and postmortem CT imaging [16,17]. From a forensic perspective, autopsy remains the gold standard for the evaluation of injury patterns. Postmortem CT imaging can be a useful addition, especially for the evaluation of osseous injuries to the facial bones, spine, and extremities [18]. Thus, in Switzerland, postmortem CT scans are routinely obtained in these cases. Using ISS data obtained from congruously unique postmortem whole-body CT data and autopsies of prehospital trauma victims within a nine-year period, we were able to evaluate injury patterns, trauma mechanisms and corresponding causes of death and to identify potentially survivable relations. Only few studies evaluated prehospital death in trauma victims in the past decades [19–25].

Potentially treatable injuries in the prehospital phase included all injuries categorized by an AIS ≤ 5. Exemplary, for the head/neck region, these range from cerebral concussion (AIS = 1), via skull fracture (AIS = 2), traumatic aneurysm (AIS = 3), artery occlusion (AIS = 4), to brainstem contusion (AIS = 5). In contrast, prehospital medical treatment was not carried out in trauma victims presenting with the appearance of certain signs of death such as livor mortis or injuries not compatible with life. While the former may rather be expectable in intentional infliction (suicides, homicides), the latter are implied by the greatest possible injury as categorized by an AIS = 6 (such as decapitation, massive scull destruction, total severance of the aorta, avulsed liver, or torso transection).

We confirmed earlier findings of predominantly male, middle-aged patients dying from trauma in the prehospital environment [19–21,23,25], with the predominant trauma mechanism being MVA [21,23,25,26]. In our cohort, suicide was the second-most common trauma mechanism. As committed suicide by trauma is intended to result in death (e.g., maximal trauma, avoidance of public detection), appropriate rationale for (non-) timely initiation of (in-) adequate therapy might be negligible. Likewise, it demonstrates the comparative potential in the rescue of mechanistic scenarios not implying similar preconditions.

Recently, the acceptance of a potentially historical trimodal temporal distribution of trauma mortality has been questioned and might have to be corrected towards a rather unimodal distribution relative to posttraumatic days [6]. In a cohort of 277 victims of road traffic injuries, Pfeifer et al. reported on a mortality rate of 78% within the first six hours.

Furthermore, they were able to show an association between different injury patterns and temporal mortality distribution.

Our findings of a high percentage of lethal sports accidents have not yet been reported. These are especially worrying given the relatively lower ISS and younger age of these patients. The lower ISS in sports-related deaths essentially arising from exsanguination and MOF implicates preventability (inadequate primary treatment or long transportation times) and contrasts with earlier findings, where MOF related deaths were reported to be attributable to the in-hospital mortality of predominantly older trauma victims [12]. Differences in pre-clinical mortality might be explicable in view of geographical diversity [6]. Exemplarily, the reported median time of 2–3 h to death from hemorrhagic shock substantiates the dependability of surviving on geographics and transport times [27,28]. However, given the predominance of mountain sports accidents in our cohort, shortening search and rescue times might confront with the security of the emergency personnel.

Similar to our findings, earlier reports on injury patterns in prehospital trauma deaths showed a prevalence of >50 to >80% for head and neck and chest injuries [19,20,25,26]. Severity characterization of injuries to different body regions has hardly been performed. Ryan et al. [20] reported the most severe injury was most commonly located either in the head or chest region. Falconer [26] reported the head/neck region to be the single largest number of AIS 6 scores, which is reflected by the comparatively highest AIS scores in this region in our study. For each increasing AIS severity category of head and neck injury, we found the odds of dying from CNS injury to be multiplied by 2.7. Over the past 30 years, CNS injury continues to be the main cause of death in prehospitally deceased [12] as well as in polytraumas admitted to the hospital [4,6,29]. Except for the head and neck trauma severity and lethality of CNS injury, our multivariate analysis did not productively result in clear relations of injury severities to selected body regions and the prediction of a specific cause of death. This might be secondary to the coexistence of multiple causes of death or the great severity of injuries to multiple body regions.

To date, ISS values of prehospitally deceased trauma patients have only been reported in few studies [20,23]. While Hussain et al. found the majority of trauma related prehospital deaths in the ISS range of 21–50 (61.2%), Ryan et al. showed the main part to have an ISS of 75 (37%). This is in line with our results (43.9% having an ISS of 75).

The relative number of patients dying in the prehospital setting with the maximum ISS of 75 seems to increase in the past decades. In 1994, Hussain et al. found 19.1% of their study cohort to have the maximum ISS of 75 [23]. Later, Papadopoulos et al. found an AIS-6 injury (ISS = 75 by definition) in 35% of patients in their cohort [22]. Ryan et al. investigated injury patterns and preventability in prehospital motor vehicle crash fatalities and found 37% of the study population to have the maximum ISS of 75 [20]. In this study, there were 44% of prehospital deaths having an ISS of 75.

This might have two reasons: On the one hand, early treatment and transport time might have improved and thus the relative number of patients surviving the prehospital phase increases compared to those with lethal injury. This would be in line with the low number of patients with an ISS < 16 in our cohort (1.5%). On the other hand, and in light of the high incidence of lethal MVA, the energy of trauma mechanisms in trauma victims might have increased.

The performance of the ISS to quantify injury severity and potential survivability remains questionable, especially, when considering the representation of multiple injuries to the same body region [1]. In line with the recent polytrauma definition, an ISS-only based approach alone cannot specify the really critically ill trauma patients [30]. Sampalis et al. [14] proposed ISS groupings to classify survivability (survivable ISS < 24; potentially survivable ISS 25–49; non-survivable ISS > 49). Age has been repeatedly shown to influence ISS based mortality prediction [15,31] and was therefore integrated in the LD50 consideration according to Bull [15,30]. Especially in patients with severe injuries, ISS might not be a valid instrument to predict mortality [32].

Defining preventable death from limited patient data remains a challenge and proposed rates of preventability have to be interpreted carefully given their methodological formation. Depending on the resorted threshold being submaximal injury, ISS < 49 or ISS < LD50, or an expert panel, potential survivability rates in trauma victims reportedly range from 15–47% (9–56% in this study) [19–24]. Our results demonstrate some clear trends regardless of the threshold: While non-survivability was determined essentially by CNS injury, trauma victims sustaining potentially survivable injuries primarily died from airway compromise and MOF. As expected, and in line with our multivariate analysis, injuries to the head and neck region were significantly more severe in maximal and unsurvivable injuries.

To our knowledge, this study is the first to use postmortem ISS obtained from autopsies combined with whole-body CT scans of an adequate sample size for analysis of prehospital death in trauma victims. Another strength is the long period of the study. Thus, we were able to provide a detailed breakdown of the injuries that led to death.

Nevertheless, the heterogenous character of injury patterns and the coexistence of several causes of death in 40% of cases limits their attributability. A further limitation of the data acquisition is that no information about any prehospital management is available. However, given the high rate of definitively unsurvivable trauma (44% of cases presenting with an ISS = 75) combined with the aforementioned heterogeneity of injury patterns, it remains questionable whether further analysis of individual prehospital treatment might gain any insights for preclinical rescue personnel.

5. Conclusions

Traumatic prehospital death is most commonly secondary to MVA. In these patients, (lethal) injuries predominate in the head/neck and chest region. CNS injury is the most common cause of death and is associated with the severity of injuries to the head and neck.

All estimation of preventable death rate from limited data must be a rough approximation. Whatever value is adopted, it is certain there is still potential for improvement in the rescue of polytraumas as there is an appreciable amount of victims dying from stoppable or reversible causes at presumably survivable overall injury severity.

Author Contributions: Conceptualization and methodology, J.G., C.E.A., W.-D.Z., M.J.B.K. and J.D.B.; validation, W.-D.Z., M.J.B.K. and J.D.B.; formal analysis, J.G. and C.E.A.; investigation, J.D.B., H.B. and W.-D.Z.; resources, W.-D.Z.; data curation, J.G., H.B., W.-D.Z. and J.D.B.; writing—original draft preparation, J.G., C.E.A., W.-D.Z., M.J.B.K. and J.D.B.; writing—review and editing, J.G., C.E.A., H.-C.P., H.B., W.-D.Z., M.J.B.K. and J.D.B.; visualization, J.G. and J.D.B.; supervision, C.E.A., W.-D.Z., M.J.B.K. and J.D.B.; project administration, W.-D.Z., M.J.B.K. and J.D.B. All authors have read and agreed to the published version of the manuscript.

Funding: This research received no external funding.

Institutional Review Board Statement: The study was conducted according to the guidelines of the Declaration of Helsinki. Usage of the acquired data was approved by the local ethics committee of the canton of Bern, Switzerland.

Informed Consent Statement: Patient consent was waived. No consent could be obtained for the injury patterns examined prior to data collection.

Data Availability Statement: The data presented in this study are available on request from the corresponding author. The data are not publicly available due to privacy reasons.

Conflicts of Interest: The authors declare no conflict of interest.

References

1. Pape, H.-C.; Lefering, R.; Butcher, N.; Peitzman, A.; Leenen, L.; Marzi, I.; Lichte, P.; Josten, C.; Bouillon, B.; Schmucker, U.; et al. The definition of polytrauma revisited. *J. Trauma Acute Care Surg.* **2014**, *77*, 780–786. [CrossRef]
2. Pfeifer, R.; Tarkin, I.S.; Rocos, B.; Pape, H.-C. Patterns of mortality and causes of death in polytrauma patients—Has anything changed? *Injury* **2009**, *40*, 907–911. [CrossRef]

3. Butcher, N.E.; Balogh, Z.J. Update on the definition of polytrauma. *Eur. J. Trauma Emerg. Surg.* **2014**, *40*, 107–111. [CrossRef]
4. Van Breugel, J.M.M.; Niemeyer, M.J.S.; Houwert, R.M.; Groenwold, R.H.H.; Leenen, L.P.H.; Van Wessem, K.J.P. Global changes in mortality rates in polytrauma patients admitted to the ICU—A systematic review. *World J. Emerg. Surg.* **2020**, *15*, 55. [CrossRef]
5. El Mestoui, Z.; Jalalzadeh, H.; Giannakopoulos, G.F.; Zuidema, W.P. Incidence and etiology of mortality in polytrauma patients in a Dutch level I trauma center. *Eur. J. Emerg. Med.* **2017**, *24*, 49–54. [CrossRef] [PubMed]
6. Pfeifer, R.; Teuben, M.; Andruszkow, H.; Barkatali, B.M.; Pape, H.-C. Mortality Patterns in Patients with Multiple Trauma: A Systematic Review of Autopsy Studies. *PLoS ONE* **2016**, *11*, e0148844. [CrossRef] [PubMed]
7. Gedeborg, R.; Chen, L.-H.; Thiblin, I.; Byberg, L.; Melhus, H.; Michaëlsson, K.; Warner, M. Prehospital injury deaths—Strengthening the case for prevention. *J. Trauma Inj. Infect. Crit. Care* **2012**, *72*, 765–772. [CrossRef] [PubMed]
8. Baker, S.P.; O'Neill, B.; Haddon, W., Jr.; Long, W.B. The injury severity score: A method for describing patients with multiple injuries and evaluating emergency care. *J. Trauma Acute Care Surg.* **1974**, *14*, 187–196. [CrossRef]
9. Palmer, C. Major Trauma and the Injury Severity Score—Where Should We Set the Bar? *Annu. Proc. Assoc. Adv. Automot. Med.* **2007**, *51*, 13–29. [PubMed]
10. Copes, W.S.; Champion, H.R.; Sacco, W.J.; Lawnick, M.M.; Keast, S.L.; Bain, L.W. The Injury Severity Score Revisited. *J. Trauma Inj. Infect. Crit. Care* **1988**, *28*, 69–77. [CrossRef]
11. Lansink, K.W.W.; Gunning, A.C.; Leenen, L.P.H. Cause of death and time of death distribution of trauma patients in a Level I trauma centre in the Netherlands. *Eur. J. Trauma Emerg. Surg.* **2013**, *39*, 375–383. [CrossRef]
12. Søreide, K.; Krüger, A.J.; Vårdal, A.L.; Ellingsen, C.L.; Søreide, E.; Lossius, H.M. Epidemiology and Contemporary Patterns of Trauma Deaths: Changing Place, Similar Pace, Older Face. *World J. Surg.* **2007**, *31*, 2092–2103. [CrossRef]
13. Chiara, O.; Scott, J.D.; Cimbanassi, S.; Marini, A.; Zoia, R.; Rodriguez, A.; Scalea, T. Trauma deaths in an Italian urban area: An audit of pre-hospital and in-hospital trauma care. *Injury* **2002**, *33*, 553–562. [CrossRef]
14. Sampalis, J.S.; Boukas, S.; Nikolis, A.; Lavoie, A. Preventable death classification: Interrater reliability and comparison with ISS-based survival probability estimates. *Accid. Anal. Prev.* **1995**, *27*, 199–206. [CrossRef]
15. Bull, J.; Dickson, G. Injury scoring by TRISS and ISS/Age. *Injury* **1991**, *22*, 127–131. [CrossRef]
16. Donchin, Y.; Rivkind, A.I.; Bar-Ziv, J.; Hiss, J.; Almog, J.; Drescher, M. Utility of postmortem computed tomography in trauma victims. *J. Trauma Inj. Infect. Crit. Care* **1994**, *37*, 552–556. [CrossRef]
17. Jalalzadeh, H.; Giannakopoulos, G.F.; Berger, F.H.; Fronczek, J.; van de Goot, F.R.; Reijnders, U.J.; Zuidema, W.P. Post-mortem imaging compared with autopsy in trauma victims—A systematic review. *Forensic Sci. Int.* **2015**, *257*, 29–48. [CrossRef] [PubMed]
18. Scholing, M.; Saltzherr, T.P.; Jin, P.H.P.F.K.; Ponsen, K.J.; Reitsma, J.B.; Lameris, J.S.; Goslings, J.C. The value of postmortem computed tomography as an alternative for autopsy in trauma victims: A systematic review. *Eur. Radiol.* **2009**, *19*, 2333–2341. [CrossRef]
19. Davis, J.S.; Satahoo, S.S.; Butler, F.K.; Dermer, H.; Naranjo, D.; Julien, K.; Van Haren, R.M.; Namias, N.; Blackbourne, L.H.; Schulman, C.I. An analysis of prehospital deaths. *J. Trauma Acute Care Surg.* **2014**, *77*, 213–218. [CrossRef]
20. Ryan, M.; Stella, J.; Chiu, H.; Ragg, M. Injury patterns and preventability in prehospital motor vehicle crash fatalities in Victoria. *Emerg. Med. Australas.* **2004**, *16*, 274–279. [CrossRef]
21. Limb, D.; McGowan, A.; Fairfield, J.E.; Pigott, T.J. Prehospital deaths in the Yorkshire Health Region. *Emerg. Med. J.* **1996**, *13*, 248–250. [CrossRef] [PubMed]
22. Papadopoulos, I.N.; Bukis, D.; Karalas, E.; Katsaragakis, S.; Stergiopoulos, S.; Peros, G.; Androulakis, G. Preventable Prehospital Trauma Deaths in a Hellenic Urban Health Region. *J. Trauma Inj. Infect. Crit. Care* **1996**, *41*, 864–869. [CrossRef] [PubMed]
23. Hussain, L.M.; Redmond, A.D. Are pre-hospital deaths from accidental injury preventable? *BMJ* **1994**, *308*, 1077–1080. [CrossRef]
24. Stocchetti, N.; Pagliarini, G.; Gennari, M.; Baldi, G.; Banchini, E.; Campari, M.; Bacchi, M.; Zuccoli, P. Trauma care in Italy: Evidence of in-hospital preventable deaths. *J. Trauma Inj. Infect. Crit. Care* **1994**, *36*, 401–405. [CrossRef]
25. Pfeifer, R.; Schick, S.; Holzmann, C.; Graw, M.; Teuben, M.; Pape, H.-C. Analysis of Injury and Mortality Patterns in Deceased Patients with Road Traffic Injuries: An Autopsy Study. *World J. Surg.* **2017**, *41*, 3111–3119. [CrossRef]
26. Falconer, J. Preventability of pre-hospital trauma deaths in southern New Zealand. *N. Z. Med. J.* **2010**, *123*, 11–19. [PubMed]
27. Berbiglia, L.; Lopez, P.P.; Bair, L.; Ammon, A.; Navas, G.; Keller, M.; Diebel, L.N. Patterns of early mortality after trauma in a neighborhood urban trauma center: Can we improve outcomes? *Am. Surg.* **2013**, *79*, 764–767. [CrossRef] [PubMed]
28. Holcomb, J.B.; Tilley, B.C.; Baraniuk, S.; Fox, E.E.; Wade, C.E.; Podbielski, J.M.; Del Junco, D.J.; Brasel, K.J.; Bulger, E.M.; Callcut, R.A.; et al. Transfusion of Plasma, Platelets, and Red Blood Cells in a 1:1:1 vs. a 1:1:2 Ratio and Mortality in Patients with Severe Trauma. *JAMA* **2015**, *313*, 471–482. [CrossRef]
29. Laudi, S.; Donaubauer, B.; Busch, T.; Kerner, T.; Bercker, S.; Bail, H.; Feldheiser, A.; Haas, N.; Kaisers, U. Low incidence of multiple organ failure after major trauma. *Injury* **2007**, *38*, 1052–1058. [CrossRef]
30. Paffrath, T.; Lefering, R.; Flohe, S. How to define severely injured patients?—An Injury Severity Score (ISS) based approach alone is not sufficient. *Injury* **2014**, *45*, S64–S69. [CrossRef]
31. Chiang, W.-K.; Huang, S.-T.; Chang, W.; Huang, M.-Y.; Chien, D.-K.; Tsai, C.-H. Mortality Factors Regarding the Injury Severity Score in Elderly Trauma Patients. *Int. J. Gerontol.* **2012**, *6*, 192–195. [CrossRef]
32. Deng, Q.; Tang, B.; Xue, C.; Liu, Y.; Liu, X.; Lv, Y.; Zhang, L. Comparison of the Ability to Predict Mortality between the Injury Severity Score and the New Injury Severity Score: A Meta-Analysis. *Int. J. Environ. Res. Public Health* **2016**, *13*, 825. [CrossRef] [PubMed]

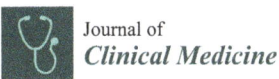

Article

Trauma Team Activation: Which Surgical Capability Is Immediately Required in Polytrauma? A Retrospective, Monocentric Analysis of Emergency Procedures Performed on 751 Severely Injured Patients

Daniel Schmitt [1,2,*], Sascha Halvachizadeh [1,2], Robin Steinemann [1,2], Kai Oliver Jensen [1,2], Till Berk [1,2], Valentin Neuhaus [1,2], Ladislav Mica [1,2], Roman Pfeifer [1,2], Hans Christoph Pape [1,2] and Kai Sprengel [1,2,3]

1. Department of Trauma, University Hospital Zurich (USZ), Raemistrasse 100, 8091 Zurich, Switzerland; sascha.halvachizadeh@usz.ch (S.H.); robin.steinemann@uzh.ch (R.S.); kaioliver.jensen@usz.ch (K.O.J.); till.berk@usz.ch (T.B.); valentin.neuhaus@usz.ch (V.N.); ladislav.mica@usz.ch (L.M.); roman.pfeifer@usz.ch (R.P.); hans-christoph.pape@usz.ch (H.C.P.); kai.sprengel@uzh.ch (K.S.)
2. Faculty of Medicine, University of Zurich (UZH), Raemistrasse 71, 8006 Zurich, Switzerland
3. Hirslanden Clinic St. Anna, St. Anna-Strasse 32, 6006 Lucerne, Switzerland
* Correspondence: daniel.schmitt@usz.ch; Tel.: +41-442-551-111

Abstract: There has been an ongoing discussion as to which interventions should be carried out by an "organ specialist" (for example, a thoracic or visceral surgeon) or by a trauma surgeon with appropriate general surgical training in polytrauma patients. However, there are only limited data about which exact emergency interventions are immediately carried out. This retrospective data analysis of one Level 1 trauma center includes adult polytrauma patients, as defined according to the Berlin definition. The primary outcome was the four most common emergency surgical interventions (ESI) performed during primary resuscitation. Out of 1116 patients, 751 (67.3%) patients (male gender, 530, 74.3%) met the inclusion criteria. The median age was 39 years (IQR: 25, 58) and the median injury severity score (ISS) was 38 (IQR: 29, 45). In total, 711 (94.7%) patients had at least one ESI. The four most common ESI were the insertion of a chest tube (48%), emergency laparotomy (26.3%), external fixation (23.5%), and the insertion of an intracranial pressure probe (ICP) (19.3%). The initial emergency treatment of polytrauma patients include a limited spectrum of potential life-saving interventions across distinct body regions. Polytrauma care would benefit from the 24/7 availability of a trauma team able to perform basic potentially life-saving surgical interventions, including chest tube insertion, emergency laparotomy, placing external fixators, and ICP insertion.

Keywords: polytrauma; emergency surgery; trauma team competence; trauma system; life-saving intervention

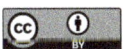

1. Introduction

Trauma is among the leading causes of morbidity and mortality in the working population [1]. Prehospital, a differentiated triage system of severely injured patients' increased survival rates [2,3] have led to the development of trauma centers, trauma networks, and national trauma registries [4–6]. Furthermore, the deployment of trauma teams has constantly improved survival [7,8]. Local institutional trauma guidelines define the members of the trauma team and the algorithms for trauma team activation [9,10]. Selected institutions have the luxury of activating an interdisciplinary trauma team, including an anesthesiologist, radiologist, neurosurgeon, and a trauma surgeon with surgical competences of the whole body [7].

There has been an ongoing discussion, especially in German speaking countries, as to which level of thoracoabdominal interventions a general surgeon is capable of providing as primary care to polytrauma patients, especially due to changes in the training of medical specialists [11,12]. In particular, whether thoracoabdominal interventions should be performed by an "organ specialist" (for example, a thoracic or visceral surgeon) who is present in the resuscitation area, or by a trauma surgeon with the appropriate general surgical training and the skills required for damage control surgery [13]. The principle of interdisciplinary collaboration under the direction of a general trauma surgeon is currently the basis of major trauma centers [14].

Unfortunately, there is only limited information about the life-saving surgeries that are immediately carried out.

To improve trauma systems and training adequately, an overview of the most common emergency interventions for severely injured patients is required. Therefore, the aim of this study was to describe the most commonly performed emergency surgical interventions (ESI) on polytrauma patients and their impact on morbidity and mortality.

2. Materials and Methods

This retrospective cohort study strictly follows the Strengthening the Reporting of Observational Studies in Epidemiology (STROBE) Statement [15].

This study was conducted at one academic Level 1 trauma center, utilizing a retrospective database of polytrauma patients. The database included demographics, injury severity and distribution, vital parameters, laboratory values that were routinely assessed during medical treatment, in-hospital mortality, and complications, with a follow-up of 30 days. All patients received a whole-body computed tomography (WBCT) upon arrival in the trauma bay.

This study includes data of polytrauma patients over a period of 16 years who fulfilled the criteria of the Berlin definition of polytrauma. Furthermore, patients with data regarding type of ESI, injury distribution, and complications were included. Secondarily transferred patients, patients with end-of life treatment, or patients with a signed "do not resuscitate" (DNR) form were excluded. The study population was stratified into patients requiring emergency surgical interventions (Group ESI) and patients without emergency surgical intervention (Group non-ESI).

The primary outcome of this study was to describe the four most common ESI and their impact on the course of the polytrauma patient. ESI included all surgical interventions that were performed within 24 h of admission. The four most common ESI were summarized, including each of the most relevant specific procedures. Injury severity was measured utilizing the ISS [16], while injury distribution and local injury severity were stratified according the Abbreviated Injury Scale (AIS) [17]. This study only analyzed injuries with an AIS of 3 or higher. The neurological status was assessed using the Glasgow Coma Scale (GCS) [18].

The course of the polytrauma patients was assessed by in-hospital mortality and 30-day major complications, including pneumonia, sepsis, bacteremia, and infections requiring medical or surgical treatment. All variables were collected during routine medical treatment of the polytrauma patients. The vital parameters and laboratory results were measured on arrival, while AIS and ISS were calculated based on the information given on the patients discharge papers. An a-priori sample size calculation was not warranted since this study analyzed maximum available datasets. The vital parameters and laboratory results were chosen in reference to the Berlin definition of polytrauma.

Data were tested for normal distribution using the Shapiro–Wilk normality test. Continuous variables were summarized as median and interquartile range (IQR, 25th–75th percentile). Categorical variables were displayed with count and percentage. Group comparisons with two partners of continuous variables was performed using the Student's *t*-test (normal distribution) or the Mann–Whitney U-test (skewed distribution). Comparisons of categorical variables were performed using the Pearson Chi-squared test. Statistical significance was set at a *p*-value of <0.05. All calculations were performed using R Core Team (2018) (R:A language and environment for statistical computing, R Foundation for

Statistical Computing, Vienna, Austria, URL: https://www.R-project.org/ (accessed on 16 August 2021)).

3. Results

3.1. Study Population

The utilized database contains the records of 3663 patients, with 1116 (30.5%) patients meeting the Berlin definition of polytrauma. After removing the patients that were secondarily transferred, received end-of life treatment, or presented with missing data, 751 (67.3%) patients were included in our study (Figure 1).

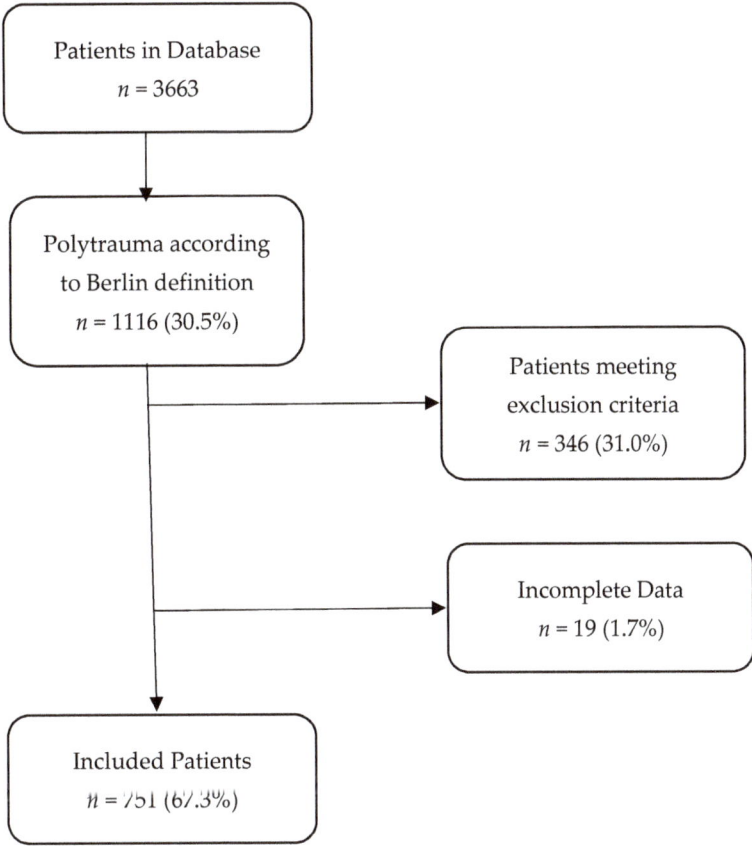

Figure 1. Flowchart of patient selection.

The median age of the study population was 39 years (25, 48), with 558 (74.3%) patients being male. The median ISS was 38 (29, 45 (25th, 75th percentile)) and patients had a median GCS of 3 (3, 12) points. The median entry lactate level of all included patients was 3 mmol/l (2, 5), and the median entry arterial pressure (MAP) of all included patients was 87 mmHg (70, 100). Group ESI included 711 patients (94.5%) and Group non-ESI had 40 (5.5%) (Table 1).

Table 1. Demographics and injury description of the study population.

	ESI	Non-ESI	p-Value
n	711	40	
Age (years)	38.0 (25, 56)	62 (43, 75)	<0.001
Male, n (%)	530 (74.5)	28 (70.0)	n.s.
ISS (points)	38 (29, 45)	34 (27, 38)	0.043
GCS (points)	7 (3, 13)	11 (6, 14)	<0.001
Lactate admission (mmol/L)	3 (2, 5)	3 (1, 4)	n.s.
MAP admission (mmHg)	85 (70, 100)	95 (75, 107)	n.s.
Heartrate admission (1/min)	100 (84, 115)	85 (74, 104)	0.011
Hematocrit admission (%)	30 (22, 36)	36 (32, 39)	<0.001
Hemoglobin admission (g/L)	10 (8, 12)	12 (10, 14)	0.015
Base excess admission (mmol/L)	−6/−9, −3)	−5 (−7, −2)	0.104
Body temperature (°C)	35 (34, 36)	35 (35, 37)	0.49

n = number; ESI = Emergency Surgical Intervention; ISS = Injury Severity Score; GCS = Glasgow Coma Scale; MAP = Mean Arterial Pressure; n.s. = not significant.

3.2. Injury Mechanism, Severity, and Distribution

The most common injury mechanism was a motor vehicle accident (n = 447, 59.5%). In total, 2238 injuries with an AIS of 3 or higher were documented. The most common injury with an AIS of 3 or higher was that at the thorax (n = 591, 26.4%), followed by the head (n = 535, 23.9%), the extremities (n = 351, 15.7%) and the abdomen (n = 312, 13.9%).

Group ESI included patients with significantly higher AIS head (p < 0.001), AIS abdomen (p = 0.007), and AIS extremity (p = 0.007). The AIS for the face, thorax, spine, pelvis, and integument were similarly distributed among these groups (Table 2).

Table 2. Comparison of injury severity and injury distribution according to AIS.

	ESI	Non-ESI	
n	711	40	
AIS Head (points), n (%)			<0.001
3	122 (17.2)	12 (30.0)	
4	149 (21.0)	7 (17.5)	
5	228 (32.1)	7 (17.5)	
6	6 (0.8)	4 (10.0)	
AIS Face (points), n (%)			0.075
3	72 (10.2)	10 (25.0)	
4	27 (3.8)	1 (2.5)	
5	2 (0.3)	0 (0.0)	
AIS Thorax (points), n (%)			0.723
3	368 (51.8)	23 (57.5)	
4	137 (19.3)	5 (12.5)	
5	54 (7.6)	2 (5.0)	
6	2 (0.3)	0 (0.0)	
AIS Abdomen (points), n (%)			0.007
3	72 (0.2)	8 (20.0)	
4	139 (19.7)	2 (5.0)	
5	90 (12.7)	1 (2.5)	
AIS Spine (points), n (%)			0.464
3	95 (13.5)	8 (20.0)	
4	11 (1.6)	0 (0.0)	
5	23 (3.3)	0 (0.0)	
6	1 (0.1)	0 (0.0)	
AIS Extremity (points), n (%)			0.007
3	249 (35.4)	6 (15.0)	
4	66 (9.4)	1 (2.5)	
5	31 (4.4)	0 (0.0)	
AIS Pelvis (points), n (%)			0.318
3	117 (6.7)	7 (17.5)	
4	28 (4.0)	0 (0.0)	
5	15 (2.1)	0 (0.0)	
AIS Integument (points), n (%)			0.055
3	20 (2.9)	1 (2.5)	
4	6 (0.9)	0 (0.0)	
5	2 (0.3)	1 (2.5)	

AIS = Abbreviated Injury Scale; ESI = Emergency Surgical Intervention.

3.3. Most Common ESI

In total, 69 different surgical interventions were performed in our study population, and 832 surgical interventions were documented in the database. Out of these, the most common ESI were emergency thoracotomy (n = 341, 41%), followed by damage-control laparotomy (n = 187, 22.5%), the external fixation of an extremity (n = 167, 20.1%), and insertion of an ICP monitor (n = 137, 16.5%) (Table 3). More elaborate surgical procedures such as lung wedge resection (n = 7) or nephrectomy (n = 6) were not taken into account, as they were very rare in the observed timespan.

Table 3. The most common surgical interventions within 24 h.

Emergency Thoracotomy, n (%)		341 (41.0)
	Chest tube	191 (56.0)
	Open CPR	35 (10.3)
	Thoracic packing	24 (7.0)
Emergency Laparotomy, n (%)		187 (22.5)
	Abdominal packing	98 (52.4)
	Splenectomy	63 (33.7)
	Pelvic packing	34 (18.2)
External Fixation, n (%)		167 (20.1)
	Upper extremity	40 (23.9)
	Lower extremity	134 (80.2)
	Pelvis	20 (12.0)
ICP monitor, n (%)		137 (16.5)

n = Number; CPR = Cardiopulmonary resuscitation; ICP = Intracranial pressure probe.

3.4. Complications

In total, complications such as infection, pneumonia, sepsis, or bacteremia were documented 783 times. The mortality of the included study population was 34.4%. The most common cause of death was traumatic brain injury (n = 127, 49.0%), followed by hemorrhagic shock (n = 82, 31.7%), multiple organ failure and systemic inflammatory response syndrome (SIRS) (n = 37, 14.3%), and others (n = 13, 5.0%). The most common complications were infection (n = 309, 39.5%), followed by pneumonia (n = 207, 26.4%), sepsis (n = 179, 22.9%), and bacteremia (n = 88, 11.2%). The rate of complications in Group ESI versus Group non-ESI was comparable (44.1% vs. 45.7% p = n.s.). Furthermore, the distribution of the rate of each assessed complication was comparable among those groups (Table 4).

Table 4. Distribution of 30-day complications.

	ESI	Non-ESI	p-Value
	711	40	
Infection, n (%)	294 (41.5)	15 (38.5)	n.s.
Pneumonia, n (%)	195 (28.8)	12 (34.3)	n.s.
Sepsis, n (%)	170 (24.1)	9 (23.1)	n.s.
Bacteremia, n (%)	85 (12.8)	3 (8.6)	n.s.
In-hospital mortality, n (%)	248 (34.8)	11 (27.5)	n.s.

n = Number; n.s. = not significant; ESI = Emergency Surgical Intervention.

4. Discussion

Polytrauma management substantially benefits from interdisciplinary teamwork, with an experienced leader heading the group. However, the specific training and medical education required of the trauma team members is still controversially discussed. The aim of this study was to summarize the most common surgical emergency interventions for polytrauma patients and to further analyze the impact of ESI on morbidity and mortality. This study revealed the following points:

1. Most polytrauma patients required an emergency surgical intervention within 24 h of admission;
2. Chest tube insertion, damage-control laparotomy, placing an external fixator on the extremities, and insertion of an intracranial pressure probe accounted for the most common potentially life-saving emergency surgical interventions;
3. Morbidity and mortality were not affected by emergency surgical interventions.

The distribution of injury severity is comparable to other hospitals in Western Europe [19,20].

The study population of this study represent "borderline" or "in extremis" polytrauma cases [21–23]. The presented mortality is comparable to current literature, where a mortality of 15–40% is described for patients that count as intermediate or high-risk according to the PolyTrauma Grading Score [24]. A multicenter study of The UK National Surgical Collective from 2017 found that 21.7% of patients who had general surgery developed sepsis, which is in the range of our results [25]. In current literature, the most commonly performed damage-control surgery on the trunk is laparotomy for abdominal packing at 56.5% [26]. Approximately 30% of penetrating and up to 15% of blunt-chest trauma require surgical treatment via thoracotomy or thoracoscopy, excluding the insertion of chest tubes alone [27]. Regarding chest tube insertion, there are rates of up to 93% for chest tube insertion in blunt thoracic trauma described in [28].

Following this definition, some sort of ESI are warranted. Furthermore, the current study population showed pathophysiologic relevant changes that are associated with the requirement of life-saving interventions [29]. While the role and strategies of fracture fixation in polytrauma have been described in numerous studies [30], only a few studies have investigated strategies for surgical interventions in the thorax and abdomen that exceeded the damage-control approach [31]. A growing body of literature has investigated damage-control principles, both in abdominal trauma [32,33] and thoracic trauma [28,34], and their effect on the outcome of polytrauma patients. It appears evident that the adequate treatment of thoracic and abdominal injuries is equally important as the treatment of fractures. Current medical advancements encourage minimal invasive procedures to control hemorrhage [35]. An increasing number of traumatic hepatic and splenic injuries are treated non-operatively [36,37] or with the support of interventional radiology (e.g., coiling) [38,39]. With evolving minimally invasive techniques or the non-operative treatment of solid organ lesions, there might be a higher threshold for the indication to perform damage-control laparotomy [40,41].

Limitations

In the utilized database, there was only limited information about non-operative procedures. Nevertheless, the use of interventional radiologic procedures is an important topic in relation to polytrauma patients and is a part of future research in our trauma center.

There is a significant difference of age between Group ESI and non-ESI that we cannot explain with our study. This finding might be due to different trauma mechanisms. However, the ISS of both groups is similar. One might explain it with the calculation of the ISS, since it is calculated according to different regions of the body; it is not possible to distinguish between multiple injuries of one body region and it does not indicate the need for emergency surgery.

Patients who received an external fixation of long bone fractures might have required this intervention due to severe soft tissue damage, but are included in Group ESI. One might argue that the placement of an external fixator is not always a life-saving emergency surgical intervention. However, we feel that this intervention might improve the outcome of polytrauma patients who are in extremis, or in stable patients with deranged soft tissue [42].

In our Level 1 trauma center, an emergency surgical intervention is usually executed by a general surgeon; only an intracranial pressure probe is performed by a neurosurgeon. If morbidity and mortality change, whether a general surgeon or an organ specialist performs the emergency surgical intervention cannot be answered with our database.

This was a single-center study conducted at a Level 1 trauma center with more seriously injured patients compared to smaller hospitals. Moreover, there are different systems and different approaches for treating polytraumatized patients in the resuscitation area. We still think that the results are interesting for other major trauma systems to use in the training of medical personnel in the resuscitation area, with focus on the ESI.

5. Conclusions

Polytrauma patients often require surgical emergency intervention within the first 24 h after admission. The most commonly performed emergency procedures include thoracotomy, emergency laparotomy, external fixation of fractures of an extremity, and the insertion of an intracranial pressure probe. Polytrauma management would benefit from round-the-clock expertise in these most potentially life-saving interventions, with a limited variety provided by either an on-call "organ specialists" or a capable trauma team member with knowledge in general surgery.

Author Contributions: D.S.: Data curation, formal analysis, interpretation of data, writing—original draft. S.H.: Formal analysis, interpretation of data, writing—review and editing. R.S.: Data curation, writing—review and editing. K.O.J.: Writing—review and editing. T.B.: Writing—review and editing. V.N.: Writing—review and editing. L.M.: Writing—review and editing. R.P.: Writing—review and editing. H.C.P.: Writing—review and editing. K.S.: Conceptualization, formal analysis, investigation, methodology, project administration, supervision, validation, visualization, writing—review and editing. All authors have read and agreed to the published version of the manuscript.

Funding: This research received no external funding.

Institutional Review Board Statement: The study was conducted according to the guidelines of the Declaration of Helsinki and approved by the Institutional Review Board (StV 1-2008). Due to the retrospective nature of this study, an additional consent to participate was not required.

Informed Consent Statement: Not applicable.

Data Availability Statement: All data of this submission are available from the Dryad Digital Repository.

Conflicts of Interest: K.S. discloses the following relationships: Advisory Board for Committee on Emergency Medicine, Intensive Care, and Trauma Management of the German Trauma Society; Member of the Non-permanent Council of the German Trauma Society. Grant/Research support from: Medtronic, DePuySynthes, CarboFix. Speaker/teacher for: Medtronic, DePuySynthes, Stöckli Medical. All other authors declare that they have no competing interests.

References

1. Haagsma, J.A.; Graetz, N.; Bolliger, I.; Naghavi, M.; Higashi, H.; Mullany, E.C.; Abera, S.F.; Abraham, J.P.; Adofo, K.; Alsharif, U.; et al. The global burden of injury: Incidence, mortality, disability-adjusted life years and time trends from the Global Burden of Disease study 2013. *Inj. Prev.* **2016**, *22*, 3–18. [CrossRef]
2. Driscoll, P.A.; Vincent, C.A. ORGANIZING AN EFFICIENT TRAUMA TEAM. *Injury-Int. J. Care Inj.* **1992**, *23*, 107–110. [CrossRef]
3. Haas, B.; Stukel, T.A.; Gomez, D.; Zagorski, B.; De Mestral, C.; Sharma, S.V.; Rubenfeld, G.D.; Nathens, A.B. The mortality benefit of direct trauma center transport in a regional trauma system: A population-based analysis. *J. Trauma Acute Care Surg.* **2012**, *72*, 1510–1515; discussion 1515–1517. [CrossRef]
4. Gillott, A.R.; Thomas, J.M.; Forrester, C. Development of a statewide trauma registry. *J. Trauma* **1989**, *29*, 1667–1672. [CrossRef]
5. Cameron, P.A.; Gabbe, B.J.; McNeil, J.J.; Finch, C.F.; Smith, K.L.; Cooper, D.J.; Judson, R.; Kossmann, T. The trauma registry as a statewide quality improvement tool. *J. Trauma* **2005**, *59*, 1469–1476. [CrossRef] [PubMed]
6. Jensen, K.O.; Heyard, R.; Schmitt, D.; Mica, L.; Ossendorf, C.; Simmen, H.P.; Wanner, G.A.; Werner, C.M.L.; Held, L.; Sprengel, K. Which pre-hospital triage parameters indicate a need for immediate evaluation and treatment of severely injured patients in the resuscitation area? *Eur. J. Trauma Emerg. Surg.* **2019**, *45*, 91–98. [CrossRef]
7. Ringen, A.H.; Hjortdahl, M.; Wisborg, T. Norwegian trauma team leaders—training and experience: A national point prevalence study. *Scand. J. Trauma Resusc. Emerg. Med.* **2011**, *19*, 54. [CrossRef] [PubMed]
8. Champion, H.R.; Sacco, W.J.; Copes, W.S. Improvement in outcome from trauma center care. *Arch. Surg.* **1992**, *127*, 333–338; discussion 338. [CrossRef] [PubMed]

9. Wang, C.-J.; Yen, S.-T.; Huang, S.-F.; Hsu, S.-C.; Ying, J.C.; Shan, Y.-S. Effectiveness of trauma team on medical resource utilization and quality of care for patients with major trauma. *BMC Health Serv. Res.* **2017**, *17*, 505. [CrossRef] [PubMed]
10. Waydhas, C.; Trentzsch, H.; Hardcastle, T.C.; Jensen, K.O.; Group, W.-T.T.S. Survey on worldwide trauma team activation requirement. *Eur. J. Trauma Emerg. Surg.* **2020**. [CrossRef] [PubMed]
11. Ciesla, D.J.; Moore, E.E.; Cothren, C.C.; Johnson, J.L.; Burch, J.M. Has the trauma surgeon become house staff for the surgical subspecialist? *Am. J. Surg.* **2006**, *192*, 732–737. [CrossRef]
12. Achatz, G.; Perl, M.; Stange, R.; Mutschler, M.; Jarvers, J.S.; Munzberg, M. How many generalists and how many specialists does othopedics and traumatology need? *Unfallchirurg* **2013**, *116*, 29–33. [CrossRef]
13. Watson, J.J.; Nielsen, J.; Hart, K.; Srikanth, P.; Yonge, J.D.; Connelly, C.R.; Kemp Bohan, P.M.; Sosnovske, H.; Tilley, B.C.; van Belle, G.; et al. Damage control laparotomy utilization rates are highly variable among Level I trauma centers: Pragmatic, Randomized Optimal Platelet and Plasma Ratios findings. *J. Trauma Acute Care Surg.* **2017**, *82*, 481–488. [CrossRef]
14. Moore, T.A.; Simske, N.M.; Vallier, H.A. Fracture fixation in the polytrauma patient: Markers that matter. *Injury* **2019**, *51*, S10–S14. [CrossRef]
15. von Elm, E.; Altman, D.G.; Egger, M.; Pocock, S.J.; Gotzsche, P.C.; Vandenbroucke, J.P.; Initiative, S. The Strengthening the Reporting of Observational Studies in Epidemiology (STROBE) Statement: Guidelines for reporting observational studies. *Int. J. Surg.* **2014**, *12*, 1495–1499. [CrossRef] [PubMed]
16. Baker, S.P.; O'Neill, B.; Haddon, W.; Long, W.B. The injury severity score: A method for describing patients with multiple injuries and evaluating emergency care. *J. Trauma* **1974**, *14*, 187–196. [CrossRef]
17. Haasper, C.; Junge, M.; Ernstberger, A.; Brehme, H.; Hannawald, L.; Langer, C.; Nehmzow, J.; Otte, D.; Sander, U.; Krettek, C.; et al. The Abbreviated Injury Scale (AIS). *Unfallchirurg* **2010**, *113*, 366–372. [CrossRef] [PubMed]
18. Teasdale, G.; Jennett, B. Assessment of coma and impaired consciousness: A practical scale. *Lancet* **1974**, *304*, 81–84. [CrossRef]
19. Schulz-Drost, S.; Finkbeiner, R.; Lefering, R.; Grosso, M.; Krinner, S.; Langenbach, A.; Dgu, T.T. Lung Contusion in Polytrauma: An Analysis of the TraumaRegister DGU. *Thorac. Cardiovasc. Surg.* **2019**. [CrossRef]
20. Heim, C.; Bosisio, F.; Roth, A.; Bloch, J.; Borens, O.; Daniel, R.T.; Denys, A.; Oddo, M.; Pasquier, M.; Schmidt, S.; et al. Is trauma in Switzerland any different? Epidemiology and patterns of injury in major trauma—A 5-year review from a Swiss trauma centre. *Swiss Med. Wkly.* **2014**, *144*, w13958. [CrossRef] [PubMed]
21. Pape, H.C.; Giannoudis, P.V.; Krettek, C.; Trentz, O. Timing of fixation of major fractures in blunt polytrauma: Role of conventional indicators in clinical decision making. *J. Orthop. Trauma* **2005**, *19*, 551–562. [CrossRef]
22. Vallier, H.A.; Wang, X.F.; Moore, T.A.; Wilber, J.H.; Como, J.J. Timing of Orthopaedic Surgery in Multiple Trauma Patients: Development of a Protocol for Early Appropriate Care. *J. Orthop. Trauma* **2013**, *27*, 543–551. [CrossRef]
23. Halvachizadeh, S.; Baradaran, L.; Cinelli, P.; Pfeifer, R.; Sprengel, K.; Pape, H.-C. How to detect a polytrauma patient at risk of complications: A validation and database analysis of four published scales. *PLoS ONE* **2020**, *15*, e0228082. [CrossRef]
24. Hildebrand, F.; Lefering, R.; Andruszkow, H.; Zelle, B.A.; Barkatali, B.M.; Pape, H.C. Development of a scoring system based on conventional parameters to assess polytrauma patients: PolyTrauma Grading Score (PTGS). *Injury* **2015**, *46* (Suppl. S4), S93–S98. [CrossRef]
25. Blencowe, N.S.; Strong, S.; Blazeby, J.; Daniels, R.; Peden, C.; Lim, J.; Messenger, D.; Stark, H.; Richards, S.; Rogers, C.; et al. Multicentre observational study of adherence to Sepsis Six guidelines in emergency general surgery. *Br. J. Surg.* **2017**, *104*, E165–E171. [CrossRef]
26. Roberts, D.J.; Bobrovitz, N.; Zygun, D.A.; Ball, C.G.; Kirkpatrick, A.W.; Faris, P.D.; Stelfox, H.T. Indications for use of damage control surgery and damage control interventions in civilian trauma patients: A scoping review. *J. Trauma Acute Care Surg.* **2015**, *78*, 1187–1196. [CrossRef] [PubMed]
27. Refaely, Y.; Koyfman, L.; Friger, M.; Ruderman, L.; Saleh, M.A.; Sahar, G.; Shaked, G.; Klein, M.; Brotfain, E. Clinical Outcome of Urgent Thoracotomy in Patients with Penetrating and Blunt Chest Trauma: A Retrospective Survey. *Thorac Cardiovasc. Surg.* **2018**, *66*, 686–692. [CrossRef]
28. Beshay, M.; Mertzlufft, F.; Kottkamp, H.W.; Reymond, M.; Schmid, R.A.; Branscheid, D.; Vordemvenne, T. Analysis of risk factors in thoracic trauma patients with a comparison of a modern trauma centre: A mono-centre study. *World J. Emerg. Surg.* **2020**, *15*, 45. [CrossRef] [PubMed]
29. Vassallo, J.; Fuller, G.; Smith, J.E.J. Relationship between the Injury Severity Score and the need for life-saving interventions in trauma patients in the UK. *Emerg. Med. J.* **2020**, *37*, 502–507. [CrossRef]
30. Pape, H.; Leenen, L. Polytrauma management-What is new and what is true in 2020? *J. Clin. Orthop. Trauma* **2020**, *12*, 88–95. [CrossRef] [PubMed]
31. Brenner, M.; Hicks, C. Major Abdominal Trauma: Critical Decisions and New Frontiers in Management. *Emerg. Med. Clin. N. Am.* **2018**, *36*, 149–160. [CrossRef] [PubMed]
32. Kuza, C.; Hirji, S.; Englum, B.; Ganapathi, A.; Speicher, P.; Scarborough, J.E. Pancreatic injuries in abdominal trauma in US adults: Analysis of the National Trauma Data Bank on Management, Outcomes, and Predictors of Mortality. *Scand. J. Surg.* **2020**, *109*, 193–204. [CrossRef]
33. Ferrah, N.; Cameron, P.; Gabbe, B.; Fitzgerald, M.; Martin, K.; Beck, B. Trends in the nature and management of serious abdominal trauma. *World J. Surg.* **2019**, *43*, 1216–1225. [CrossRef]

34. Horst, K.; Andruszkow, H.; Weber, C.D.; Pishnamaz, M.; Herren, C.; Zhi, Q.; Knobe, M.; Lefering, R.; Hildebrand, F.; Pape, H.C. Thoracic trauma now and then: A 10 year experience from 16,773 severely injured patients. *PLoS ONE* **2017**, *12*, e0186712. [CrossRef] [PubMed]
35. Halvachizadeh, S.; Mica, L.; Kalbas, Y.; Lipiski, M.; Canic, M.; Teuben, M.; Cesarovic, N.; Rancic, Z.; Cinelli, P.; Neuhaus, V. Zone-dependent acute circulatory changes in abdominal organs and extremities after resuscitative balloon occlusion of the aorta (REBOA): An experimental model. *Eur. J. Med Res.* **2021**, *26*, 10. [CrossRef] [PubMed]
36. Teuben, M.; Spijkerman, R.; Blokhuis, T.; Pfeifer, R.; Teuber, H.; Pape, H.-C.; Leenen, L. Nonoperative management of splenic injury in closely monitored patients with reduced consciousness is safe and feasible. *Scand. J. Trauma Resusc. Emerg. Med.* **2019**, *27*, 108. [CrossRef] [PubMed]
37. Raza, M.; Abbas, Y.; Devi, V.; Prasad, K.V.; Rizk, K.N.; Nair, P.P. Non operative management of abdominal trauma—A 10 years review. *World J. Emerg. Surg.* **2013**, *8*, 14. [CrossRef]
38. Markogiannakis, H.; Sanidas, E.; Messaris, E.; Michalakis, I.; Kasotakis, G.; Melissas, J.; Tsiftsis, D. Management of blunt hepatic and splenic trauma in a Greek level I trauma centre. *Acta Chir. Belg.* **2006**, *106*, 566–571. [CrossRef]
39. Austin, M.T.; Diaz, J.J.; Feurer, I.D.; Miller, R.S.; May, A.K.; Guillamondegui, O.D.; Pinson, C.W.; Morris, J.A. Creating an emergency general surgery service enhances the productivity of trauma surgeons, general surgeons and the hospital. *J. Trauma* **2005**, *58*, 906–910. [CrossRef]
40. Demetriades, D.; Velmahos, G. Technology-driven triage of abdominal trauma: The emerging era of nonoperative management. *Annu. Rev. Med.* **2003**, *54*, 1–15. [CrossRef]
41. Groven, S.; Gaarder, C.; Eken, T.; Skaga, N.O.; Naess, P.A. Abdominal injuries in a major Scandinavian trauma center—Performance assessment over an 8year period. *J. Trauma Manag. Outcomes* **2014**, *8*, 9. [CrossRef] [PubMed]
42. Pfeifer, R.; Kalbas, Y.; Coimbra, R.; Leenen, L.; Komadina, R.; Hildebrand, F.; Halvachizadeh, S.; Akhtar, M.; Peralta, R.; Fattori, L.; et al. Indications and interventions of damage control orthopedic surgeries: An expert opinion survey. *Eur. J. Trauma Emerg. Surg.* **2020**. [CrossRef] [PubMed]

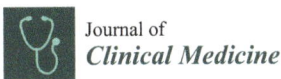

Article

Comparison of Injury Patterns between Electric Bicycle, Bicycle and Motorcycle Accidents

Emilian Spörri [1], Sascha Halvachizadeh [1], Jamison G. Gamble [2], Till Berk [1], Florin Allemann [1], Hans-Christoph Pape [1] and Thomas Rauer [1,*]

[1] Department of Trauma Surgery, University Hospital Zurich, 8091 Zurich, Switzerland; emilian.spoerri@gmail.com (E.S.); Sascha.Halvachizadeh@usz.ch (S.H.); till.berk@usz.ch (T.B.); Florin.Allemann@usz.ch (F.A.); hans-christoph.pape@usz.ch (H.-C.P.)
[2] St. George's University School of Medicine, St. George, Grenada; jg120gamble@gmail.com
* Correspondence: thomas.rauer@usz.ch

Abstract: Background: Electric bicycles (E-bikes) are an increasingly popular means of transport, and have been designed for a higher speed comparable to that of small motorcycles. Accident statistics show that E-bikes are increasingly involved in traffic accidents. To test the hypothesis of whether accidents involving E-bikes bear more resemblance to motorcycle accidents than conventional bicyclists, this study evaluates the injury pattern and severity of E-bike injuries in direct comparison to injuries involving motorcycle and bicycle accidents. Methods: In this retrospective cohort study, the data of 1796 patients who were treated at a Level I Trauma Center between 2009 and 2018 due to traffic accident, involving bicycles, E-bikes or motorcycles, were evaluated and compared with regard to injury patterns and injury severity. Accident victims treated as inpatients at least 16 years of age or older were included in this study. Pillion passengers and outpatients were excluded. Results: The following distribution was found in the individual groups: 67 E-bike, 1141 bicycle and 588 motorcycle accidents. The injury pattern of E-bikers resembled that of bicyclists much more than that of motorcyclists. The patients with E-bike accidents were almost 14 years older and had a higher incidence of moderate traumatic brain injuries than patients with bicycle accidents, in spite of the fact that E-bike riders were nearly twice as likely to wear a helmet as compared to bicycle riders. The rate of pelvic injuries in E-bike accidents was twice as high compared with bicycle accidents, whereas the rate of upper extremity injuries was higher following bicycle accidents. **Conclusion:** The overall E-bike injury pattern is similar to that of cyclists. The differences in the injury pattern to motorcycle accidents could be due to the higher speeds at the time of the accident, the different protection and vehicle architecture. What is striking, however, is the higher age and the increased craniocerebral trauma of the E-bikers involved in accidents compared to the cyclists. We speculate that older and untrained people who have a slower reaction time and less control over the E-bike could benefit from head protection or practical courses similar to motorcyclists.

Keywords: E-bike injuries; polytrauma; outcome; injury pattern comparison

1. Introduction

E-bikes, marketed as a clean alternative to cars with low energy consumption, have become a popular mode of transport with increasing interest [1]. Due to an increasing number of E-bike accidents [2], the topic of accident prevention and safety has been raised too. In Switzerland, the percentage of E-bikes sold as a percentage of all bicycles sold increased from 3.9% in 2008 to 32.2% in 2018 [3]. The trend started in China, where about 90% of all E-bikes were registered in 2011 [4] and where most of the early studies on E-bike accidents originated [5–7].

According to the motor assistance, E-bikes can reach speeds of up to 25 km/h or 45 km/h, hence they are able to reach higher velocities with less effort when compared with conventional bicycles [8]. Accordingly the rise in number and use of E-bikes led to a substantial increase in E-bike related traffic accidents [9]. Some studies have focused on crash characteristics [10], experience surveys [10,11] or riding behavior [12]. Others dealt with injury severity [1,13–16] or injury patterns occurring from E-bike accidents [9,13–16].

To date, only a few studies comparing E-bike related injuries with those suffered by conventional bicyclists or motorcyclists are available. A previous study, evaluating the injury severity of E-Bikers compared to conventional bicyclists, in police-recorded accidents without comparison of injury patterns, showed diverging results in injury severity [1].

The aim of this study was to evaluate the patterns and severity of E-bike injuries in comparison to findings in conventional bicycle and motorcycle accidents to further fill the gap of available literature on E-bike injuries. It is hypothesized that E-bike accidents have more similarity with motorcycle accidents than with conventional bicyclists due to higher speed.

2. Materials and Methods

This study was designed as a monocentric retrospective cohort study and was approved by the local institutional review board (PB_2016-01888). It follows the Strengthening the Reporting of Observational Studies in Epidemiology (STROBE) guidelines for reporting observational studies [17].

2.1. Setting

This study includes patients that were treated due to a road traffic accident at an academic Level I Trauma Center between 2009 and 2018. All medical data were collected from the electronical medical records during the hospitalization and analyzed retrospectively. Patients were followed-up until discharge from the hospital.

2.2. Inclusion and Exclusion Criteria

Patients were included in this study if they were treated following a road traffic accident including E-bikes, bicycles or motorcycles. Further, patients were 16 years and older. Patients who were hit by a bike, or pillion passengers were excluded from this study. Patients' data with more than 10% missing values were excluded from this study. Further, patients with injuries resulting from a motorized standing scooter accident were excluded. Patients who had an accident abroad were excluded, with the exception of patients transferred to our hospital from neighboring countries within 24 h of the accident. Patients who underwent elective surgery after a bike accident without first presenting to our hospital for initial treatment were also excluded. Outpatients were excluded due to a lack of detailed information on accident mechanism and medical clarification.

All patients were stratified according to the vehicle driven during the injury into: Group E-Bike (E), Group Bicycle (B), or Group Motorcycle (M).

The bicycle group contained conventional bicycles and mountain bikes. The E-Bike group included both E-Bikes with motor assistance up to 25 km/h and those with assistance up to 45 km/h, as it was not possible to retrospectively distinguish between these two types of assistance from the available data set. In the group of motorcycles, in addition to classic motorcycles, mopeds were also included.

2.3. Search Strategy

The patients were identified using the appropriate International Classification of Diseases (ICD) Code of transportation accidents (ICD V99) in the computerized patient database. From this pool only conventional bicycle, E-bike and motorcycle accidents were selected. The medical database enabled instantaneous retrieval of past diagnostic reports, scores, treatment and other relevant documents to analyze. Knowing that not all possible rider accidents had the right ICD Code nor every report had accurate information about vehicle or accident type, patients with incomplete documentation were called and interviewed.

2.4. Data Collection

Data collected included sex, age, helmet use, collision or self-accident, anatomic region of injury, injury severity regarding the Injury Severity Score (ISS) [18], dislocated/open fractures regarding the radiology report and initial Glasgow Coma Scale (GCS) [19]. Size data were asked for during hospital stay. Outcomes included treatment, intensive care unit (ICU), mortality and duration of hospital stay. Early onset surgery and late onset surgery, which was performed at least 48 h after the accident respectively planned as an elective procedure, were summarized in one group. Anatomic regions were divided to upper extremity, lower extremity, thorax, abdomen, pelvis, spine (cervical, thoracic, lumbar, sacral), head, face and skin. According to the ISS [18] the injuries were classified as minor or major trauma. The cut-off point for a major trauma was settled as ISS over 15. Traumatic brain injuries (TBI) were further classified into mild (initial GCS-Score 13–15), moderate (initial GCS-Score 9–12) and severe (initial GCS-Score 3–8).

2.5. Statistical Analysis

The primary analysis of this work bases on descriptive statistics in order to present comparative measures among the three groups. Continuous variables are presented as mean with standard deviation (SD), categorical variables as numbers and percentage. Comparison of the three groups (E/B/M) was initially performed with Kruskal Wallis test in cases, where data distribution appeared nonuniform. The additional risk of suffering from specific injuries were calculated and presented with odds ratio (OR) and 95% confidence interval (95% CI).

A p-value of less than or equal to 0.05 was considered as statistically significant. Statistical analysis was performed using R (R Core Team (2020). R: A language and environment for statistical computing. R Foundation for Statistical Computing, Vienna, Austria. URL https://www.R-project.org/ accessed on 28 July 2021).

3. Results

Out of 3932 eligible patients, 1796 met the inclusion criteria, 67 (3.7%) had E-bike related injuries, 1141 (64%) had bicycle related injuries and 588 (33%) had motorcycle related injuries.

The average age at the time of injury was 56 years for E-bikers, which was the oldest group by far, compared to 42 years for the bicyclists and 41 years for the motorcyclists. The male-to-female ratio in total was 3.2 to 1. Motorcyclists had the highest male rate with 88% (n = 515) followed by the bicyclists with 72% (n = 816) and the E-bikers with the lowest of 61% (n = 41, Table 1).

Table 1. Demographics.

	Bicycle n = 1141	E-Bike n = 67	Motorcycle n = 588
Age (years) (SD)	42.1 (16.0)	56.0 (15.2)	40.8 (15.3)
BMI (kg/m^2) (SD)	23.8 (3.4)	25.0 (3.8)	25.7 (4.1)
Sex (male) (%)	816 (71.5%)	41 (61.2%)	515 (87.6%)

Motorcyclists had the significantly highest collision proportion with 41% (n = 243). The lowest collision proportion were the E-bikers with only 13% (n = 9), meaning they had the highest self-accident proportion. Helmet use was established for 73% (n = 49) of the E-bikers whereas only 38% (n = 429) of the bicyclists wore a helmet. Generally, motorcyclists almost always wore a helmet 96% (n = 243), as it is mandatory in Switzerland. Standing out in terms of injury severity with the highest rate in major traumas 39% (n = 230), dislocated fractures 60% (n = 353), open fractures 16% (n = 96), paralysis 2.9% (n = 17) and mortality

2.6% (n = 15) were the motorcyclists (Table 2). E-bike driver were more commonly subject of collison, rather than self-inflicted accidents as compared with bicyclists (OR 1.64, 95%CI 1.31 to 2.1, p < 0.001).

Table 2. Accident Type and Severity.

	Bicycle n = 1141	E-Bike n = 67	Motorcycle n = 588
Collision	264 (23.1%)	9 (13.4%)	243 (41.3%)
Helmet use	429 (37.6%)	49 (73.1%)	564 (95.9%)
Major trauma	207 (18.1%)	13 (19.4%)	230 (39.1%)
Dislocated fractures	425 (37.2%)	30 (44.8%)	353 (60.0%)
Open fractures	31 (2.7%)	1 (1.5%)	96 (16.3%)
Paralysis	13 (1.1%)	1 (1.5%)	17 (2.9%)
Mortality	14 (1.2%)	1 (1.5%)	15 (2.6%)

Head injuries were seen more often in bicycle (64%) and E-bike (66%) accidents compared to motorcycle accidents with 47%. Motorcyclists also had the lowest rate of facial injuries at 19%, compared with bicyclists and E-bikers with 42% and 40% respectively. On the other hand, lower extremity (55%), thoracic (51%), abdominal (18%) and spinal injuries (24%) were all significantly more frequent in motorcyclists. Upper extremity injuries (48% and 41%) were more prevalent than lower extremity injuries (28% and 25%) in E-bikers and bicyclists. In contrast, motorcyclists had an antipodal rate with a higher frequency of lower extremity injuries (55%) than upper extremity injuries (43%). The injury localization shows clear similarities between E-bikers and conventional bicyclists. Exceptions can be recognized in terms of thoracic and pelvic injuries. Bicyclists have a higher rate in thoracic injuries (37% vs. 25%) whereas E-bikers were more likely to experience pelvic injuries (13% vs. 7%). The risk of suffering from a pelvic injury was nearly twice as high following an E-bike accident when compared with bicycle (OR 1.95, 95%CI 1.01 to 4.08, p = 0.0093). However, E-bike driver were less likely to suffer from upper extremity injuries when compared with bicyclists (OR 0.80, 95%CI 0.67 to 0.98, p = 0.035). A complete list of injury localization is provided in Table 3.

Table 3. Injury Localization.

	Bicycle n = 1141	E-Bike n = 67	Motorcycle n = 588
Head	731 (64.1%)	44 (65.7%)	275 (46.8%)
Face	479 (42.0%)	27 (40.3%)	112 (19.0%)
Thorax	427 (37.4%)	18 (26.9%)	300 (51.0%)
Abdomen	81 (7.1%)	3 (4.5%)	107 (18.2%)
Pelvis	84 (7.4%)	9 (13.4%)	99 (16.8%)
Spine total	167 (14.6%)	11 (16.4%)	142 (24.1%)
Upper extremities	472 (41.4%)	32 (47.8%)	251 (42.7%)
Lower extremities	279 (24.5%)	19 (28.4%)	326 (55.4%)

Motorcyclists had the fewest traumatic brain injuries (TBI) respectively (resp.) head injuries with 47% compared to E-bikers with 66% and bicyclists with 64%. The rate of moderate TBI was found to be significantly higher among E-bikers at 10%. In addition, the initial GCS-Score of less than 15 at the accident site was seen the most in the E-bike group by far. For more details about traumatic brain injury see Table 4.

Table 4. Traumatic Brain Injury.

	Bicycle n = 1141	E-Bike n = 67	Motorcycle n = 588
TBI total	731 (64.1%)	44 (65.7%)	275 (46.8%)
Mild TBI	645 (56.5%)	35 (52.2%)	213 (36.2%)
Moderate TBI	45 (3.9%)	7 (10.4%)	28 (4.8%)
Severe TBI	41 (3.6%)	2 (3.0%)	34 (5.8%)
Initial GCS <15	239 (20.9%)	26 (38.8%)	129 (21.9%)

Motorcyclists were found to have a hospital stay nearly twice as long (10 days) as compared to bicyclists (5 days) and E-bikers (6) days. The same pattern is seen for surgical procedures required (74%) and intensive care unit stay (ICU) required (29%) due to consequences of the initial accident only, where motorcyclists clearly take the lead. Wound care without surgery after an E-bike accident was performed in 48% of the cases, 43% after a bicycle accident and 33% after a motorcycle accident. Following a hospital stay 10% of the bicyclists, 12% of the E-bikers and 27% of the motorcyclists went to a stationary rehabilitation center. Only a few patients were transferred to another hospital respectively regionalized (Table 5).

Table 5. Hospitalization.

	Bicycle n = 1141	E-Bike n = 67	Motorcycle n = 588
Required ICU stay	148 (13.0%)	11 (16.4%)	173 (29.4%)
Required Surgery	590 (51.7%)	35 (52.2%)	434 (73.8%)
Wound care	491 (43.0%)	32 (47.8%)	196 (33.3%)
Hospital stay (days) (SD)	5.0 (6.7)	5.9 (5.5)	10.2 (10.3)
Discharged home	993 (87.0%)	54 (80.6%)	385 (65.5%)
Rehabilitation	109 (9.6%)	8 (11.9%)	160 (27.2%)
Relocation/Transfer	25 (2.2%)	4 (6.0%)	28 (4.8%)

4. Discussion

The main aim of this study was to investigate the characteristics of E-bike accidents compared to bicycles and motorcycles with the question of wether the injury pattern of E-Bike accidents is more similar to that of motorcycle accidents or more similar to that of bicycle accidents.

This study has revealed the following main results:

1. Injury patterns in E-bike accidents are more comparable to those of bicyclists than to those of motorcyclists.
2. The rate of pelvic injuries in E-bike accidents is twice as high compared with bicycle accidents, whereas the rate of upper extremity injuries was higher following bicycle accidents.
3. E-bikers who sustained injuries were older than bicycle or motorcycle riders.

Technology has produced a number of recreational vehicles over the past few decades. The literature follows exposing the dangers and pitfalls of riding without proper safety precautions in most vehicle types. Attention has now turned to a novel class of two-wheel vehicle. As the scientific community works to catch up with the fast-paced rate of technological advancements in transportation technologies such as E-bikes, trends in the data, such as those presented in this study, will lay the groundwork to educate, advise and eventually enact policies and precautions aimed at reducing and preventing E-bike related injuries. Another major topic is the growing availability of bike sharing programs, especially E-bike sharing. Gross et al. [14], Baschera et al. [16] and DiMaggio et al. [9] compared E-bike accidents with other two-wheel vehicular related traumas. Gross et al. [14] compared resulting injuries between children and adults from E-bike accidents whereas, Baschera et al. [16] compared traumatic brain injuries caused by E-bike and bicycle accidents.

In accordance with the results of Gross et al. [14] the assumption was that E-bike accidents are similar to motorcycle accidents in terms of injury patterns. However, the results of this study could not reproduce these results and showed conversely that the injury patterns in E-bike accidents are more comparable to those of bicyclists than to those of motorcyclists. E-bike users, reported to the hospital, are less frequently male as compared with conventional bicycle and motorcycle users. We found that the majority of cases involved middle-aged victims, which is in accordance with previous studies [1,13,16]. Whereas conventional bicycle or motorcycle accident victims were found to be considerably younger [20]. Self-accidents of E-bikers were higher than those seen with bicyclists and motorcyclists, which may be attributed to higher age, likely longer reaction times and a higher mental workload in difficult traffic situation [8]. Due to the retrospective nature of the present study, no statements could be made regarding either the speed of the E-bike riders at the time of the accident or any accident partners in non-self-inflicted accidents due to a lack of documentation. This limits the generalizability and significance of the results of the present study. In line with a recent study confirming that e-bikers ride faster than conventional cyclists [8], this could also be assumed for the present study and could account for an influence on injury distribution. Greater TBI rates in E-bikers compared to conventional bicyclists was found, despite the fact that E-bikers wore helmets almost twice as often as bicyclists. In addition, the E-bikers initial GCS-Score indicated abnormal resp. under 15 almost twice as often as bicyclists.

Overall, the injury patterns in E-bike accidents are more comparable to those of bicyclists than to those of motorcyclists. However, while the rates of spinal cord injury, severe traumatic brain injury, and upper extremity injury were comparable in all three groups, the rate of pelvic injury in E-bike accidents was comparable to that of motorcycle riders.

In this study, the percentage in E-bikers who experienced major trauma (19%) and patients requiring surgery (46%) was higher than that described by Papoutsi et al. (13% resp. 26%) and lower than Gross et al. regarding the percentage of major trauma (35%) [13,14]. Weiss et al. postulated the risk of an accident increases with age, but not with bicycle type [21]. This study confirms that this is different for higher or more severe accident rates. The percentage of TBI (66% in E-bikers and 64% in bicyclists) is very similar to the study of Baschera et al. (69% resp. 59%) [16]. Other studies have described TBI in under 40% of cyclists [6,22]. These big differences can be explained due to different definitions of TBI or data collection methods. The most common injury occurring in motorcycle accidents are lower extremity injury, in 55% of the cases, same incidence as in Fletcher et al. [23].

One strength of this study is that it was conducted at a Level I Trauma Center, with wide variations in injury severity. Victims from rural and urban accidents are included. The source of information is from a detailed patient database. Other studies relied on in field EMS personnel reports, insurance claim reports or questionnaire-based survey datasets only. While the number of E-bike accidents may not be as high as other modes of transportation, it is directly proportional to bicycle and motorcycle accident rates, warranting further examination. An analysis of the national road traffic accident statistics showed a total of 20,022 patients involved in accidents in 2020: Of these, 3565 were motorcyclists, 1690 E-bike riders and 3637 bicyclists [24]. Given the retrospective nature of this study, it is possible that the number of E-bikers was under reported, thus not providing a completely clear picture on the actual number of e-bike users. Attempting to summarizing all two-wheeled vehicles in use on the streets in only 3 groups is a very pragmatic approach. Furthermore, this study was limited to adults 16 years of age or older, as children are treated at a separate hospital. Furthermore, being that this study was conducted at a Level 1 trauma center, it is not only a strength it is also an important limitation. It is possible that we saw a higher level of more severe E-bike related trauma than might be seen at lower-level trauma centers. E-biker with less serious injuries may have been treated at hospitals with more limited trauma care, resulting in a selection bias for more serious injuries in this study. In this study, patients from rural and urban settings of a major European city were included. Types of injury may be different with different terrain and traffic in other parts of the country, which may also represent a selection bias.

Future studies should include data from hospitals of varying trauma center levels.

5. Conclusions

The overall E-bike injury pattern is similar to that of cyclists. The difference in the injury pattern of motorcycle accidents could be due to the higher speeds at the time of the accidents, the different protective clothing and architecture of the vehicle. What is striking, however, is the higher age and the increased craniocerebral trauma of the E-bikers involved in an accident compared to the cyclists. In our opinion older and untrained people may have slower reaction times and less control over the E-bike, which are now faster due to the motorized support of the E-bike. This population could benefit from head protection or practical courses similar to that of motorcyclists. The innovation of environmentally friendly transportation brings benefits and novel, indisputable injury risks. Further studies are needed to compare the different types of E-bikes with more detailed data. Data from E-bike share companies would also bring more transparency in terms of the relationship between accidents and commercial use.

Author Contributions: Conceptualization, E.S. and T.R.; methodology, E.S. and T.R.; software, E.S. and T.R.; validation, E.S., T.R. and H.-C.P.; formal analysis, E.S., S.H. and T.R.; data curation, E.S.; writing—original draft preparation, E.S.; writing—review and editing, J.G.G., T.B., F.A., S.H., H.-C.P. and T.R.; visualization, E.S. and T.R.; supervision, T.R. All authors have read and agreed to the published version of the manuscript.

Funding: This research received no external funding.

Institutional Review Board Statement: This study was conducted according to the guidelines of the Declaration of Helsinki, and with the approval of the cantonal ethic commission Zurich (PB_2016-01888).

Informed Consent Statement: General consent was obtained or accepted from all subjects enrolled in the study as approved by the Zurich Cantonal Ethics Committee (PB_2016-01888).

Data Availability Statement: Data is accessible on reasonable request.

Conflicts of Interest: The authors declare no conflict of interest.

References

1. Weber, T.; Scaramuzza, G.; Schmitt, K.U. Evaluation of e-bike accidents in Switzerland. *Accid. Anal. Prev.* **2014**, *73*, 47–52. [CrossRef] [PubMed]
2. Unfallstatistik Strassenverkehr 2014–2018. Bundesamt für Strassen (ASTRA). 2019. Available online: https://www.newsd.admin.ch/newsd/message/attachments/56382.pdf (accessed on 20 June 2020).
3. Entwicklung Schweizer Fahrrad- und E-Bike-Markt 2005–2019. Schweizer Fachstelle für Velo und E-Bike. 2020. Available online: https://www.velosuisse.ch/wp-content/uploads/2020/11/Gesamt_2005--2019_Veloverkaufsstatistik_Schweizer_Markt.pdf (accessed on 20 June 2020).
4. China Electric Bicycle Industrie Report, 2010–2011. Research in China. 2011. Available online: http://www.researchinchina.com/Htmls/Report/2011/6134.html (accessed on 20 June 2020).
5. Feng, Z.; Raghuwanshi, R.P.; Xu, Z.; Huang, D.; Zhang, C.; Jin, T. Electric-bicycle-related injury: A rising traffic injury burden in China. *Inj. Prev.* **2010**, *16*, 417–419. [CrossRef] [PubMed]
6. Hu, F.; Lv, D.; Zhu, J.; Fang, J. Related risk factors for injury severity of e-bike and bicycle crashes in Hefei. *Traffic Inj. Prev.* **2014**, *15*, 319–323. [CrossRef] [PubMed]
7. Zhang, X.; Cui, M.; Gu, Y.; Stallones, L.; Xiang, H. Trends in electric bike-related injury in China, 2004–2010. *Asia Pac. J. Public Health* **2015**, *27*, Np1819–Np1826. [CrossRef] [PubMed]
8. Vlakveld, W.P.; Twisk, D.; Christoph, M.; Boele, M.; Sikkema, R.; Remy, R.; Schwab, A.L. Speed choice and mental workload of elderly cyclists on e-bikes in simple and complex traffic situations: A field experiment. *Accid. Anal. Prev.* **2015**, *74*, 97–106. [CrossRef] [PubMed]
9. DiMaggio, C.J.; Bukur, M.; Wall, S.P.; Frangos, S.G.; Wen, A.Y. Injuries associated with electric-powered bikes and scooters: Analysis of US consumer product data. *Inj. Prev.* **2020**, *26*, 524–528. [CrossRef] [PubMed]

10. Hertach, P.; Uhr, A.; Niemann, S.; Cavegn, M. Characteristics of single-vehicle crashes with e-bikes in Switzerland. *Accid. Anal. Prev.* **2018**, *117*, 232–238. [CrossRef] [PubMed]
11. Dozza, M.; Bianchi Piccinini, G.F.; Werneke, J. Using naturalistic data to assess e-cyclist behavior. *Transp. Res. Part F Traffic Psychol. Behav.* **2016**, *41*, 217–226. [CrossRef]
12. MacArthur, J.; Dill, J.; Person, M. Electric Bikes in North America:Results of an Online Survey. *Transp. Res. Rec.* **2014**, *2468*, 123–130. [CrossRef]
13. Papoutsi, S.; Martinolli, L.; Braun, C.T.; Exadaktylos, A.K. E-bike injuries: Experience from an urban emergency department-a retrospective study from Switzerland. *Emerg. Med. Int.* **2014**, *2014*, 850236. [CrossRef] [PubMed]
14. Gross, I.; Weiss, D.J.; Eliasi, E.; Bala, M.; Hashavya, S. E-Bike-Related Trauma in Children and Adults. *J. Emerg. Med.* **2018**, *54*, 793–798. [CrossRef] [PubMed]
15. Tenenbaum, S.; Weltsch, D.; Bariteau, J.T.; Givon, A.; Peleg, K.; Thein, R.; Group, I.T. Orthopaedic injuries among electric bicycle users. *Injury* **2017**, *48*, 2140–2144. [CrossRef] [PubMed]
16. Baschera, D.; Jäger, D.; Preda, R.; Z'Graggen, W.J.; Raabe, A.; Exadaktylos, A.K.; Hasler, R.M. Comparison of the Incidence and Severity of Traumatic Brain Injury Caused by Electrical Bicycle and Bicycle Accidents—A Retrospective Cohort Study from a Swiss Level I Trauma Center. *World Neurosurg.* **2019**, *126*, e1023–e1034. [CrossRef] [PubMed]
17. von Elm, E.; Altman, D.G.; Egger, M.; Pocock, S.J.; Gøtzsche, P.C.; Vandenbroucke, J.P. The Strengthening the Reporting of Observational Studies in Epidemiology (STROBE) Statement: Guidelines for reporting observational studies. *Int. J. Surg.* **2014**, *12*, 1495–1499. [CrossRef] [PubMed]
18. Osler, T.; Baker, S.P.; Long, W. A modification of the injury severity score that both improves accuracy and simplifies scoring. *J. Trauma* **1997**, *43*, 922–925. [CrossRef] [PubMed]
19. Teasdale, G.; Jennett, B. Assessment of coma and impaired consciousness—A practical scale. *Lancet* **1974**, *2*, 81–84. [CrossRef]
20. Yelon, J.A.; Harrigan, N.; Evans, J.T. Bicycle trauma: A five-year experience. *Am. Surg.* **1995**, *61*, 202–205. [PubMed]
21. Weiss, R.; Juhra, C.; Wieskötter, B.; Weiss, U.; Jung, S.; Raschke, M. [How Probable is it That Seniors Using an E-Bike Will Have an Accident?—A New Health Care Topic, Also for Consulting Doctors]. *Z. Orthop. Unfall.* **2018**, *156*, 78–84. [PubMed]
22. Zibung, E.; Riddez, L.; Nordenvall, C. Helmet use in bicycle trauma patients: A population-based study. *Eur. J. Trauma Emerg. Surg. Off. Publ. Eur. Trauma Soc.* **2015**, *41*, 517–521. [CrossRef] [PubMed]
23. Fletcher, C.; Mcdowell, D.; Thompson, C.; James, K. Predictors of hospitalization and surgical intervention among patients with motorcycle injuries. *Trauma Surg. Acute Care Open* **2019**, *4*, e000326. [CrossRef] [PubMed]
24. Bundesamt für Statistik BFS. Verunfallte Personen nach Verkehrsmittel, 2020: ASTRA—Strassenverkehrsunfälle (SVU). 2020. Available online: https://www.bfs.admin.ch/bfs/de/home/statistiken/mobilitaet-verkehr/unfaelle-umweltauswirkungen/verkehrsunfaelle/strassenverkehr.html (accessed on 21 July 2021).

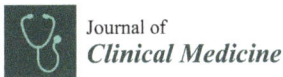

Article

The GERtality Score: The Development of a Simple Tool to Help Predict in-Hospital Mortality in Geriatric Trauma Patients

Julian Scherer [1], Yannik Kalbas [1], Franziska Ziegenhain [1], Valentin Neuhaus [1], Rolf Lefering [2], Michel Teuben [1], Kai Sprengel [1], Hans-Christoph Pape [1] and Kai Oliver Jensen [1,*]

[1] Department of Traumatology, University Hospital of Zürich, 8091 Zürich, Switzerland; julian.scherer@usz.ch (J.S.); yannik.kalbas@usz.ch (Y.K.); franziska.ziegenhain@usz.ch (F.Z.); valentin.neuhaus@usz.ch (V.N.); michel.teuben@usz.ch (M.T.); kai.sprengel@usz.ch (K.S.); hans-christoph.pape@usz.ch (H.-C.P.)
[2] Institute for Research in Operative Medicine (IFOM), University of Witten/Herdecke, 58453 Cologne, Germany; Rolf.Lefering@uni-wh.de
* Correspondence: kaioliver.jensen@usz.ch; Tel.: +41-442551111

Citation: Scherer, J.; Kalbas, Y.; Ziegenhain, F.; Neuhaus, V.; Lefering, R.; Teuben, M.; Sprengel, K.; Pape, H.-C.; Jensen, K.O. The GERtality Score: The Development of a Simple Tool to Help Predict in-Hospital Mortality in Geriatric Trauma Patients. *J. Clin. Med.* **2021**, *10*, 1362. https://doi.org/10.3390/jcm10071362

Academic Editor: Roman Pfeifer

Received: 8 February 2021
Accepted: 22 March 2021
Published: 25 March 2021

Publisher's Note: MDPI stays neutral with regard to jurisdictional claims in published maps and institutional affiliations.

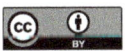

Copyright: © 2021 by the authors. Licensee MDPI, Basel, Switzerland. This article is an open access article distributed under the terms and conditions of the Creative Commons Attribution (CC BY) license (https://creativecommons.org/licenses/by/4.0/).

Abstract: Feasible and predictive scoring systems for severely injured geriatric patients are lacking. Therefore, the aim of this study was to develop a scoring system for the prediction of in-hospital mortality in severely injured geriatric trauma patients. The TraumaRegister DGU® (TR-DGU) was utilized. European geriatric patients ($\geq$65 years) admitted between 2008 and 2017 were included. Relevant patient variables were implemented in the GERtality score. By conducting a receiver operating characteristic (ROC) analysis, a comparison with the Geriatric Trauma Outcome Score (GTOS) and the Revised Injury Severity Classification II (RISC-II) Score was performed. A total of 58,055 geriatric trauma patients (mean age: 77 years) were included. Univariable analysis led to the following variables: age $\geq$ 80 years, need for packed red blood cells (PRBC) transfusion prior to intensive care unit (ICU), American Society of Anesthesiologists (ASA) score $\geq$ 3, Glasgow Coma Scale (GCS) $\leq$ 13, Abbreviated Injury Scale (AIS) in any body region $\geq$ 4. The maximum GERtality score was 5 points. A mortality rate of 72.4% was calculated in patients with the maximum GERtality score. Mortality rates of 65.1 and 47.5% were encountered in patients with GERtality scores of 4 and 3 points, respectively. The area under the curve (AUC) of the novel GERtality score was 0.803 (GTOS: 0.784; RISC-II: 0.879). The novel GERtality score is a simple and feasible score that enables an adequate prediction of the probability of mortality in polytraumatized geriatric patients by using only five specific parameters.

Keywords: geriatric trauma; scoring; polytrauma; ISS; AIS; geriatric patients; orthogeriatric

1. Introduction

The elderly population increases worldwide and subsequently the number of geriatric trauma patients rises as well [1]. Geriatric patients require special medical attention due to the higher risks for mortality and morbidity related to frailty, reduced physiological compensation mechanisms after trauma, polypharmacy and preexisting comorbidities, both in high-energy trauma cases as well as in low-energy trauma situations [2–6].

Prediction model based outcome scores are useful tools for judging patients' status and to guide medical decision making. Especially in trauma, there is a need for adequate (mortality) prediction models to optimize post-resuscitation triage and the determination of initial therapy until transfer to the intensive care unit (ICU) in severely injured patients. Several trauma outcome scores have been developed in which patients' age is also addressed. The RISC-II (Revised Injury Severity Classification II) and the newly published GTOS (Geriatric Trauma Outcome Score) seem to predict mortality in elderly poly-traumatized patients quite accurately. However, these scores highly rely on Injury Severity Score (ISS) judgments, which are known for their suboptimal inter-observer reliability [7–9]. Unlike the GTOS, the RISC-II was not specifically developed and validated for mortality prediction of the elderly severely injured patient, but is considered to be the most accurate prediction model for severely injured patients in German speaking countries. The Geriatric Trauma Outcome Score is composed of the following parameters: patient's age, the ISS and red blood cell transfusion requirements, whereas more factors, 15 in total, are required to calculate the RISC-II score [10]. Thus, the GTOS system includes less factors, which has practical benefits; however, the RISC-II score has been shown to be more accurate [11]. The aim of the current study was to develop a feasible and accurate novel score (the GERtality score) which combines simplicity with high accuracy for the prediction of in-hospital mortality in geriatric trauma patients.

2. Experimental Section

2.1. The TraumaRegister DGU®

The TraumaRegister DGU® of the German Trauma Society (Deutsche Gesellschaft für Unfallchirurgie, DGU) was founded in 1993. The aim of this multi-center database is the pseudonymized and standardized documentation of severely injured patients.

Data are collected prospectively in four consecutive time phases from the site of the accident until discharge from hospital: (A) Pre-hospital phase, (B) Emergency room and initial surgery, (C) Intensive care unit and (D) Discharge. The documentation includes detailed information on demographics, injury pattern, comorbidities, pre- and in-hospital management, course on intensive care unit, relevant laboratory findings including data on transfusion and the outcome of each individual. The inclusion criterion is admission to hospital via emergency room with subsequent ICU/ICM (intensive care medicine) care or reaching the hospital with vital signs and dying before admission to ICU.

The infrastructure for documentation, data management, and data analysis is provided by AUC—Academy for Trauma Surgery (AUC—Akademie der Unfallchirurgie GmbH), a company affiliated to the German Trauma Society. The scientific leadership is provided by the Committee on Emergency Medicine, Intensive Care and Trauma Management (Sektion NIS) of the German Trauma Society. The participating hospitals submit their data pseudonymized into a central database via a web-based application. Scientific data analysis is approved according to a peer review procedure laid down in the publication guideline of TraumaRegister DGU®.

The participating hospitals are primarily located in Germany (90%), but a rising number of hospitals in other countries contribute data as well (at the moment from Austria, Belgium, China, Finland, Luxembourg, Slovenia, Switzerland, The Netherlands, and the United Arab Emirates). Currently, approx. 33,000 cases from more than 650 hospitals are entered into the database per year.

Participation in TraumaRegister DGU® is voluntary. For hospitals associated with TraumaNetzwerk DGU®, however, the entry of at least a basic data set is obligatory for reasons of quality assurance [12].

In order to gain data for the development of the new GERtality score, data from the TraumaRegister DGU® from 1 January 2008 to 31 December 2017 were used.

The present study is in line with the publication guidelines of the TraumaRegister DGU® and registered as TR-DGU project ID 2017-048.

2.2. Inclusion and Exclusion Criteria

The aim of this study was to develop a new mortality prediction model for severely injured geriatric patients. We excluded all patients below the age of 65 years, non-European hospitals, and patients with minor trauma (maximum Abbreviated Injury Score (AIS) of 1 or 2 without admission to the ICU). Patients with missing data regarding blood transfusion, as well as transfer in or early transfer out of the hospital, were also excluded from this study. Therefore, we selected all patients aged ≥ 65 years with an AIS of 2 or less who required intensive care treatment and all patients with an AIS of 3 or more from the TR-DGU. The following parameters were included: patients' age, sex, ISS, maximum Abbreviated Injury

Score (AIS) [13], pre-hospital and in-hospital diagnostics, initial and further treatment, trauma characteristics and the patients' outcome.

2.3. Statistical Analysis

In the first step, patients' data were dichotomized and the specific odds of all relevant variables (age, sex, American Society of Anesthesiologists (ASA) [14], trauma mechanism, Glasgow Coma Scale (GCS), maximum AIS, PRBCs (Packed Red Blood Cells) given prior to ICU admission, systolic blood pressure ≤ 90 mmHg) for in-hospital mortality were calculated in a univariable way. This was performed due to an expected mortality of at least 25% or more for every single parameter. Secondly, relevant variables were added to the new GERtality score and subsequently compared to the RISC-II, GTOS, maximum AIS, ISS and age by conducting a receiver operating characteristic (ROC) analysis.

3. Results

The TR-DGU included 289,698 patients from 2008 to 2017, of which 58,055 patients met the inclusion criteria. A PRISMA flowchart is provided in Figure 1. The mean age of all patients was 77 years, and 58% were males. Baseline characteristics are shown in Table 1.

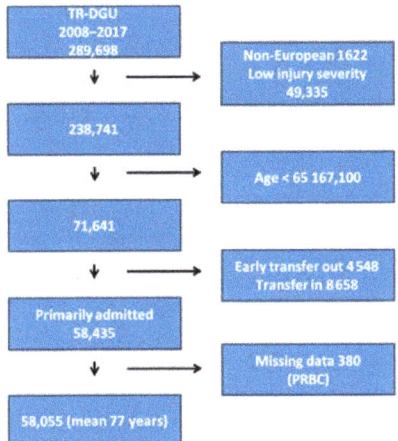

Figure 1. Inclusion flow of selected patients from the TraumaRegister DGU® (TR-DGU). PRBC, Packed Red Blood Cells.

Table 1. Basic data of 58,055 geriatric trauma patients.

Measurement	Unit	Value
Age	years	77.2/77 (7.6)
Male sex	n (%)	33,483 (57.8%)
Injury Severity Score (ISS)	points	19.2/17 (11.8)
Number of injuries	n	4.2/4 (2.6)
Penetrating trauma	n (%)	1426 (2.6%)
Mechanism: traffic	n (%)	19,910 (35.1%)
Mechanism: low fall (<3 m)	n (%)	25,218 (45.0%)
Mechanism: high fall	n (%)	7727 (13.6%)
Severe head injury (AIS ≥ 3)	n (%)	26,504 (45.7%)
Treated on intensive care unit	n (%)	51,166 (88.1%)
Ventilated on ICU	n (%)	22,486 (38.7%)
Length of stay in hospital	days	16.6/12 (16.7)
Hospital mortality	n (%)	12,969 (22.3%)

Continuous measurements are presented as mean/median (SD). AIS, Abbreviated Injury Scale, ICU, intensive care unit.

GERtality score development:

We analyzed different parameters as sole predictors for in-hospital mortality. In a first step, relevant aspects with known prognostic relevance were defined: age, concomitant diseases, severity of head injury, relevant other injuries, and bleeding. Within each subarea, potential predictors were considered and compared. For continuous measures, cut-off values were derived to reach a mortality of ~30% or more. The final decision for a certain criterion was based on a multivariate odds ratio (OR) > 2.0 (Table 2).

Table 2. Mortality rates and odds ratios of specific variables.

Variable	Subgroups	No. of Patients	Mortality Rate	Odds Ratio (OR)	95% CI of OR
Age	≥80 years <80 years	21,810 (38%) 36,245	31.5% 16.8%	2.27	2.18–2.36
Max. AIS	4 or more 2–3	25,924 (45%) 32,131	38.7% 9.2%	6.25	5.97–6.54
Blood transfusion	yes no	4813 (8%) 53,242	43.4% 20.4%	2.99	2.81–3.17
ASA	3/4 1/2	20,235 (41%) 28,269	29.1% 16.4%	2.09	2.00–2.18
GCS	3–13 14–15	22,559 (41%) 32,719	42.2% 8.8%	7.61	7.27–7.89

ASA, American Society of Anesthesiologists, GCS, Glasgow Coma Scale, CI, confidence interval.

The following patient specific parameters were suitable for the new GERtality score:
- Age ≥ 80 years
- Maximum AIS in any body region ≥4
- PRBCs received prior to admission to the ICU
- ASA ≥ 3
- GCS < 14

To calculate the new score, each finding, if present, adds up one additional point to the GERtality score. Thus, the new score ranges from 0 to 5 points (Figure 2).

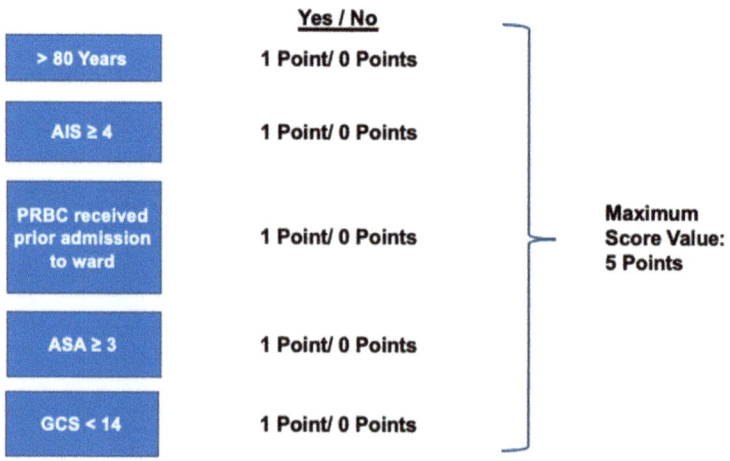

Figure 2. Relevant variables for the GERtality score. ASA, American Society of Anesthesiologists, GCS, Glasgow Coma Scale.

The maximum GERtality score showed an in-hospital mortality rate of 72.4% compared to 65.1% with patients scoring 4 points on the GERtality score and 47.5% with a total score of 3 points. The mortality with a score of 0 was 1.6% (Figure 3).

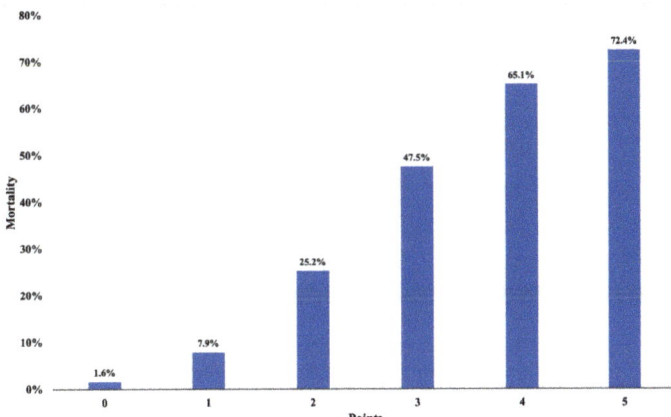

Figure 3. Observed in-hospital mortality rate based on GERtality score calculation.

GERtality score comparison:

The final ROC analysis of our patient collective showed an AUC (area under the curve) for the new GERtality score of 0.803 (CI (confidence interval) 0.799–0.807). The complex RISC-II score with its 15 variables showed an AUC of 0.879 (CI 0.876–0.883), whereas the Geriatric Trauma Outcome Score had an AUC of 0.784 (CI 0.780–0.789). Individual variables showed an AUC of 0.772 (CI 0.767–0.776) for the maximum AIS score, 0.753 (CI 0.748–0.757) for the Injury Severity Score, and 0.633 (CI 0.627–0.638) for age (Figure 4).

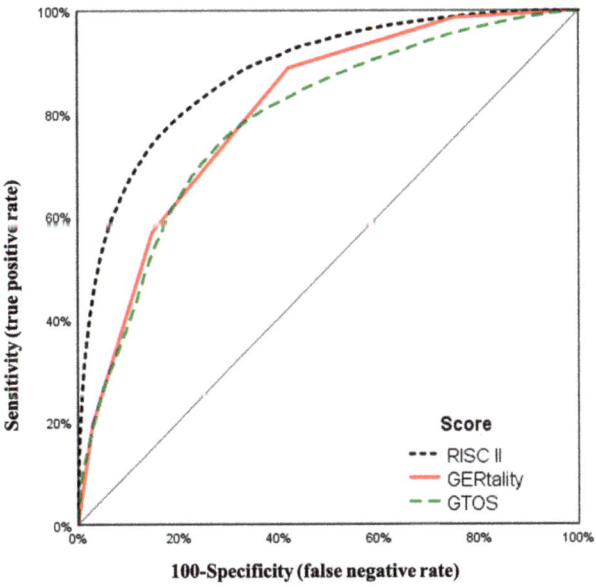

Figure 4. ROC (receiver operating characteristic) analysis.

4. Discussion

Trauma scoring systems are important instruments for the optimization of clinical decision making, the determination of outcome and the standardization of clinical studies [15,16]. Several successful trauma outcome scores have been developed in the last few decades, such as the Trauma Injury Severity Score (TRISS), APACHE-II-Score, Revised Trauma Score (RTS) and the Revised Injury Severity Classification (RISC) Score [17–20]. However, extrapolation to the geriatric population has limitations and, therefore, to date, only a few feasible scores for the prediction of mortality in geriatric trauma patients exist. To our knowledge, only two scoring systems were explicitly developed for mortality prediction after trauma in the geriatric population: namely, the new Geriatric Trauma Outcome Score (GTOS) and the very recently published Elderly Mortality after Trauma Score (EMAT) [21]. Unfortunately, we were not able to evaluate the EMAT Score because the registry data do not include all parameters used in the scoring system. The well-established Revised Injury Severity Classifications-Score II (RISC-II), although not especially developed for geriatric patients, is believed to also calculate mortality in elderly patients the most adequately and is considered the gold standard in trauma outcome prediction. The GTOS uses the patient's age, ISS and PRBCs for estimating the mortality of geriatric patients using the following rather intricate formula to calculate the possibility of death:

$$\text{age} + (2.5 \times \text{ISS}) + 22 \text{ (if given PRBCs)}$$

The GTOS predicts a chance of mortality of 50% with a score of 177 and a chance of 99% with a score of 310 [10].

The RISC-II, which was introduced in 2014, requires 15 different variables to predict mortality adequately [11]. The RISC-II, among other scoring systems, is believed to predict mortality the most accurately. Originally, this scoring system was not developed for the mortality prediction of geriatric patients, and with its carefully adjusted and weighted 15 variables, it is difficult to be calculated at the bedside.

The EMAT score contains two scoring models: the quick elderly mortality after trauma score, which should be used at the initial presentation of the patient, and the full EMAT score for calculation after radiological evaluation. The qEMAT score can be calculated with eight variables, including systolic blood pressure, pulse rate higher than 120 bpm or lower than 50 bpm, GCS, penetrating injury, congestive heart failure, liver cirrhosis and chronic renal failure, whereas the fEMAT requires 26 variables to be calculated. In this mortality prediction model, each positive variable adds up points (e.g., systolic blood pressure < 90 mmHg = 17 points and heart rate below 50 bpm = 7 points) and can then be calculated by a mobile application which is provided freely by the authors. One of the limitations of this scoring system is that it was developed and validated using a geriatric population (>65 years of age). However, age was not used as an independent factor for mortality. The EMAT also does not address severe bleeding due to trauma as a leading cause of death in severely injured patients and, as a result, the need for blood transfusions [22]. Furthermore, we believe that the EMAT is not suitable for the European population since the incidence of penetrating traumatic injuries is much lower than in the U.S. [23]. In addition, in order to calculate the EMAT, full patients' history, including co-morbidities, has to be provided, which often is not possible in the event of acute trauma [24].

Therefore, we aimed to develop a new scoring system which is easy and fast to calculate at site, but still predicts mortality in geriatric patients adequately.

In the collective of 58,055 patients used in this study, the AUC for the accuracy of mortality prediction of the GTOS was 0.784 and 0.879 of the RISC-II, whereas the novel GERtality score showed an accuracy of 0.803. These findings show that the RISC-II score is a highly accurate prediction score, but also has severe practical limitations which affect its feasibility. The RISC-II score combines a total of 15 different patient related variables which are rather unhandy to calculate on site. The GTOS, on the other hand, is relatively easy to calculate as it only uses three variables (age, ISS and received PRBS), but it had a slight disadvantage in accuracy towards the GERtality score. Furthermore, the RISC-II was made for post hoc calculation in databases and would require a computer, while the GERtality score intends to provide a simple point system to gain a quick and simple overview shortly after the admission of the patient.

It is well known that the parameters age, ISS and GCS are positive predictors for death [25,26]. In a study from a western European trauma ICU investigating the changes in outcome of severe trauma patients over a period of 15 years, age, hemorrhagic shock, GCS and the ISS were positive predictors of death [27]. Age, as a variable, combines an age-related decrease in immune defense as well as age-related comorbidities [28–33]. Frailty syndrome contributes to increased vulnerability in geriatric patients after severe trauma [34]. Generally, the treatment of unstable geriatric trauma patients does not differ a lot from non-geriatric trauma patients, but due to associated postoperative morbidities and complications in frail patients, for example, diagnostic laparoscopy should be preferred over open diagnostic laparotomy in hemodynamically stable patients [35]. Frailty is defined as clinically recognizable declines in the physiologic reserve of multiple organ systems as well as a decline in coping mechanisms for everyday life stressors [36,37]. This definition suggests that frailty is not defined by chronological age, but studies have shown a clear correlation between increasing FI (Frailty Index) and age in Europeans. However, frailty is a stronger predictor for mortality than chronological age [37].

In order to address comorbidities, we used the ASA classification as a variable in the GERtality score. As anticipated, this study shows that there is a strong association between age over 80 years and the probability of death after trauma. It may be interesting to focus on specific factors related to trauma mortality in octogenarians in further studies.

It is also known that outpatient anticoagulants are associated with a higher likelihood of PRBC transfusions [38]. One of the leading causes of death in trauma patients is hemorrhage related irreversible shock [22]. This is underlined by the current study as an association between the need for blood transfusion and the probability of death in elderly severely injured patients was found.

To sum up, the novel GERtality score combines the five most important variables associated with death after trauma in the elderly: age above 80 years, GCS < 14, maximum AIS $\geq$ 4, need for blood transfusion prior to ICU admission, and ASA $\geq$ 3. The newly developed score might help improve quality assurance, identifying the early need for transfusion/coagulation correction and decision making on further treatment for the polytraumatized geriatric patient. Before a decision on treatment, knowledge of calculated mortality odds can be advantageous, especially in usually complex ethical questions, which arise in geriatric patients frequently.

There are some limitations present in this study. In general, the quality of registry data is considered inferior due to lacking data verification. Furthermore, we were unable to calculate the frailty index, which is considered to be a good predictor for mortality in geriatric patients. The TR-DGU does not document the patient's Frailty Index, and as a consequence, we decided to utilize the chronological age in combination with the ASA Score in our dataset.

As mentioned above, outpatient anticoagulant medication has a strong correlation with PRBC transfusions. Unfortunately, the use of anticoagulants was not assessed in this dataset because it was introduced as a novel parameter in the registry since 2015. In this study, we did not yet validate the developed score.

5. Conclusions

The new GERtality score seems to be a feasible and adequate in-hospital mortality prediction model for severely injured geriatric trauma patients. The score includes only five easily assessable patient variables, which makes it practical and simple to calculate. Further studies should validate the novel GERtality score on different datasets.

Author Contributions: Conceptualization, J.S. and K.O.J.; Data curation, R.L.; Formal analysis, J.S., R.L. and K.O.J.; Methodology, J.S., R.L. and K.O.J.; Software, J.S. and R.L.; Supervision, K.O.J.; Validation, J.S., R.L. and K.O.J.; Visualization, J.S.; Writing—original draft, J.S.; Writing—review and editing, Y.K., F.Z., V.N., R.L., M.T., K.S., H.-C.P. and K.O.J. All authors have read and agreed to the published version of the manuscript.

Funding: This research received no external funding.

Institutional Review Board Statement: This registry study did not require approval by an ethical committee or review board.

Informed Consent Statement: Not applicable.

Data Availability Statement: Data is accessible on reasonable request.

Acknowledgments: The authors would like to thank A. Broughton, as a native speaker, for reviewing and correcting the English language in this manuscript.

Conflicts of Interest: The authors declare no conflict of interest.

References

1. World Health Organization. *Ageing and Health*; 2020. Available online: https://www.who.int/news-room/fact-sheets/detail/ageing-and-health (accessed on 16 December 2020).
2. Hukkelhoven, C.W.P.M.; Steyerberg, E.W.; Rampen, A.J.J.; Farace, E.; Habbema, J.D.F.; Marshall, L.F.; Murray, G.D.; Maas, A.I.R. Patient age and Outcome FOLLOWING Severe Traumatic brain Injury: An Analysis of 5600 patients. *J. Neurosurg.* **2003**, *99*, 666–673. [CrossRef]
3. Demetriades, D.; Sava, J.; Alo, K.; Newton, E.; Velmahos, G.C.; Murray, J.A.; Belzberg, H.; Asensio, J.A.; Berne, T.V. Old age as a criterion for trauma team activation. *J. Trauma* **2001**, *51*, 754–756; discussion 756–757. [CrossRef] [PubMed]
4. Joseph, B.; Zangbar, B.; Pandit, V.; Kulvatunyou, N.; Haider, A.; O'Keeffe, T.; Khalil, M.; Tang, A.; Vercruysse, G.; Gries, L.; et al. Mortality after trauma laparotomy in geriatric patients. *J. Surg. Res.* **2014**, *190*, 662–666. [CrossRef] [PubMed]
5. Con, J.; Friese, R.S.; Long, D.M.; Zangbar, B.; O'Keeffe, T.; Joseph, B.; Rhee, P.; Tang, A.L. Falls from ladders: Age matters more than height. *J. Surg. Res.* **2014**, *191*, 262–267. [CrossRef] [PubMed]
6. Peterer, L.; Ossendorf, C.; Jensen, K.O.; Osterhoff, G.; Mica, L.; Seifert, B.; Werner, C.M.L.; Simmen, H.-P.; Pape, H.-C.; Sprengel, K. Implementation of new standard operating procedures for geriatric trauma patients with multiple injuries: A single level I trauma centre study. *BMC Geriatr.* **2019**, *19*, 359. [CrossRef] [PubMed]
7. Champion, H.R.; Copes, W.S.; Sacco, W.J.; Lawnick, M.M.; Keast, S.L.; Bain, L.W.; E Flanagan, M.; Frey, C.F. The Major Trauma Outcome Study: Establishing national norms for trauma care. *J. Trauma* **1990**, *30*, 1356–1365. [CrossRef] [PubMed]
8. Maduz, R.; Kugelmeier, P.; Meili, S.; Döring, R.; Meier, C.; Wahl, P. Major influence of interobserver reliability on polytrauma identification with the Injury Severity Score (ISS): Time for a centralised coding in trauma registries? *Injury* **2017**, *48*, 885–889. [CrossRef] [PubMed]
9. Pothmann, C.E.M.; Baumann, S.; Jensen, K.O.; Mica, L.; Osterhoff, G.; Simmen, H.-P.; Sprengel, K. Assessment of polytraumatized patients according to the Berlin Definition: Does the addition of physiological data really improve interobserver reliability? *PLoS ONE* **2018**, *13*, e0201818. [CrossRef] [PubMed]
10. Zhao, F.Z.; Wolf, S.E.; Nakonezny, P.A.; Minhajuddin, A.; Rhodes, R.L.; Paulk, M.E.; Phelan, H.A. Estimating Geriatric Mortality after Injury Using Age, Injury Severity, and Performance of a Transfusion: The Geriatric Trauma Outcome Score. *J. Palliat. Med.* **2015**, *18*, 677–681. [CrossRef]
11. Lefering, R.; Huber-Wagner, S.; Nienaber, U.; Maegele, M.; Bouillon, B. Update of the trauma risk adjustment model of the TraumaRegister DGU: The Revised Injury Severity Classification, version II. *Crit Care* **2014**, *18*, 476. [CrossRef]
12. Deutsche Gesellschaft für Orthopädie und Unfallchirurgie. *Traumaregister DGU®*. 2019. Available online: www.traumaregister-dgu.de (accessed on 30 November 2020).
13. Haasper, C.; Junge, M.; Ernstberger, A.; Brehme, H.; Hannawald, L.; Langer, C.; Nehmzow, J.; Otte, D.; Sander, U.; Krettek, C.; et al. The Abbreviated Injury Scale (AIS). Options and problems in application. *Unfallchirurg* **2010**, *113*, 366–372. [PubMed]
14. Doyle, D.J.; Garmon, E.H. *American Society of Anesthesiologists Classification (ASA Class)*; StatPearls: Treasure Island, FL, USA, 2019.
15. Abu-Hanna, A.; Lucas, P.J. Prognostic models in medicine. AI and statistical approaches. *Methods Inf. Med.* **2001**, *40*, 1–5.
16. Laun, R.A.; Schröder, O.; Schoppnies, M.; Röher, H.D.; Ekkernkamp, A.; Schulte, K.M. Transforming growth factor-beta1 and major trauma: Time-dependent association with hepatic and renal insufficiency. *Shock* **2003**, *19*, 16–23. [CrossRef] [PubMed]
17. Wagner, D.P.; Draper, E.A. Acute physiology and chronic health evaluation (APACHE II) and Medicare reimbursement. *Health Care Financ. Rev.* **1984**, *Suppl*, 91–105.
18. Boyd, C.R.; Tolson, M.A.; Copes, W.S. Evaluating trauma care: The TRISS method. Trauma Score and the Injury Severity Score. *J. Trauma* **1987**, *27*, 370–378. [CrossRef] [PubMed]
19. Champion, H.R.; Sacco, W.J.; Copes, W.S.; Gann, D.S.; Gennarelli, T.A.; Flanagan, M.E. A revision of the Trauma Score. *J. Trauma* **1989**, *29*, 623–629. [CrossRef] [PubMed]

20. Lefering, R. Development and validation of the revised injury severity classification score for severely injured patients. *Eur. J. Trauma Emerg. Surg.* **2009**, *35*, 437–447. [CrossRef] [PubMed]
21. Morris, R.S.; Milia, D.; Glover, J.; Napolitano, L.M.; Chen, B.; Lindemann, E.; Hemmila, M.R.; Stein, D.; Kummerfeld, E.; Chipman, J.; et al. Predictors of elderly mortality after trauma: A novel outcome score. *J. Trauma Acute Care Surg.* **2020**, *88*, 416–424. [CrossRef]
22. O'Reilly, D.; Mahendran, K.; West, A.; Shirley, P.; Walsh, M.; Tai, N. Opportunities for improvement in the management of patients who die from haemorrhage after trauma. *Br. J. Surg.* **2013**, *100*, 749–755. [CrossRef] [PubMed]
23. Lustenberger, T.; Talving, P. Focus on challenges and advances in the treatment of patients with penetrating injuries. *Eur. J. Trauma Emerg. Surg.* **2016**, *42*, 661–662. [CrossRef] [PubMed]
24. Howard, B.M.; Kornblith, L.Z.; Conroy, A.S.; Burlew, C.C.; Wagenaar, A.E.; Chouliaras, K.; Hill, J.R.; Carrick, M.M.; Mallory, G.R.; Watkins, J.R.; et al. The found down patient: A Western Trauma Association multicenter study. *J. Trauma Acute Care Surg.* **2015**, *79*, 976–982. [CrossRef]
25. Randolph, A.G.; Guyatt, G.H.; Richardson, W.S. Prognosis in the intensive care unit: Finding accurate and useful estimates for counseling patients. *Crit. Care Med.* **1998**, *26*, 767–772. [CrossRef] [PubMed]
26. Matthes, G.; Seifert, J.; Bogatzki, S.; Steinhage, K.; Ekkernkamp, A.; Stengel, D. Age and survival likelihood of polytrauma patients. "Local tailoring" of the DGU prognosis model. *Unfallchirurg* **2005**, *108*, 288–292.
27. Di Saverio, S.; Gambale, G.; Coccolini, F.; Catena, F.; Giorgini, E.; Ansaloni, L.; Amadori, N.; Coniglio, C.; Giugni, A.; Biscardi, A.; et al. Changes in the outcomes of severe trauma patients from 15-year experience in a Western European trauma ICU of Emilia Romagna region (1996–2010). A population cross-sectional survey study. *Langenbecks Arch. Surg.* **2014**, *399*, 109–126. [CrossRef]
28. Broos, P.L.O.; D'Hoore, A.; Vanderschot, P.; Rommens, P.M.; Stappaerts, K.H. Multiple trauma in elderly patients. Factors influencing outcome: Importance of aggressive care. *Injury* **1993**, *24*, 365–368. [PubMed]
29. Broos, P.L.; D'Hoore, A.; Vanderschot, P.; Rommens, P.M.; Stappaerts, K.H. Multiple trauma in patients of 65 and over. Injury patterns. Factors influencing outcome. The importance of an aggressive care. *Acta Chir. Belg.* **1993**, *93*, 126–130. [PubMed]
30. Dzankic, S.; Pastor, D.; Gonzalez, C.; Leung, J.M. The prevalence and predictive value of abnormal preoperative laboratory tests in elderly surgical patients. *Anesth Analg.* **2001**, *93*, 301–308.
31. Frankenfield, D.; Cooney, R.N.; Smith, J.S.; Rowe, W.A. Age-related differences in the metabolic response to injury. *J. Trauma* **2000**, *48*, 49–56; discussion 56–57. [CrossRef]
32. Knies, R.C., Jr. Assessment in geriatric trauma: What you need to know. *Int. J. Trauma Nurs.* **1996**, *2*, 85–91. [CrossRef]
33. Leung, J.M.; Dzankic, S. Relative importance of preoperative health status versus intraoperative factors in predicting postoperative adverse outcomes in geriatric surgical patients. *J. Am. Geriatr. Soc.* **2001**, *49*, 1080–1085. [CrossRef] [PubMed]
34. Chen, X.; Mao, G.; Leng, S.X. Frailty syndrome: An overview. *Clin. Interv. Aging* **2014**, *9*, 433–441. [PubMed]
35. Di Saverio, S.; Birindelli, A.; Podda, M.; Segalini, E.; Piccinini, A.; Coniglio, C.; Frattini, C.; Tugnoli, G. Trauma laparoscopy and the six w's: Why, where, who, when, what, and how? *J. Trauma Acute Care Surg.* **2019**, *86*, 344–367. [CrossRef] [PubMed]
36. Fried, L.P.; Hadley, E.C.; Walston, J.D.; Newman, A.B.; Guralnik, J.M.; Studenski, S.; Harris, T.B.; Ershler, W.B.; Ferrucci, L. From bedside to bench: Research agenda for frailty. *Sci. Aging Knowl. Environ.* **2005**, *2005*, pe24. [CrossRef] [PubMed]
37. Romero-Ortuno, R.; Kenny, R.A. The frailty index in Europeans: Association with age and mortality. *Age Ageing* **2012**, *41*, 684–689. [CrossRef] [PubMed]
38. Ang, D.; Kurek, S.; McKenney, M.; Norwood, S.; Kimbrell, B.; Barquist, E.; Liu, H.; O'Dell, A.; Ziglar, M.; Hurst, J. Outcomes of Geriatric Trauma Patients on Preinjury Anticoagulation: A Multicenter Study. *Am. Surg.* **2017**, *83*, 527–535. [CrossRef] [PubMed]

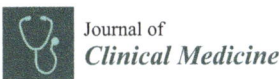

Review

The Pathophysiology and Management of Hemorrhagic Shock in the Polytrauma Patient

Alison Fecher [1], Anthony Stimpson [1], Lisa Ferrigno [2] and Timothy H. Pohlman [3],*

1. Division of Acute Care Surgery, Lutheran Hospital of Indiana, Fort Wayne, IN 46804, USA; amfecher@gmail.com (A.F.); agstimpson@lhn.net (A.S.)
2. Department of Surgery, UCHealth, University of Colorado-Denver, Aurora, CO 80045, USA; lisalouferrigno@yahoo.com
3. Surgery Section, Woodlawn Hospital, Rochester, IN 46975, USA
* Correspondence: tpohlman606@gmail.com

Abstract: The recognition and management of life-threatening hemorrhage in the polytrauma patient poses several challenges to prehospital rescue personnel and hospital providers. First, identification of acute blood loss and the magnitude of lost volume after torso injury may not be readily apparent in the field. Because of the expression of highly effective physiological mechanisms that compensate for a sudden decrease in circulatory volume, a polytrauma patient with a significant blood loss may appear normal during examination by first responders. Consequently, for every polytrauma victim with a significant mechanism of injury we assume substantial blood loss has occurred and life-threatening hemorrhage is progressing until we can prove the contrary. Second, a decision to begin damage control resuscitation (DCR), a costly, highly complex, and potentially dangerous intervention must often be reached with little time and without sufficient clinical information about the intended recipient. Whether to begin DCR in the prehospital phase remains controversial. Furthermore, DCR executed imperfectly has the potential to worsen serious derangements including acidosis, coagulopathy, and profound homeostatic imbalances that DCR is designed to correct. Additionally, transfusion of large amounts of homologous blood during DCR potentially disrupts immune and inflammatory systems, which may induce severe systemic autoinflammatory disease in the aftermath of DCR. Third, controversy remains over the composition of components that are transfused during DCR. For practical reasons, unmatched liquid plasma or freeze-dried plasma is transfused now more commonly than ABO-matched fresh frozen plasma. Low-titer type O whole blood may prove safer than red cell components, although maintaining an inventory of whole blood for possible massive transfusion during DCR creates significant challenges for blood banks. Lastly, as the primary principle of management of life-threatening hemorrhage is surgical or angiographic control of bleeding, DCR must not eclipse these definitive interventions.

Keywords: polytrauma; hemorrhage; shock; resuscitation; coagulopathy; oxygen transport; endotheliopathy; microcirculation; macrocirculation

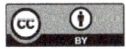

1. Introduction

For the polytrauma patient, brain injury is the most common cause of early death followed by acute blood loss as the second most common cause of early death [1,2]. In the U.S., 150,000 people die each year due to injury and many of these deaths occur in relatively younger individuals, which causes an aggregate loss of productive life of over 3.3 million years [3]. This results in an annual cost to society of USD 2.34 billion in today's dollars from lost wages and medical costs. In prospective studies that examine resuscitation after trauma the median time to hemorrhagic death is 2.0 to 2.6 h [4–7]. Hemorrhage is the most common cause of shock in the injured, and a substantial number of trauma patients will arrive at hospital with profound physiologic disturbances due to acute circulatory failure. Dr. Samuel D Gross, regarded as one of the most innovative and influential surgeons of the

19th century described shock simply as, " ... a rude unhinging of the machinery of life". Indeed, this remarkable characterization of hemorrhagic shock remains as informative today as certainly it was over 175 years ago [8].

The polytrauma victim with significant hemorrhage suffers a life-threatening acute reduction in oxygen delivery (DO_2) to tissue. DO_2 depends on both an adequate circulating blood volume representing sufficient oxygen carrying capacity, and effective cardiovascular function to maintain the circulation of blood to capillary beds in the periphery.

Furthermore, between 25% to 35% of hemorrhaging patients will develop a biochemically evident coagulopathy (trauma-induced coagulopathy; TIC) before arrival to the emergency department, which can manifest clinically as either hypercoagulable or hypocoagulable states, or both. In the polytrauma patient the presence of TIC is associated with higher transfusion requirements, increased I.C.U. and hospital length of stay (LOS), prolonged requirement for mechanical ventilation, an increase in the incidence of multiorgan dysfunction, and, most concerning of all, a threefold to fourfold higher rate of mortality [9–13]. TIC has deleterious effects independent of injury severity, level of shock, degree of acidosis or depth of hypothermia [14].

Here we examine important pathophysiologic concepts of hemorrhagic shock, and we describe resuscitation strategies for the patient with acute, life-threatening blood loss. Detailed explanations of the complex molecular and cellular aspects of shock and trauma exceed the scope of this review. However, specific advances toward a more complete understanding of hemorrhagic shock at these basic levels may significantly alter future clinical approaches to the polytrauma patient.

2. Pathophysiology of Hemorrhagic Sock

Oxygen Delivery/Utilization Imbalance

The pathophysiology of hemorrhagic shock involves a decrease in systemic DO_2 to a level less than what is needed to maintain cellular function (VO_2). DO_2 equals the rate of blood flow, which is cardiac output (Q; normal = 5–6 L/min) multiplied by the content of oxygen bound to hemoglobin (Hgb) in a volume of blood (normal: male = 20.7 mL O_2/dL; female = 18.4 mL O_2/dL). A normal DO_2 is approximately 1000 to 1250 mL O_2/min in males, and approximately 925 to 1100 mL O_2/min for females. If oxygen delivery is insufficient, tissue hypoxia develops resulting in anaerobic metabolism and production of lactate.

An important variable in oxygen transport physiology not often considered because it is seldom measured is the oxygen binding affinity of Hgb, expressed as p50 and depicted by oxy-hemoglobin dissociation (OHD) curves (Figure 1A–C). This property of Hgb determines the extent of peripheral oxygen offloading and therefore the quantity of oxygen available for tissue oxygenation. Acidosis shifts the OHD curve to the right (referred to as the Bohr effect) and increases the offloading of oxygen. Conversely, hypothermia shifts the curve to the left tends to decrease offloading of oxygen in the periphery. Acidosis and hypothermia are frequent homeostatic disturbances that complicate resuscitation. Depending on the magnitude of either one at any one moment during resuscitation, offloading of oxygen from Hgb may be enhanced or impeded [15]. These considerations may explain in part variability of responses to resuscitation of different patients. Additionally, of interest is the possibility of enhancing end-organ oxygen availability in patients with compromised oxygen transport by a pharmacological increase in p50 [16].

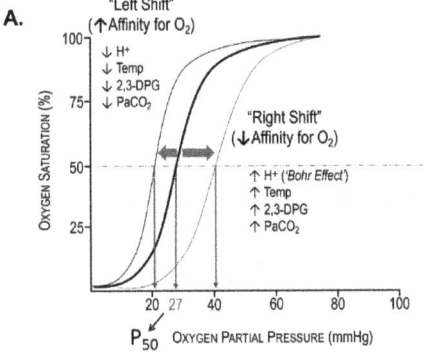

Figure 1. (**A**) OHD curve which relates the saturation of Hgb (*y*-axis) to the degree of partial pressure of oxygen to which Hgb is exposed (*x*-axis). The pO$_2$ that saturates $\frac{1}{2}$ of Hgb is referred to as p50, which in this example p50 = 27 mmHg. The p50 is the conventional measure of affinity of Hgb for oxygen. The lower the p50 the higher the affinity of Hgb for oxygen. The 'steep' portion of the oxyHgb dissociation curve is in the range of pO$_2$ that exists in systemic capillaries (thus a small decrease in systemic capillary pO$_2$ can result in the release of large amounts of oxygen for diffusion to, and uptake by cells). As shown in the figure, several factors increase the affinity of Hgb for oxygen (leftward shift; ↓p50) or decrease affinity (rightward shift; ↑p50). Biochemically, H+ is a heterotropic allosteric inhibitor of Hgb, whereas O$_2$ is a homeotropic allosteric activator of Hgb. (**B**) Hypothermia and acidosis have opposing effects on p50. Lower temperature shifts the curve to the left increasing Hgb affinity for oxygen and decreasing offloading in capillaries; low pH (increase in H+) decreases the affinity of Hgb for oxygen (Bohr effect) increasing oxygen availability to reverse anaerobic metabolism. A trauma patient may be, and often is hypothermic and acidotic (and coagulopathic). Whether there is a significant change in p50 can be calculated using the Hill–Langmuir equation. (**C**): Hypothetical oxygen transport variables of a normal subject (Temp = 37 °C; p50 = 25 mmHg) and a subject with hypothermia (Temp = 31 °C; p50 = 20 mmHg), before and after compensation. The p50 at 31 °C and pH = 7.4 is calculated using the Hill–Langmuir equation. A venous blood gas is obtained through a Swan Catheter introducer (7.5Fr) with the tip in the superior vena cava reveals in the hypothermic subject, central venous oxygen saturation (ScvO$_2$) = 85%. This reflects the fact that hypothermia increases the affinity of Hgb for oxygen, shifting the Hgb dissociation curve to the left.

A ScvO$_2$ of 85% would imply only 15% of the delivered 1000 mL of oxygen (DO$_2$) prior to compensation is being offloaded, which is approximately 150 mL/min, well below VO$_2$ (250 mL/min). The hypothermic patient can compensate by increasing cardiac output and hence DO$_2$. Assume that stroke volume is unchanged (although a well-known consequence of tachycardia is a reduction in stroke volume), and cardiac output increases by an increase in heart rate (HR) from 72 beats/min to 120 beats/min (a 40% increase in HR causing a substantial increase in myocardial oxygen demand).

Systemic oxygen utilization (VO$_2$), approximately 250 mL O$_2$/min, is the amount of oxygen consumed each minute by all metabolic processes in the body. The physiologic relationship of VO$_2$ to DO$_2$ is expressed as the oxygen extraction ratio (O$_2$ER),

$$O_2ER = \frac{VO_2}{DO_2}$$

VO$_2$ and thus O$_2$ER differ significantly among different organ systems. For example, extraction ratios measured in the in the heart, liver, and kidney, are 60%, 45% and 15% respectively. Predictably, a higher O$_2$ER is associated with greater DO$_2$ dependency.

O$_2$ER provides an important compensatory mechanism offsetting reductions in DO$_2$ due to acute blood loss and a decrease in cardiac output. An initial reduction in DO$_2$ is offset by an increase in O$_2$ER that maintains VO$_2$ constant. In this hemodynamic state, the value of VO$_2$ is flow-independent. As a compensatory mechanism for blood volume loss, O$_2$ER-mediated flow-independence of VO$_2$ may result in a deceptive clinical presentation of hemodynamic stability (compensated hemorrhagic shock), although as much as 30 percent of blood volume may have been lost. As cardiac output and thus DO$_2$ continue to decline with ongoing hemorrhage, O$_2$ER will increase until eventually the amount of oxygen that can be extracted plateaus (O$_2$ER = 60–70% for most tissues). From this point, any further decrease in DO$_2$ will cause VO$_2$ to decline such that the value of VO$_2$ is now flow-dependent. The value of DO$_2$ that represents the boundary between flow-independent VO$_2$ and flow-dependent VO$_2$ is designated DO$_{2\,CRIT}$. Any DO$_2$ < DO$_{2\,CRIT}$ is associated with a decrease in VO$_2$ and impaired oxygen-dependent cellular processes as metabolism shifts from aerobic to anaerobic pathways.

DO$_{2\,CRIT}$ marks the onset of lactic acidosis and the beginning of an accumulating oxygen debt [17] (Figure 2). Without effective resuscitation, ongoing hemorrhage progresses to decompensated shock, characterized by hemodynamic instability and diminished blood flow that cannot maintain life-sustaining physiologic processes; and then to refractory shock, representing exhaustion of physiological reserves, hemodynamic collapse, vital organ dysfunction and subsequent failure, and ultimately, death.

Therefore, a principal objective of care for the polytrauma patient in shock is to restore DO$_2$ to a level (DO$_2 \approx$ 350–450 mL O$_2$/min/m^2) such that, to a first approximation, DO$_2$ > DO$_{2\,CRIT}$. However, targeting even higher, supranormal values for DO$_2$ (DO$_2$ > 600 mL O$_2$/min/m^2) with aggressive fluid administration predisposes to secondary complications of volume overload. Higher values of DO$_2$ likely will not improve survival and, in fact, is associated with detrimental patient outcomes [18].

DO$_2$ can be determined from the Hgb concentration, SaO$_2$ and stroke volume (hence, cardiac output). Stroke volume can be obtained non-invasively, expeditiously, and to a reasonable degree of accuracy [19] by transthoracic echocardiographic measurement of blood flow velocity at the left ventricular outflow track [20–22]. VO$_2$ can be estimated as 125 mL/min/m^2 × BSA (BSA m^2 = 0.007184 × (W)$^{0.425}$ kg × (H)$^{0.725}$ cm), determined by indirect calorimetry, or calculated using the Fick equation [23]. However, DO$_{2\,CRIT}$ is not an exact transition point from flow-independent to flow-dependent VO$_2$ [24] and varies considerably from one organ system to another. Moreover, direct point-of-care measurement of many critical parameters of oxygen transport generally are neither practical, nor feasible during resuscitation. Nevertheless, we believe familiarity with the physiology of oxygen delivery/utilization balance, and an appreciation for the meaning of O$_2$ER and

$DO_{2\,CRIT}$, establishes an important conceptual foundation that informs critical decisions typically required during resuscitation.

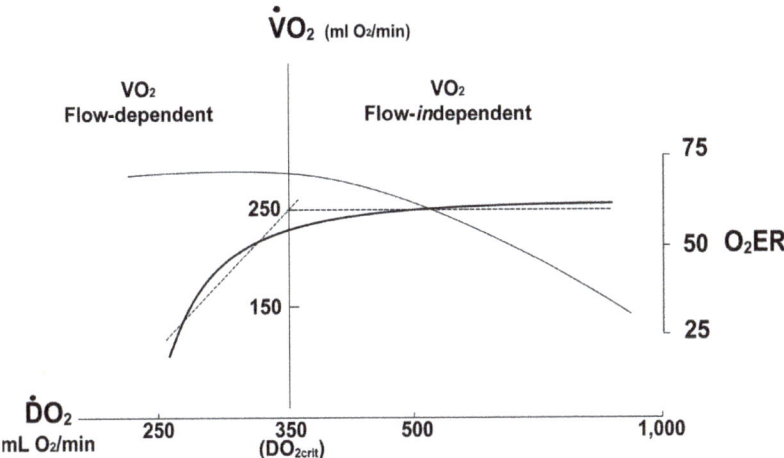

Figure 2. $DO_{2\,CRIT}$ defines shock. As DO_2 (solid black line) decreases secondary to a fall in cardiac output, drop in Hgb concentration, or both, O_2ER (solid grey line) increases to maintain VO_2 constant until extraction is maximized. At this point, designated as $DO_{2\,CRIT}$ (also referred to as the anaerobic threshold), VO_2 begins to decrease with further decreases in DO_2. When $DO_2 > DO_{2\,CRIT}$ t, VO_2 is flow-independent; when $DO_2 < DO_{2\,CRIT}$, VO_2 becomes flow-dependent. In addition, $DO_{2\,CRIT}$ is associated with the onset of lactate formation and accumulation. Thus, shock can be defined conceptually as the presence of DO_2 less than $DO_{2\,CRIT}$, producing a reduction in VO_2. Normal $DO_2 = 800$ mL $O_2/min/m^2$; normal $VO_2 = 200$ mL $O_2/min/m^2$; normal $O_2ER = 25\%$.

3. Trauma-Induced Coagulopathy

In 2003, Brohi and colleagues identified an acquired coagulopathy in trauma patients recognized as distinct from the coagulation abnormalities caused by dilution during resuscitation [13]. Trauma-induced defects in hemostasis occur in approximately 25 to 65 percent of injured patients who are more likely to be in shock and to have the highest injury severity scores. TIC is associated with increased early transfusion requirements, the development of organ failure, and higher mortality [25]. Mechanistically trauma-induced coagulopathy (TIC), as presently defined, represents a gamut of observed abnormalities in clot formation, fibrinolysis or in any one of several hemostatic pathways that control these two processes.

TIC is associated with diffuse injury to the endothelium (or, endotheliopathy). Trauma-induced endotheliopathy is characterized as a systemic disturbance of microvascular endothelial cell function thought to be caused by exposure to the high levels of circulating catecholamines [26–31], and a diverse array of extracellular stimuli, including cytokines such as IL-6 and TNF-α [32]. An important pathologic feature of trauma-induced endotheliopathy is microvascular thrombus formation that blocks flow and oxygen offloading from Hgb in capillary circuits. Shock-induced endotheliopathy occurs together with shedding of the adjacent endothelial glycocalyx. The endothelial glycocalyx is an indistinct layer rich in syndecan-1, hyaluronic acid, heparan sulfate and chondroitin sulfate. The glycocalyx contributes to endothelial cell permeability and function by restricting the movement of fluid and proteins from blood to the interstitium, modulating sheer stress, and controlling inflammatory cell-endothelial cell interactions and associated thrombotic and inflammatory reactions [33]. Shedding of the glycocalyx removes these homeostatic functions and releases proteoglycans that bind and activate endogenous anticoagulant proteins including antithrombin, tissue factor pathway inhibitor (TFPI), and heparin sulfate-like moieties, which essentially heparinize the bleeding trauma patient [34].

TIC also includes fibrinogen depletion and disseminated intravascular coagulation [35–39]. Von Willebrand factor dysfunction may also occur after trauma and is classified as part of TIC. Furthermore, certain qualitative platelet defects develop in trauma patients, particularly in those with head injuries [40–44]. In addition to these coagulopathies trauma patients will demonstrate distinct patterns of dysfunction in the fibrinolytic system ranging from fulminant hyperfibrinolysis to fibrinolysis shutdown, with profound implications for resuscitation strategies.

3.1. Specific Defects in Hemostasis Induced by Trauma

3.1.1. Upregulated Protein C Expression

Thrombomodulin (TM) is an endothelial cell surface receptor that binds thrombin. Thrombin-TM interactions promote thrombin-mediated activation of soluble vitamin K-dependent protein C, a reaction that is accelerated by binding of protein C to a co-localizing endothelial cell surface receptor, endothelial cell protein C receptor (EPCR). Activated protein C together with protein S (protein S is named after Seattle the city of its discovery [45]) proteolytically degrades coagulation cofactors VIII and V. Consequently, activations of coagulation factors IX and X are suppressed and thrombin generation from prothrombin terminates [46,47]. In addition to down regulating clot formation, activated protein C/protein S promotes clot lysis by blocking an important inhibitor of fibrinolysis, PAI-1 (plasminogen activation inhibitor-1). Although, thrombin when bound to TM increases anticoagulant activity through activation of protein C, thrombin-TM interactions also promote antifibrinolytic activity by thrombin-mediated activation of TAFI (thrombin-activatable fibrinolysis inhibitor). Activated TAFI interferes with plasminogen binding to fibrin clots, which is required for plasminogen conversion to plasmin by plasminogen activators [48]. Additionally, it is noteworthy that TAFI functions in control of inflammatory processes by modulating complement anaphylatoxin C5a activity [49]. Thus, the clinical variability of TIC may be related in part to the development of endotheliopathy and the countervailing activities induced by upregulated expression of TM.

3.1.2. Von Willebrand Factor

Von Willebrand factor (VWF) is a high-molecular-weight adhesive glycoprotein that plays an essential role in primary hemostasis by promoting platelet adhesion to the subendothelium and platelet plug formation at the sites of vascular injury [50] VWF is increased in plasma and bronchoalveolar lavage (BAL) fluid of patients with acute injury and is predictive of the development of acute respiratory distress syndrome [51]. VWF stored in endothelial cell Weibel–Palade bodies and platelet α-granules after being synthesized in both cell types. VWF ultra-large multimers (ULVWFs) are released from endothelial cells following trauma possibly through systemic endothelial cell activation by IL-1, IL-8, and TNF-α [52]. ULVWFs are then rapidly cleaved to active units by circulating ADAMTS13. Dysregulation of VWF/ADAMTS13 is hypothesized to have a role in propagation of shock-induced endotheliopathy, coagulopathy, and systemic auto-inflammatory reactions. However, despite reports on clinical association between dysregulation of VWF/ADAMTS-13 and poor outcomes of patients with severe trauma, this phenomenon has not been explained mechanistically.

Hypothermia affects all aspects of hemostasis including both procoagulant and anticoagulant activities. However, VWF-platelet glycoprotein receptor Ib-IX-V interactions appear to be the most sensitive to lower temperature [53].

3.1.3. Hypofibrinogenemia

Congenital fibrinogen disorders are rare bleeding disorders affecting either the quantity (afibrinogenemia and hypofibrinogenemia) or the quality (dysfibrinogenemia) or both (hypodysfibrinogenemia) of fibrinogen [54]. Acquired hypofibrinogenemia (depending how it is defined) has been reported in up to 40% of hypotensive trauma patients [55–57]. In many cases fibrinogen is the first coagulation component to fall to critical levels [58], and the extent of hypofibrinogenemia correlates with injury severity [59]. Fibrinogen functions as the primary substrate for the coagulation cascade and is converted by thrombin to fibrin strands for clot formation. Fibrinogen is important also for platelet aggregation after engaging the platelet membrane receptor, GPIIb/IIIa. Fibrinogen concentrations < 230 mg/dL are associated with an increase in mortality and moderate hypofibrinogenemia is a determinate of early organ failure, negatively correlating with 24-h SOFA (sequential organ failure assessment) scores [60]. Hypofibrinogenemia is more likely observed in patients with severe extremity or pelvic fractures, who are acidotic and experiencing a long delay in transfer to a trauma center. Specific viscoelastic assays permit rapid assessment of the contribution of fibrinogen to clot strength but must be interpreted with caution [61].

3.1.4. Platelet Dysfunction

Injury, and in particular traumatic brain injury (TBI), is associated with acquired platelet dysfunction, present in nearly 30 percent of patients on admission when assessed by impedance aggregometry in response to arachidonic acid, collagen, or thrombin. Decreased platelet responsiveness to ADP secondary to downregulation of platelet $P2Y_{12}$ receptor has also been well-described [41,42,62,63]. $P2Y_{12}$ is a G-protein coupled receptor that binds adenosine diphosphate (ADP) released from platelet dense granules. Consequently down regulation of this receptor or antagonist blockade inhibits ADP-mediated platelet aggregation. $P2Y_{12}$ inhibition correlates with the severity of TBI as well as TBI-related mortality. The median percent inhibition in TBI patients (mean Glasgow Coma Scale score of 11.9) is 86 percent [42]. Additionally, in patients bearing high injury severity scores and presenting with a severe lactic acidosis (base deficit −8 mEq/L or more), ADP-mediated aggregation is nearly completely inhibited (97 percent). The mean platelet count for all these patients with acquired qualitative platelet defects is normal ($232 \times 10^3/\mu L$), and thus impedance aggregometry should be performed. The mechanism responsible for $P2Y_{12}$ down-regulation is not clearly defined.

3.2. Dysregulation of Fibrinolysis
3.2.1. Hyperfibrinolysis

Fibrin has a fundamental role in hemostasis as the product of the coagulation cascade and the principal component in clot formation and as the substrate for fibrinolysis and clot breakdown. Fibrinolysis efficiency is greatly influenced by clot structure, fibrinogen isoforms and polymorphisms, the rate of thrombin generation, the reactivity of thrombin-activated cells such as platelets, and the relative balance of activators and inhibitors of fibrinolysis [64]. Hemostasis is a tightly maintained process that involves formation of clot to arrest bleeding and lysis of clot to maintain vascular patency. Normal clot formation and deposition of fibrin promotes tissue plasminogen activator (tPA) mediated conversion of plasminogen to plasmin and activation of primary fibrinolysis limiting thrombus growth to the site of injury (Figure 3). tPA is released by fibrin-mediated enhancement of TIC can also be caused by dysregulated fibrinolytic activity [65]. Two major pathologic fibrinolytic patterns are identified in trauma patients: hyperfibrinolysis (HF) and fibrinolysis shutdown (FS). Hemorrhagic shock tends to induce hyperfibrinolysis; tissue destruction, particularly involving solid organs tends to initiate fibrinolysis shutdown [65,66].

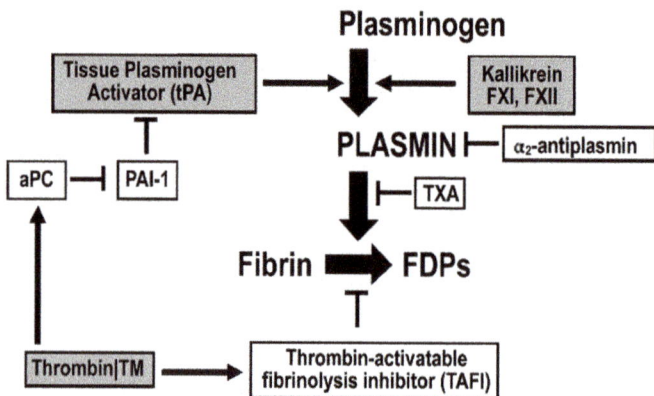

Figure 3. Pathways of plasminogen activation and inhibition. Plasminogen is synthesized by and released from the liver. To be activated to plasmin, plasminogen initially binds to lysine residues exposed on fibrin. The generation of plasmin from its precursor, plasminogen is achieved by the plasminogen activators, tissue-type type plasminogen activator (tPA), and urokinase (not depicted). Protien C, once activated by thrombin bound to thrombomodulin blocks PAI-1, the major inhibitor of tPA; therefore thrombin, through activated protein C, can promote fibrinolysis. However, thrombin-thrombimodulin interactions can also inhibit fibrinolysis through activation of TAFI (thrombin-activatable fibrinolysis inhibitor). Plasmin once formed can also cleave plasma prekallikrein (Fletcher factor) and Hageman factor (FXII) and in turn plasminogen can be activated to plasmin by these proteases. Furthermore, plasmin, can activate the complement factors, C5 and C3, while on the other hand, it can itself be inhibited by the C1-inhibitor, thereby providing a natural means to regulate this process. Excessive plasmin formation can result in hyperfibrinolysis, which increases the risk of bleeding. Tranexamic acid (TXA) blocks lysine-dependent interactions and therefore inhibits binding of plasminogen to and transfusion requirements. Plasminogen receptors located on the surface of immune cells also contain C-terminal lysine the surface of fibrin and misfolded proteins. Plasmin also activates other substrates with pro-inflammatory potential including TGF-β, a neurotrophic agent brain-derived neurotropic factor, and other proteases like the matrix metalloproteinases.

HF is a highly lethal, typically fulminant coagulopathy associated with a mortality as high as 75 percent in adults [65] and 100 percent in pediatric patients [67]. This bleeding diathesis develops in approximately 10 to 20 percent of patients who, on admission, will have a higher ISS (>15) and a significantly larger base deficit compared to polytrauma patients without HF. Additionally, hemodilution due to large prehospital crystalloid infusion volumes increase the possibility of patients developing HF compared to patients with similar ISS and base deficit who receive significantly less fluid [68]. Shock-induced endotheliopathy increases TM-mediated activation of protein C. Thus, degradation of the endogenous fibrinolytic inhibitor, PAI-1 by activated protein C results in unregulated accumulation tPA and uncontrolled tPA-mediated induction and amplification of fibrinolysis [69–72]. This hypothesis has intuitive appeal because it satisfies the principle of parsimony, frequently referred to as the natural law of Occam's razor, meaning one pathophysiological mechanism (endotheliopathy) links several hemostatic abnormalities that comprise TIC. Conversely it is suggested that lack of detectable PAI-1 activity is not caused by protein C-mediated proteolysis, but rather is secondary to PAI-1 forming covalent complexes with tPA [73].

It is also more apparent, however, from later studies that hyperfibrinolysis is not linked to defects in the coagulation cascade. This conjecture holds that primary HF (and hyperfibrinogenolysis) occurs after a massive shock-induced release of tPA from vascular endothelium. High levels of circulating tPA rapidly sequesterPAI-1 as PAI-1-tPA complexes. tPA in excess of PAI-1 then initiates and propagates systemic fibrinolytic activity by conversion of plasminogen to plasmin. Although other inhibitors and pathways of activation exist for the fibrinolytic system, tPA and PAI-1 interactions predominate [73–77].

3.2.2. Fibrinolysis Shutdown

Whereas HF is the most fulminant form of fibrinolytic dysregulation following severe trauma (ISS $\geq$ 15), it occurs in in a smaller percentage of severely injured patients (18%) compared to FS, which is observed in 46% of patients. FS is associated with macro-thromboses, resulting in stroke, deep vein thrombosis (DVT), and pulmonary embolism (PE). Additionally, microvascular thromboses can lead to multiple organ failure [78] and eventually death [79]. The mechanism of FS shutdown is thought to be due to massive release of PAI-1. PAI-1 exists in three forms in plasma: (1) free active PAI-1, (2) inactive PAI-1 complexed with t-PA and (3) latent PAI-1 (an inactive PAI-1 conformation). PAI-1 plasma levels vary more than any other component of the fibrinolytic system, likely due to the wide variety of substances that induce PAI-1 production. These include insulin, TNFα, IL-1, transforming growth factor β (TGFβ), and thrombin [80]. PAI-1 is synthesized in hepatocytes and endothelial cells. Platelets α-granules also are a prominent source of PAI-1 (and, α2-antiplasmin) in the circulation after platelet activation with thrombin. However, a mechanistic link between activated platelet PAI-1-mediated inhibition of tPA to fibrinolytic shutdown has yet to be established, whereas platelet dysfunction has been associated with hyperfibrinolysis.

4. Management of the Polytrauma Victim

4.1. Pre-Hospital Care

4.1.1. Physician-Staffed EMS Response

Twelve percent of trauma deaths may be preventable with advanced resuscitative interventions, which would likely require the presence of physicians in the field or highly trained paramedics [81]. Inclusion of emergency medicine physicians or trauma surgeons in pre-hospital trauma care is, however, controversial. A physician-staffed EMS response to trauma increases the complexity of the care provided at the scene, and this will invariably prolong to some degree scene and total prehospital times. An association between longer scene times and increased mortality in severely injured patients has been demonstrated [82]. Noncompressible bleeding in the abdomen is rapidly fatal, with mortality increasing approximately 1% for each 3 min delay to damage control laparotomy [83]. There are also data to suggest that there is no association between prehospital time and mortality in polytrauma patients [84,85], and that specific patients may benefit more by undergoing advanced airway and chest procedures rather than just faster transport to a trauma center [86]. However, the best prehospital strategies for certain subgroups such as rural trauma patients, patients with multiple blunt force-induced injuries, and perhaps patients undergoing complicated extrications remain unclear [87].

In Germany EMS dispatch is structured on a rendezvous-system between ambulances staffed with paramedics and a vehicle with an emergency physician. The decision to involve the EMS physician is made selectively in an EMS dispatch center. Recently, a telemedicine system was implemented that permits paramedics to consult physicians at anytime. Paramedic-tele-EMS physician consults can bridge the time gap between diagnosis and treatment for patients with life-threatening injuries until the EMS physician arrives at the scene. Furthermore, several potentially life-threatening cases could be handled by a tele-EMS physician as they did not require any invasive interventions that needed to be performed by an onsite EMS physician. Consequently, telemedicine systems establish a higher quality of emergency medical care at an earlier stage [88].

4.1.2. Prehospital Transfusion

Various observations suggest early initiation of resuscitation in the prehospital environment could possibly reduce excessive mortality [89]. To address this issue, two RCTs, the Control of Major Bleeding After Trauma trial (COMBAT (NCT01838863); an individual patient randomized. single-center study design), and the Prehospital Air Medical Plasma trial (PAMPer (NCT01818427); a pragmatic, multicenter, cluster-randomized, phase 3 superiority study design) [90] examined the use of plasma for resuscitation in the prehospital setting. Whereas the COMBAT trial showed that resuscitation with thawed plasma instead of saline for patients in hemorrhagic shock during ground transport (generally with short transport times) did not reduce mortality, the PAMPer trial, in contrast, demonstrated the administration of thawed plasma for hemorrhagic shock during helicopter transport reduced 30-day mortality by 30 percent (23.3% vs. 33.0%; $p = 0.03$) [90]. A post hoc combined analysis of the data from the COMBAT and PAMPer trials revealed that patients who received prehospital plasma transfusion had significantly reduced 28-day mortality compared with standard care, when prehospital transport times were longer than 20 min [91].

Use of whole blood for resuscitation of hemorrhagic shock in the pre-hospital setting has also been examined. A recent study demonstrated that trauma patients who received prehospital LTOWB transfusion had a greater improvement hemodynamically and showed a reduction in early mortality compared to patients who were not transfused, even though the cohort being transfused were in more advanced stages of hemorrhagic shock [92].

4.1.3. Empiric Administration of Tranexamic Acid (TXA)

The Clinical Randomization of an Antifibrinolytic in Significant Haemorrhage-2 (CRASH-2), a pragmatic, randomized, placebo-controlled phase 3 study that involved 274 hospitals in 40 countries, enrolled 20,127 subjects over a five-year period, May 2005 to January 2010, and was funded in part by a major pharmaceutical company that manufacture TXA. The study assessed the effect of TXA on mortality, vascular occlusion events and receipt of blood transfusion following trauma. The study detected a small but statistically significant decrease in 28-day, all-cause mortality deaths of 1.5% in study subjects treated with TXA (1463/10,060 (14.5%) TXA group vs. 1613/10,067 (16.0%) placebo group); death to hemorrhage was reduced 0.8% (489/10,060 (4.9%) vs. 574/10,067 (5.7%)) [93]. In this study of an antifibrinolytic drug, fibrinolytic activity was not measured. Although concerns about CRASH-2 design and methodology persist [94], the results of the study became widely accepted as definitive, and TXA became recognized as the "anti-hemorrhage" drug carried on many ambulances and medical helicopters [95]. In fact, data confirm the effectiveness of TXA when selectively administered to seriously injured patients (mean ISS $\geq$ 30) during the prehospital phase of care [96,97].

However, in the trauma patient, different states of fibrinolysis other than hyperfibrinolysis can be identified, including inhibition of fibrinolysis and fibrinolysis shutdown representing an inhibition beyond physiologic levels after activation of fibrinolytic pathways [77]. Further inhibition by TXA of a system already demonstrating diminished fibrinolytic activity may increase mortality when given to patients maintaining low but still physiologic levels of fibrinolysis [98], or TXA may precipitate FS in those patients [76]. Thus, inhibition of fibrinolysis in severely injured patients requires careful consideration, recognizing that in certain circumstances TXA can adversely affect survival [65]. Arguably, nonselective administration of TXA to trauma patients is not indicated.

Although TXA is considered primarily an inhibitor of fibrinolysis, it is suggested that early TXA administration also blocks protease-mediated glycocalyx degradation thereby preventing endotheliopathy and associated hemostatic defects [76,99,100].

4.2. Hospital Management of the Polytrauma Patient

4.2.1. Initial Assessment

Assessment is commonly based on clinical experience and a set of basic parameters including, level of consciousness, systolic blood pressure (SPB), diastolic blood pressure (DPB), heart rate (HR), respiratory rate, capillary filling time, and capnometry [101]. Hypotension is considered the relevant hemodynamic abnormality in a patient with acute blood loss. However, hypotension is a late finding and suggests physiologic reserves are nearly depleted or have been exhausted. Additionally, hypotension fails to predict the presence of a significant injury or a more immediate requirement for advanced interventions. Shock Index (SI), defined as, HR/SBP may provide a stronger prediction of significant injury [102]. A normal index is essentially < 1.0; thus, whenever the HR is numerically more than the SBP, the patient is in shock. SI $\geq$ 1.5 is reported to predict massive transfusion for a trauma patient with reasonable sensitivity [103]. A yet more sensitive metric for shock is the modified SI, which is determined by HR/(mean arterial blood pressure); a modified SI $\geq$ 1.3 indicates a hypodynamic state [104]. The ROPE index is defined as HR/pulse pressure. From the example above, ROPE index = 110/(94−60) = 3.2. This index indicates shock when $\geq$2.2 and has the potential to be an early indicator of blood loss [105].

For ongoing hemorrhage, the decision to initiate a major resuscitation including massive transfusion is often at the discretion of the trauma surgeon. Twenty-four different scoring systems predict the need for massive transfusion (MT) for a patient with the potential for hemorrhagic shock. Massive transfusion is generally defined as the transfusion of 10 more units of blood within a 24 period; it is also be defined as 3 units of blood per hour (critical administration threshold) [106]. Of scores that use clinical assessment, laboratory values, and ultrasound results, the Modified Traumatic Bleeding Severity Score exhibits the most precision, while the Trauma Associated Severe Hemorrhage score is the most well validated [107]. Recently, a definition of massive transfusion that takes into account the use of whole blood was created that identifies early mortality more accurately than other definitions [108]. Although not widely utilized, noninvasive measurement of muscle oxygenation based on optical spectroscopy may provide the most direct measure of shock and is potentially the best indicator with respect to sensitivity and specificity for massive transfusion [109–112].

4.2.2. Damage Control Resuscitation (DCR)

Application of evidence-based principles of DCR improves survival in injured patients, although survival of patients with the most severe hemorrhage associated with hypotension is not necessarily improved over older strategies of resuscitation [113]. DCR principles include compressible hemorrhage control; hypotensive resuscitation; avoidance of the overuse of crystalloids and colloids; prevention or correction of acidosis, hypothermia, and hypocalcemia; and hemostatic resuscitation (early use of a balanced amount of red blood cells (RBCs), plasma, and platelets) [114]. DCR can be accomplished using (1) transfusion of whole blood, (2) transfusion of blood components in equal volumes, or (3) transfusion of components directed by results of viscoelastic assay (so-called goal-directed DCR). Notably during DCR microcirculatory function and metabolic cellular function are not measured specifically, directly or continuously in a way that informs decisions in a realistic clinical context. Availability of plasma and platelets is limited in some environments. In these situations, the use of low titer, type O whole blood, thawed or liquid plasma, cold stored platelets or reconstituted freeze-dried plasma can be used as substitutes. Of interest, cold-stored platelets may be superior to room temperature platelets in hemostatic potential [115].

- Resuscitation with whole blood

In 1969, with the advent of component separation of blood at hand, Dr. Francis Moore, former surgeon-in-chief at the Peter Bent Brigham and recipient of the Samuel Gross Medal of the American Surgical Association, published this opinion on resuscitation, "For the restoration of homeostasis after acute massive hemorrhage, it appears that fresh compatible whole blood is the ideal transfusion." [116]. Restoration of adequate blood volume and correction of trauma-induced defects in hemostasis can be accomplished with transfusion of low titer (anti-A antibodies, anti-B antibodies < 1:256), type O, Rh-negative, whole blood (LTOWB). The use of LTOWB for trauma patients has expanded substantially in U.S level 1 and 2 trauma centers from 2018 to 2020, which includes an increase in the use of Rh-positive LTOWB in females of child-bearing years [117,118]. Benefits of LTOWB-based resuscitation include possibly an increase in survival compared to component-based resuscitation [119,120], reduced donor exposure, all elements critical to hemorrhage control are contained in one product in physiologic amounts [118], and that transfusion of younger red blood cells occurs [119] because of shorter storage times. Length of storage time for whole blood remains debated, although data show significant degradation of the hemostatic potential of whole blood after 14 days of storage [121]. Leukoreduction of LTOWB does not appear to afford any distinct clinical benefit over non-leukoreduced units [122]. Additionally, resuscitation with whole blood may be a better option for exsanguinating hemorrhage in certain parts of the world where there is a lack of well-equipped blood banks and insufficient availability of blood products [123]. However, the percentage of all donors who are eligible to donate RhD-negative LTOWB (male, group O, RhD-negative, and have low titer anti-A and -B) is only 3% RhD-alloimmunization rate is approximately 21% [124].

Successful experience with fresh whole blood by the US military is well documented [125]. Recent studies suggest that LTOWB in resuscitation of civilian trauma is associated with a reduction in post-emergency department transfusions and increase likelihood of 24-h and 28-day survival [120,126]. Conversely, other data suggest that, although safe, resuscitation with LTOWB does not significantly improve survival compare to component-based resuscitation [127,128], and LTOWB does not reduce blood product utilization, as first hypothesized [120]. Arguably, existing studies on LTOWB-based resuscitation are limited for the most part, and a more rigorous, high quality investigation to address the effectiveness of LTOWB may be warranted [117,119,129].

- Fixed Component Ratio-based DCR

The 2015 Pragmatic, Randomized Optimal Platelet and Plasma Ratios (PROPPR) trial established use of balanced blood component transfusions for resuscitation of hemorrhagic shock. This study involving 12 major US. Trauma centers showed resuscitation with blood components transfused in a fixed ratio of 1:1:1 (plasma:PLTs:pRBCs) reduced mortality caused by exsanguination at 24 h when compared to transfusion of components in a fixed ratio of 1:1:2 (9.6% vs. 14.6%) [130]. In both groups, platelets were transfused first followed by plasma alternating with pRBCs. Components transfused 1:1:1 deliver a blood substitute that is anemic, thrombocytopenic and hypocoagulable [131].

Platelets are separated from a unit of fresh whole blood by apheresis or centrifugation. Platelets are customarily stored in the blood bank at room temperature (20–24 °C) for up to 5 days. Platelets stored at this temperature incur a substantial risk of bacterial contamination. Transfusion of platelets stored at room temperature is associated with a greater risk of septicemia and death than transfusion of any other blood product [132]. Moreover, at room temperature, there is rapid deterioration in platelet function referred to as a platelet storage lesion, characterized by, fragmentation, activation, degranulation and aggregation together with increased glycolysis and intracellular acidosis that significantly diminish the efficacy of platelet transfusions [133]. Increased demand for platelets during DCR placed on an always-limited blood bank inventory may significantly challenge resuscitative efforts.

To circumvent these problems, platelet storage at 4 °C is being re-examined [134,135]. Platelets were originally stored at 4 °C until it was shown that the half-life of cold-stored platelets after transfusion was markedly reduced in circulation (1.3 days) compared to the half-life of platelets stored at room temperature (3.9 days) [136]. However, cold stored platelets show evidence of activation including increased thromboxane A2 production and increased surface expression of P-selectin and GPIba receptors [137]. It is suggested that because of pre-activation, cold stored platelets may be more effective than platelets stored at room temperature for hemostatic resuscitation [137]. Cold stored platelets have better adhesion and aggregation functionality than platelets kept at room temperatures, which is associated with a reduction in bleeding times [138]. The issue then becomes whether the short half-life of cold-stored platelets is still sufficient for DCR.

Transfusion of packed red cells at times in massive amounts can reestablish adequate oxygen carrying capacity, although RBC transfusions are associated with measurable risks of morbidity and mortality. After separation from whole blood, pRBC's are stored at 4 °C in a preservation additive for up to 42 days. Current blood banking procedures may not fully preserve red blood cell (RBC) function during storage, contributing to the decrease of RBC oxygen release ability [139]. The storage time of transfused blood is an independent risk factor for post-injury multiple organ failure [140,141]. During this time RBCs undergo biochemical changes collectively referred to as RBC storage lesion. In addition to developing severe metabolic imbalances, stored RBCs transform morphologically from flexible biconcave discs into rigid shapes (burr cells) that do not readily deform and obstruct flow through capillary beds [142]. Furthermore, microvascular flow is increased by nitric oxide and adenosine triphosphate released from RBCs in hypoxic conditions. Both these microvascular regulatory mediators are depleted in cold-stored RBC's.

Additionally, cold stored RBCs are depleted of erythrocyte 2,3-diphosphoglycerate (2,3-DPG). Binding of 2,3-DPG to Hgb decreases the oxygen binding affinity of Hgb (rightward shift of the oxyHgb dissociation curve; increase in p50), which facilitates offloading of oxygen from Hgb in tissue. In MT, when a patient may have predominately banked blood circulating, the time needed to synthesize and accumulate 2,3-DPG and regenerate a p50 favorable to tissue oxygenation may be excessive [143]. RBC energy metabolism progressively deteriorates, and energy-dependent redox systems fail. Increasing oxidant stress leads to accumulation of irreversibly oxidized proteins, metabolites, and lipids. Therefore, it is reasonable to consider that a significant red cell storage lesion would negatively affect outcomes in transfused trauma patients, and that fresh blood or blood with relatively a short storage time should be used. Earlier studies in the aggregate are inconclusive regarding whether age of transfused blood has any association with trauma patient outcomes [144]. In one study, an increase in the number of older PRBCs ($\geq$22 days storage) transfused during massive transfusion of trauma patients was shown, in fact, to be independently associated with increased likelihood of 24-h mortality (adjusted odds ratio = 1.05 per PRBC unit; 95% confidence interval) [145]. However, in a more recent analysis, no systematic correlation was found between storage time of transfused RBC units and in-hospital mortality of patients undergoing massive transfusion [146].

Plasma transfusion during DCR provides clotting factors and has been shown to mitigate the endotheliopathy of trauma. Protection of the endothelium may be in part due to fibrinogen and other plasma-derived proteins, although the exact mechanism of endothelial cell protection by plasma has not yet been elucidated [30,31,147]. In the U.S. the designation fresh frozen plasma (FFP) means plasma was separated and frozen within 8 h of collection; plasma produced from whole blood stored at 4 °C for up to 24 h prior to component separation is designated FP24. FFP is rapidly administered early in the course of resuscitation. However, there are technical difficulties with the timely administration of FFP, which is stored at -18 °C and requires 30 to 40 min to thaw, label and issue. Moreover, utilization of FFP is limited by a short half-life once thawed and by the fact FFP from rare blood group AB donors is used before the recipient's blood type is known. To make plasma readily available at the initiation of DCR, it may be feasible for blood banks to maintain a small inventory of plasma that has been thawed for less than 24 h, which can be issued without delay and transfused immediately while type-specific FFP is thawed.

Thawed plasma or "never-frozen" liquid plasma are two other products that can be used immediately and thereby obviate FFP and FP24 transfusion for management of TIC [148]. Coagulation factor levels are maintained in thawed plasma for up to 5 days with the exception of coagulation cofactor VIII, which falls below the lower limit of normal by the fifth day of storage [149,150]. Additionally, to preserve blood bank inventories of group AB plasma, group A thawed plasma is transfused empirically when the recipient's blood type is unknown [151–153]. The risk of an ABO blood group mismatch reaction is relatively rare since the most common encountered blood group in a recipient will be group A. Moreover, anti-B antibodies generally are low in group A plasma from certain donors, for example, North American males >50 years of age. Greater than 90% of surveyed trauma centers report using type A plasma.

Despite significant declines in some factors in liquid plasma stored for up to 40 days, fibrinogen concentration and clot strength as measured by viscoelastic assay were stable. Liquid plasma is easier to store and prepare and may be more amenable to prehospital transfusion [154].

Freeze-dried plasma (FDP), which can be stored at room temperature for 2 years is another source for clotting factors for transfusion into the hemorrhaging trauma patient. FDP is rapidly reconstituted with sterile water and can be used within minutes. The overall safety and efficacy of FDP may be equivalent to allogenic blood products based largely on observational studies; however, there are no data from larger, randomized controlled trials comparing FDP with FFP to confirm this. Furthermore, the effects of FDP on host auto-inflammatory reactions, if any, are unknown [155]. Finally, concerns regarding disease transmission, including hepatitis, with the use of pooled FDP, led to the cessation of large-scale production [156]. Interest in FDP persists in the military setting, nonetheless, and with significant improvement in donor screening, testing procedures, and pathogen reduction technology, including a photochemical pathogen inactivation process the French military continues to produce French lyophilized plasma (FLyP) [157]. Providing FFP early for civilian patients in the prehospital setting, when TIC is thought to first develop presents formidable technical and logistical challenges. Military applications of FDP suggest, however, the feasibility of plasma transfusion in civilian prehospital and early hospital settings, or in settings where FFP is unavailable [158].

Because hypofibrinogenemia is recognized to significantly complicate hemorrhagic shock, early repletion of fibrinogen [159,160] in concert with platelet, RBC and plasma transfusion is advocated. Several international guidelines for DCR specify fibrinogen infusion for plasma fibrinogen levels <150–200 mg/dL or diminished clot strength due to hypofibrinogenemia (or possibly acquired dysfibrinogenemia [161]) as indicated by viscoelastic assay [162]. In the U.S., cryoprecipitate (cryo) is the principal source of fibrinogen [163], which is produced by slowly thawing FFP. Other coagulation factors enriched in cryo include von Willebrand factor, FVIII, and FXIII, and these plausibly contribute to hemostatic resuscitation. Recent in vitro and in vivo data suggest that cryo potentially attenuates the endotheliopathy induced by hemorrhagic shock [164].

- Goal-directed DCR

A viscoelastic assay (VEA), by either thromboelastography (TEG) (Figure 4) or rotational thromboelastometry (ROTEM), assesses several parameters of fibrin formation and HF and/or FS in whole blood [165–168]. VEA-based assessment of coagulation provides a rapid, integrated measure of clot formation and dissolution in blood compared to conventional coagulation tests (CCT) of individual coagulation pathways performed on prepared plasma and therefore in the absence of platelets and red cells. In addition, VEAs can detect hyperfibrinolysis or fibrinolysis shutdown, which are not detectable by CCTs, although on occasion VEAs may fail to detect so-called occult fibrinolysis [169]. Neither VEAs, nor CCTs assess the complex influence of the endothelium on hemostatic activity.

As DCR progresses serial viscoelastic assays on a patient reliably identify particular coagulopathies and delineate fibrinolytic phenotypes within a realistic clinical context and in a timelier fashion than conventional tests of coagulation [170,171]. For example, VEA's may predict a specific need for plasma or suggest instead cryoprecipitate for TIC even before coagulopathic bleeding is evident clinically. These assays can also predict massive transfusion earlier and more accurately than clinical judgement or CCTs. Viscoelastic assay is particularly useful, for example, in suggesting the possibility of coagulopathy due to platelet dysfunction (MA < 55 on TEG) in a head injury patient with a normal platelet count. Additionally, complicating factors such as the effects of preexisting pharmacological treatment with direct oral anticoagulants can be identified by VEAs.

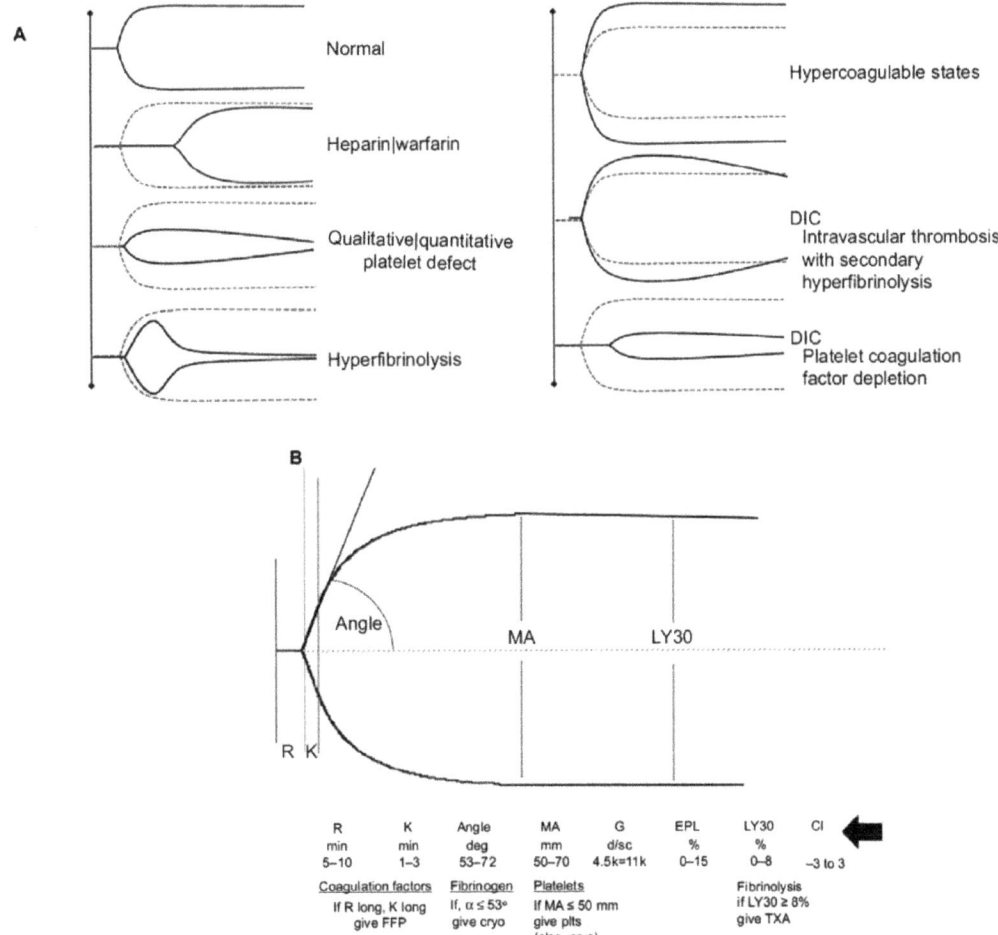

Figure 4. Thromboelastography (TEG®). (**A**) Schematic presentation of different viscoelastic tracings reflecting states of the coagulation system compared with normal. (**B**) Basic viscoelastic tracing with measured parameters and limits of normal for thromboelastography, correlated with different elements of the coagulation system (R = reaction time, K = clot formation time, angle, MA = maximum amplitude, Ly30 = percent clot lysis 30 m after MA). Viscoelastic k-time and angle correlate to some degree with fibrinogen concentration. However, the agreement between these parameters and fibrinogen levels determined by standard von Clauss assay is not sufficiently strong to be useful clinically. To overcome this limitation with TEG, the specific contributions of fibrinogen and platelets to clot strength can be determined with additional reagents (TEG; Functional Fibrinogen [Haemonetics Corp, Niles, IL, USA]). Using TEG, additional measures of clot strength can be computed. Coagulation index (CI; black arrow) is derived from R, k-time, angle, and MA, with a CI >+3.0 suggesting a hypercoagulable state and CI <−3.0 suggesting coagulopathy. The shear elastic module strength, designated G, is a computer-generated quantity that reflects an integrated measure of clot strength. Conceptually, G is considered the most informative parameter of clot strength because it reflects the contributions of the enzymatic and platelet components of hemostasis. Abbreviations: rTEG, rapid thromboelastography; DIC, disseminated intravascular coagulation; EPL, estimated percent lysis; FFP, fresh frozen plasma; Cryo, cryoprecipitate; Plts, platelets; TXA, tranexamic acid.

Viscoelastic assays such as TEG that are used to diagnose hyperfibrinolysis may take as long as 60 min before results are obtained on which to base anti-fibrinolytic therapy with TXA. Delays in TXA administration to trauma patients who are coagulopathic due to hyperfibrinolysis reduce the effectiveness of TXA [172], whereas empiric TXA administration exposes patients without hyperfibrinolysis to risks of TXA-induced VTE and organ failure [98,173]. Of more concern is the potential adverse effects of TXA administration to patients with FS [174]. A complete TEG at POC provides data certainly no sooner that CCTs performed in the laboratory. Rapid TEG accelerates the process by addition of thrombin as a initiating agent, which is accelerated faster still by the addition of plasmin. Added plasmin identifies patients at highest risk for hyperfibrinolysis within 5 min instead of 60 min, and therefore may prove useful for selective and timely administration of TXA [175]. The detection of hyperfibrinolysis can direct selective use of TXA [176] rather than empiric treatment of all trauma patients with this potentially dangerous anti-fibrinolytic. Until recently, VEAs results and the reproducibility of results were dependent on the accuracy of pipetting while performing the assay. This challenge has been obviated and accuracy improved with preloaded cartridge systems with the TEG 6S and ROTEM Sigma [170]. Neither VEAs, nor CCTs include, however, the important contribution of the endothelium to hemostasis [177]. Currently it is suggested that VEAs in DCR may improve survival and reduce blood component transfusion [168,178].

- Resuscitation with Concentrates

Several European countries provide clotting factors as concentrates. Four factor prothrombin complex concentrate (4F-PCC), is a fractionated, heat-treated, nanofiltered, lyophilized, non-activated plasma product made from pooled human donations. 4F-PCC contains the four vitamin–K dependent coagulation factors II, VII, IX and X, and protein C and protein S that also require post-synthesis vitamin K mediated carboxylation of glutamate residues. Protein C and protein S anticoagulant activities balance the procoagulant activity of PCC and reduce the incidence thromboembolic complications associated with this product.

Hypofibrinogenemia and increased fibrinogen breakdown are important findings of TIC and fibrinogen is usually the first factor to reach critically low levels in traumatic hemorrhage [179]. The presence of hypofibrinogenemia on arrival at hospital predicts massive transfusion, and is associated with an increase in morbidity and mortality [180–182]. Several studies have examined the feasibility of providing fibrinogen to severely bleeding trauma patients and have suggested that soluble fibrinogen given early during trauma resuscitation may have some clinical benefit [183–186]. Pre hospital administration of fibrinogen concentrate has been shown to improve clot stability and to prevent significant decreases in plasma fibrinogen. In the U.S., fibrinogen concentrate is used to treat bleeding and for prophylaxis of patients with congenital hypofibrinogenemia [187] but it is not approved for use in patients with acquired disorders of fibrinogen.

Fibrinogen concentrates do not contain platelet membrane microparticles. These small structures are generated in freeze-thaw cycled plasma during preparation of cryoprecipitate and are associated with thrombotic or inflammatory potential in trauma patients [188]. There are several plasma derived fibrinogen concentrates marketed world-wide for the management of acquired hypofibrinogenemia. The manufacturing processes differ suggesting that small but potentially clinically relevant differences in composition may be present including, fibronectin, vWF antigen, vitronectin, albumin, fibrinopeptide A, and plasminogen. Of note, factor XIII is detectable in different products from 0.2 U/mL to 3.9 U/mL [189]. Recent studies demonstrate the combination of added fibrinogen and factor XIII is highly effective in raising maximum clot firmness determined by viscoelastic assay [190]. Factor XIII not only generated stable clot resistance to hyperfibrinolysis but also enhanced platelet function by facilitating clot retraction. High-dose FXIII administration therapy has significant clinical impact for severe trauma. High-dose Factor XIII administration induces effective hemostasis for TIC both in vitro and in rat hemorrhagic shock models [191].

4.2.3. Secondary Assessment

We target intermediate variables of reflecting microcirculatory function such as stroke volume, mean arterial pressure, heart rate, and urine output. Modalities that can be used to monitor microcirculatory dysfunction include determination of the PCO_2 gap, in-vivo videomicroscopy using orthogonal polarization spectral imaging or sidestream dark field imaging. With NIRS, (Near Infrared Spectroscopy) of oxygenated Hgb in that tissue). The NIRS value of the Hgb oxygen concentration in a tissue is represented as StO_2 (tissue oxygen saturation) and this value can be obtained for vessels that are less than 1 mm in size.

During resuscitation, reaching satisfactory measures of macrocirculatory oxygen transport do not necessarily indicate adequate perfusion at a microvascular level or sufficient oxygenation of tissue. Additional parameters to assess include serum lactate and the oxygen saturation of central venous blood ($ScvO_2$) a surrogate for the saturation of true mixed venous blood (SvO_2) sampled from the pulmonary artery [192–194]. Because there is a lack of agreement between absolute values for SvO_2 and $ScvO_2$, the clinical utility of $ScvO_2$ has long been in question [195,196]. However, we believe trends in $ScvO_2$ can provide important and accurate information for decision making during resuscitation, although normalization of $ScvO_2$ neither excludes persistent tissue hypoperfusion, nor precludes evolution to multi-organ dysfunction and death [197]. The difference between central venous pCO_2 ($pcvCO_2$) and arterial pCO_2 ($paCO_2$), which can be referred to as "pCO_2 gap" may support deductions regarding oxygen delivery to tissues, although this parameter is applied more frequently to patients in septic shock. A deficit in tissue perfusion secondary to persisting reductions in microvascular flow, or macrovascular flow is considered as a primary cause of a pCO_2 gap (>6 mmHg) [198,199] Furthermore, measurement of $ScvO_2$, a surrogate for global tissue oxygenation, in the context of a pCO2gap, a surrogate for cardiac output (or flow), may provide a more useful assessment of the effectiveness of a resuscitation. Thus, hemorrhagic shock should show $\downarrow\downarrow ScvO_2$ with $\uparrow pCO_2$ gap associated with an $\uparrow\uparrow O_2 ER$ and $\uparrow$ lactate. Distributive shock would appear essentially the same except for $\uparrow ScvO_2$ and $\downarrow pCO_2 gap$ [200].

5. Conclusions

This review examined first, the pathophysiology of hemorrhagic shock and second, current management strategies for acute blood loss in the polytrauma patient. Hemorrhagic shock is in part characterized by a critical reduction in global oxygen delivery (DO_2) caused by an acute loss of O_2 carrying capacity such that $DO_2 < DO_{2\ CRIT}$ and O_2 consumption becomes flow-dependent. During reductions in DO_2 that do not fall below $DO_{2\ CRIT}$, oxygen availability is maintained by increased extraction of oxygen from blood delivered to the periphery. This compensatory mechanism can create a deceptive appearance of stability in the polytrauma patient who may have suffered a significant blood loss and is continuing to hemorrhage.

In addition, serious injury and hemorrhage are associated with one or more defects in coagulation, fibrinolysis, or both, which, predictably, exacerbate bleeding. Disorders of hemostasis are detectable in approximately 25–56% of polytrauma patients prior to initiating resuscitation [201]. Clot formation, centered on the generation of thrombin and fibrinolysis, centered on the generation of plasmin are two highly complex integrated plasma-based systems consisting of several proteins and endogenous inhibitors, which interact with the vascular endothelium under normal conditions and the endothelium and sub-endothelium at sites of injury. Acquired defects of hemostasis in the polytrauma patient include systemic damage to the endothelium (referred to as endotheliopathy), qualitative platelet defects (especially in patients with head injury), fibrinogen depletion, vWF dysfunction, or disorders of fibrinolysis, including fulminant hyperfibrinolysis and fibrinolytic shutdown. We have referred to these collectively as trauma-induced coagulopathy (TIC), which may manifest as either a hypocoagulable or hypercoagulabe (thrombotic) states. Precise descriptions of mechanisms responsible for most of these acquired hemostatic defects are incomplete. However, the excess mortality associated with TIC perhaps justifies close familiarity with fundamental precepts of hemorrhagic shock.

Furthermore, we have examined different aspects of DCR for the management of hemorrhagic shock in the polytrauma patient. During the last 70 years, the resuscitation of hemorrhagic shock has evolved from transfusion of whole blood; to transfusion of packed RBCs with large volumes of isotonic crystalloid; to balanced transfusion of RBCs, plasma and platelets, without crystalloid, and with or without fibrinogen replacement by transfusion of cryoprecipitate; to again transfusion of whole blood. At the same time, extension of viscoelastic assays from assessment of coagulopathies secondary to liver disease to polytrauma patients with TIC has been the basis for so-called goal-directed DCR strategies, which also include viscoelastic assessments of fibrinolysis not routinely included in conventional tests of coagulation. Acquisition of viscoelastic data (by either thromboelastography or rotational thromboelastometry) presents additional challenges during DCR, as trained personnel to perform the assay and experienced clinicians to accurately interpret the results are required.

We have described DCR in general terms as a structured approach to major trauma that integrates the principles of hemodynamic resuscitation, including massive transfusion to restore adequate O_2 delivery, hemostatic resuscitation to treat or prevent TIC, and homeostatic resuscitation to treat or prevent extreme hypothermia, divalent cation imbalances, acidosis, and anticipated left-shifts in the OHD curve. Another important component of DCR is permissive hypotension which is predicated on perceiving hemorrhagic shock as a blood flow problem and not necessarily a blood pressure problem.

We believe future DCR protocols will demonstrate the increasing use of specific concentrates such as fibrinogen concentrate, or PCCs adapted specifically to the trauma patient in place of allogenic blood components. We predict that the most successful concentrate will likely be a combination of certain concentrates that individually have minimal impact on outcomes, but synergistically improve mortality significantly, for example, a fibrinogen concentrate combined with a factor XIII concentrate.

Finally, we expect that a more complete pathophysiologic description of hemorrhagic shock will require a substantially better understanding of microcirculation function [202] and hemorrhagic shock-induced disruption of the critical role the microcirculation holds in regulation of tissue perfusion. Moreover, we anticipate that specific treatments of disorders of the microcirculation in patients in hemorrhagic shock will mean significant modification of current practices of DCR.

Author Contributions: Conceptualization, T.H.P. and A.S.; writing—review and editing, T.H.P., A.F., A.S. and L.F.; visualization, T.H.P., A.F., A.S. and L.F.; supervision, T.H.P.; project administration, T.H.P. All authors have contributed substantially to this work. All authors have read and agreed to the published version of the manuscript.

Funding: This research received no external funding.

Conflicts of Interest: The authors declare no conflict of interest.

Abbreviations

DO_2—Oxygen delivery, VO_2—oxygen consumption, OHD—oxyhemoglobin dissociation curve, Hgb—hemoglobin, O_2ER—oxygen extraction ratio, TIC—trauma-induced coagulopath, PAI-1—plasminogen activator inhibitor, TAFI—thrombin-activatable fibrinolysis inhibitor, DAMP—damage-associated molecular pattern, PAMP—pathogen-associated molecular pattern, HF—hyperfibrinolysis, FS—fibrinolysis shutdown, Ang-1,-2—anngiopoietin-1,-2, EC—endothelial cell, TM—thrombomodulin, MT—massive transfusion, LTOWB—low titer, type O, whole blood, DCR—damage control resuscitation.

References

1. Demetriades, D.; Murray, J.; Martin, M.; Velmahos, G.; Salim, A.; Alo, K.; Rhee, P. Pedestrians injured by automobiles: Relationship of age to injury type and severity. *J. Am. Coll. Surg.* **2004**, *199*, 382–387. [CrossRef]
2. Moore, F.A.; Nelson, T.; McKinley, B.A.; Moore, E.E.; Nathens, A.B.; Rhee, P.; Puyana, J.C.; Beilman, G.J.; Cohn, S.M.; StO$_2$ Study Group. Is there a role for aggressive use of fresh frozen plasma in massive transfusion of civilian trauma patients? *Am. J. Surg.* **2008**, *196*, 948–958; discussion 958–960. [CrossRef]
3. Cannon, J.W. Hemorrhagic Shock. *N. Engl. J. Med.* **2018**, *378*, 370–379. [CrossRef]
4. Tisherman, S.A.; Schmicker, R.H.; Brasel, K.J.; Bulger, E.M.; Kerby, J.D.; Minei, J.P.; Powell, J.L.; Reiff, D.A.; Rizoli, S.B.; Schreiber, M.A. Detailed description of all deaths in both the shock and traumatic brain injury hypertonic saline trials of the Resuscitation Outcomes Consortium. *Ann. Surg.* **2015**, *261*, 586–590. [CrossRef]
5. Hauser, C.J.; Boffard, K.; Dutton, R.; Bernard, G.R.; Croce, M.A.; Holcomb, J.B.; Leppaniemi, A.; Parr, M.; Vincent, J.L.; Tortella, B.J.; et al. Results of the CONTROL trial: Efficacy and safety of recombinant activated Factor VII in the management of refractory traumatic hemorrhage. *J. Trauma* **2010**, *69*, 489–500. [CrossRef]
6. Holcomb, J.B.; del Junco, D.J.; Fox, E.E.; Wade, C.E.; Cohen, M.J.; Schreiber, M.A.; Alarcon, L.H.; Bai, Y.; Brasel, K.J.; Bulger, E.M.; et al. The prospective, observational, multicenter, major trauma transfusion (PROMMTT) study: Comparative effectiveness of a time-varying treatment with competing risks. *JAMA Surg.* **2013**, *148*, 127–136. [CrossRef]
7. Fox, E.E.; Holcomb, J.B.; Wade, C.E.; Bulger, E.M.; Tilley, B.C.; Group, P.S. Earlier Endpoints are Required for Hemorrhagic Shock Trials Among Severely Injured Patients. *Shock* **2017**, *47*, 567–573. [CrossRef]
8. Mullins, R.J.; Trunkey, D.D. Samuel, D. Gross: Pioneer academic trauma surgeon of 19th century America. *J. Trauma* **1990**, *30*, 528–538. [CrossRef]
9. Maegele, M.; Lefering, R.; Yucel, N.; Tjardes, T.; Rixen, D.; Paffrath, T.; Simanski, C.; Neugebauer, E.; Bouillon, B.; AG Polytrauma of the German Trauma Society (DGU). Early coagulopathy in multiple injury: An analysis from the German Trauma Registry on 8724 patients. *Injury* **2007**, *38*, 298–304. [CrossRef]
10. MacLeod, J.B.; Lynn, M.; McKenney, M.G.; Cohn, S.M.; Murtha, M. Early coagulopathy predicts mortality in trauma. *J. Trauma* **2003**, *55*, 39–44. [CrossRef]
11. Niles, S.E.; McLaughlin, D.F.; Perkins, J.G.; Wade, C.E.; Li, Y.; Spinella, P.C.; Holcomb, J.B. Increased mortality associated with the early coagulopathy of trauma in combat casualties. *J. Trauma* **2008**, *64*, 1459–1463; discussion 1463–1465. [CrossRef]
12. Brohi, K.; Cohen, M.J.; Ganter, M.T.; Matthay, M.A.; Mackersie, R.C.; Pittet, J.F. Acute traumatic coagulopathy: Initiated by hypoperfusion: Modulated through the protein C pathway? *Ann. Surg.* **2007**, *245*, 812–818. [CrossRef]
13. Brohi, K.; Singh, J.; Heron, M.; Coats, T. Acute traumatic coagulopathy. *J. Trauma* **2003**, *54*, 1127–1130. [CrossRef]
14. Kutcher, M.E.; Howard, B.M.; Sperry, J.L.; Hubbard, A.E.; Decker, A.L.; Cuschieri, J.; Minei, J.P.; Moore, E.E.; Brownstein, B.H.; Maier, R.V.; et al. Evolving beyond the vicious triad: Differential mediation of traumatic coagulopathy by injury, shock, and resuscitation. *J. Trauma Acute Care Surg.* **2015**, *78*, 516–523. [CrossRef]
15. Ekeloef, N.P.; Eriksen, J.; Kancir, C.B. Evaluation of two methods to calculate p50 from a single blood sample. *Acta Anaesthesiol. Scand.* **2001**, *45*, 550–552. [CrossRef]
16. Srinivasan, A.J.; Morkane, C.; Martin, D.S.; Welsby, I.J. Should modulation of p50 be a therapeutic target in the critically ill? *Expert Rev. Hematol.* **2017**, *10*, 449–458. [CrossRef]
17. Leach, R.M.; Treacher, D.F. The pulmonary physician in critical care * 2: Oxygen delivery and consumption in the critically ill. *Thorax* **2002**, *57*, 170–177. [CrossRef]
18. Abdelsalam, M.; Cheifetz, I.M. Goal-directed therapy for severely hypoxic patients with acute respiratory distress syndrome: Permissive hypoxemia. *Respir. Care* **2010**, *55*, 1483–1490.
19. Mercado, P.; Maizel, J.; Beyls, C.; Titeca-Beauport, D.; Joris, M.; Kontar, L.; Riviere, A.; Bonef, O.; Soupison, T.; Tribouilloy, C.; et al. Transthoracic echocardiography: An accurate and precise method for estimating cardiac output in the critically ill patient. *Crit. Care* **2017**, *21*, 136. [CrossRef]
20. Jozwiak, M.; Monnet, X.; Teboul, J.L. Monitoring: From cardiac output monitoring to echocardiography. *Curr. Opin. Crit. Care* **2015**, *21*, 395–401. [CrossRef]
21. Cecconi, M.; De Backer, D.; Antonelli, M.; Beale, R.; Bakker, J.; Hofer, C.; Jaeschke, R.; Mebazaa, A.; Pinsky, M.R.; Teboul, J.L.; et al. Consensus on circulatory shock and hemodynamic monitoring. Task force of the European Society of Intensive Care Medicine. *Intensive Care Med.* **2014**, *40*, 1795–1815. [CrossRef]
22. Antonelli, M.; Levy, M.; Andrews, P.J.; Chastre, J.; Hudson, L.D.; Manthous, C.; Meduri, G.U.; Moreno, R.P.; Putensen, C.; Stewart, T.; et al. Hemodynamic monitoring in shock and implications for management. International Consensus Conference, Paris, France, 27–28 April 2006. *Intensive Care Med.* **2007**, *33*, 575–590. [CrossRef]
23. Narang, N.; Thibodeau, J.T.; Levine, B.D.; Gore, M.O.; Ayers, C.R.; Lange, R.A.; Cigarroa, J.E.; Turer, A.T.; de Lemos, J.A.; McGuire, D.K. Inaccuracy of estimated resting oxygen uptake in the clinical setting. *Circulation* **2014**, *129*, 203–210. [CrossRef]
24. Lubarsky, D.A.; Smith, L.R.; Sladen, R.N.; Mault, J.R.; Reed, R.L., 2nd. Defining the relationship of oxygen delivery and consumption: Use of biologic system models. *J. Surg. Res.* **1995**, *58*, 503–508. [CrossRef]
25. Kornblith, L.Z.; Moore, H.B.; Cohen, M.J. Trauma-induced coagulopathy: The past, present, and future. *J. Thromb. Haemost.* **2019**, *17*, 852–862. [CrossRef]

26. Gonzalez Rodriguez, E.; Ostrowski, S.R.; Cardenas, J.C.; Baer, L.A.; Tomasek, J.S.; Henriksen, H.H.; Stensballe, J.; Cotton, B.A.; Holcomb, J.B.; Johansson, P.I.; et al. Syndecan-1: A Quantitative Marker for the Endotheliopathy of Trauma. *J. Am. Coll. Surg.* **2017**, *225*, 419–427. [CrossRef]
27. Di Battista, A.P.; Rizoli, S.B.; Lejnieks, B.; Min, A.; Shiu, M.Y.; Peng, H.T.; Baker, A.J.; Hutchison, M.G.; Churchill, N.; Inaba, K.; et al. Sympathoadrenal Activation is Associated with Acute Traumatic Coagulopathy and Endotheliopathy in Isolated Brain Injury. *Shock* **2016**, *46*, 96–103. [CrossRef]
28. Johansson, P.; Stensballe, J.; Ostrowski, S. Shock induced endotheliopathy (SHINE) in acute critical illness—A unifying pathophysiologic mechanism. *Crit. Care* **2017**, *21*, 25. [CrossRef]
29. Ostrowski, S.R.; Henriksen, H.H.; Stensballe, J.; Gybel-Brask, M.; Cardenas, J.C.; Baer, L.A.; Cotton, B.A.; Holcomb, J.B.; Wade, C.E.; Johansson, P.I. Sympathoadrenal activation and endotheliopathy are drivers of hypocoagulability and hyperfibrinolysis in trauma: A prospective observational study of 404 severely injured patients. *J. Trauma Acute Care Surg.* **2017**, *82*, 293–301. [CrossRef]
30. Pati, S.; Potter, D.R.; Baimukanova, G.; Farrel, D.H.; Holcomb, J.B.; Schreiber, M.A. Modulating the endotheliopathy of trauma: Factor concentrate versus fresh frozen plasma. *J. Trauma Acute Care Surg.* **2016**, *80*, 576–584; discussion 584–585. [CrossRef]
31. Wu, F.; Chipman, A.; Pati, S.; Miyasawa, B.; Corash, L.; Kozar, R.A. Resuscitative Strategies to Modulate the Endotheliopathy of Trauma: From Cell to Patient. *Shock* **2020**, *53*, 575–584. [CrossRef]
32. Huber-Lang, M.; Lambris, J.D.; Ward, P.A. Innate immune responses to trauma. *Nat. Immunol.* **2018**, *19*, 327–341. [CrossRef]
33. Rahbar, E.; Cardenas, J.C.; Baimukanova, G.; Usadi, B.; Bruhn, R.; Pati, S.; Ostrowski, S.R.; Johansson, P.I.; Holcomb, J.B.; Wade, C.E. Endothelial glycocalyx shedding and vascular permeability in severely injured trauma patients. *J. Transl. Med.* **2015**, *13*, 117. [CrossRef]
34. Ostrowski, S.R.; Johansson, P.I. Endothelial glycocalyx degradation induces endogenous heparinization in patients with severe injury and early traumatic coagulopathy. *J. Trauma Acute Care Surg.* **2012**, *73*, 60–66. [CrossRef]
35. Schlimp, C.J.; Schochl, H. The role of fibrinogen in trauma-induced coagulopathy. *Hamostaseologie* **2014**, *34*, 29–39. [CrossRef]
36. Fries, D.; Martini, W.Z. Role of fibrinogen in trauma-induced coagulopathy. *Br. J. Anaesth.* **2010**, *105*, 116–121. [CrossRef]
37. Johansson, P.I.; Sorensen, A.M.; Perner, A.; Welling, K.L.; Wanscher, M.; Larsen, C.F.; Ostrowski, S.R. Disseminated intravascular coagulation or acute coagulopathy of trauma shock early after trauma? An observational study. *Crit. Care* **2011**, *15*, R272. [CrossRef]
38. Oshiro, A.; Yanagida, Y.; Gando, S.; Henzan, N.; Takahashi, I.; Makise, H. Hemostasis during the early stages of trauma: Comparison with disseminated intravascular coagulation. *Crit. Care* **2014**, *18*, R61. [CrossRef]
39. Spahn, D.R.; Bouillon, B.; Cerny, V.; Duranteau, J.; Filipescu, D.; Hunt, B.J.; Komadina, R.; Maegele, M.; Nardi, G.; Riddez, L.; et al. The European guideline on management of major bleeding and coagulopathy following trauma: Fifth edition. *Crit. Care* **2019**, *23*, 98. [CrossRef]
40. Lippi, G.; Carbucicchio, A.; Benatti, M.; Cervellin, G. The mean platelet volume is decreased in patients with mild head trauma and brain injury. *Blood Coagul. Fibrinolysis* **2013**, *24*, 780–783. [CrossRef]
41. Windelov, N.A.; Sorensen, A.M.; Perner, A.; Wanscher, M.; Larsen, C.F.; Ostrowski, S.R.; Johansson, P.I.; Rasmussen, L.S. Platelet aggregation following trauma: A prospective study. *Blood Coagul. Fibrinolysis* **2014**, *25*, 67–73. [CrossRef]
42. Wohlauer, M.V.; Moore, E.E.; Thomas, S.; Sauaia, A.; Evans, E.; Harr, J.; Silliman, C.C.; Ploplis, V.; Castellino, F.J.; Walsh, M. Early platelet dysfunction: An unrecognized role in the acute coagulopathy of trauma. *J. Am. Coll. Surg.* **2012**, *214*, 739–746. [CrossRef]
43. Sillesen, M.; Johansson, P.I.; Rasmussen, L.S.; Jin, G.; Jepsen, C.H.; Imam, A.M.; Hwabejire, J.; Lu, J.; Duggan, M.; Velmahos, G.; et al. Platelet activation and dysfunction in a large-animal model of traumatic brain injury and hemorrhage. *J. Trauma Acute Care Surg.* **2013**, *74*, 1252–1259. [CrossRef]
44. Solomon, C.; Traintinger, S.; Ziegler, B.; Hanke, A.; Rahe-Meyer, N.; Voelckel, W.; Schochl, H. Platelet function following trauma. A multiple electrode aggregometry study. *Thromb. Haemost.* **2011**, *106*, 322–330. [CrossRef]
45. Di Scipio, R.G.; Hermodson, M.A.; Yates, S.G.; Davie, E.W. A comparison of human prothrombin, factor IX (Christmas factor), factor X (Stuart factor), and protein S. *Biochemistry* **1977**, *16*, 698–706. [CrossRef]
46. Esmon, C.T.; Owen, W.G. The discovery of thrombomodulin. *J. Thromb. Haemost.* **2004**, *2*, 209–213. [CrossRef]
47. Fuentes-Prior, P.; Iwanaga, Y.; Huber, R.; Pagila, R.; Rumennik, G.; Seto, M.; Morser, J.; Light, D.R.; Bode, W. Structural basis for the anticoagulant activity of the thrombin-thrombomodulin complex. *Nature* **2000**, *404*, 518–525. [CrossRef]
48. Sillen, M.; Declerck, P.J. Thrombin Activatable Fibrinolysis Inhibitor (TAFI): An Updated Narrative Review. *Int. J. Mol. Sci.* **2021**, *22*, 3670. [CrossRef]
49. Nishimura, T.; Myles, T.; Piliponsky, A.M.; Kao, P.N.; Berry, G.J.; Leung, L.L. Thrombin-activatable procarboxypeptidase B regulates activated complement C5a in vivo. *Blood* **2007**, *109*, 1992–1997. [CrossRef]
50. Simurda, T.; Dobrotova, M.; Skornova, I.; Sokol, J.; Kubisz, P.; Stasko, J. Successful Use of a Highly Purified Plasma von Willebrand Factor Concentrate Containing Little FVIII for the Long-Term Prophylaxis of Severe (Type 3) von Willebrand's Disease. *Semin. Thromb. Hemost.* **2017**, *43*, 639–641. [CrossRef]
51. Bajaj, M.S.; Tricomi, S.M. Plasma levels of the three endothelial-specific proteins von Willebrand factor, tissue factor pathway inhibitor, and thrombomodulin do not predict the development of acute respiratory distress syndrome. *Intensive Care Med.* **1999**, *25*, 1259–1266. [CrossRef] [PubMed]

52. Zeineddin, A.; Dong, J.F.; Wu, F.; Terse, P.; Kozar, R.A. Role of Von Willebrand Factor after Injury: It May Do More Than We Think. *Shock* **2021**, *55*, 717–722. [CrossRef] [PubMed]
53. Kermode, J.C.; Zheng, Q.; Milner, E.P. Marked temperature dependence of the platelet calcium signal induced by human von Willebrand factor. *Blood* **1999**, *94*, 199–207. [CrossRef] [PubMed]
54. Casini, A.; de Moerloose, P.; Neerman-Arbez, M. Clinical Features and Management of Congenital Fibrinogen Deficiencies. *Semin. Thromb. Hemost.* **2016**, *42*, 366–374. [CrossRef] [PubMed]
55. Mengoli, C.; Franchini, M.; Marano, G.; Pupella, S.; Vaglio, S.; Marietta, M.; Liumbruno, G.M. The use of fibrinogen concentrate for the management of trauma-related bleeding: A systematic review and meta-analysis. *Blood Transfus.* **2017**, *15*, 318–324. [CrossRef] [PubMed]
56. Rourke, C.; Curry, N.; Khan, S.; Taylor, R.; Raza, I.; Davenport, R.; Stanworth, S.; Brohi, K. Fibrinogen levels during trauma hemorrhage, response to replacement therapy, and association with patient outcomes. *J. Thromb. Haemost.* **2012**, *10*, 1342–1351. [CrossRef]
57. Schochl, H.; Frietsch, T.; Pavelka, M.; Jambor, C. Hyperfibrinolysis after major trauma: Differential diagnosis of lysis patterns and prognostic value of thrombelastometry. *J. Trauma* **2009**, *67*, 125–131. [CrossRef]
58. Schlimp, C.J.; Voelckel, W.; Inaba, K.; Maegele, M.; Ponschab, M.; Schochl, H. Estimation of plasma fibrinogen levels based on hemoglobin, base excess and Injury Severity Score upon emergency room admission. *Crit. Care* **2013**, *17*, R137. [CrossRef]
59. Hagemo, J.S.; Stanworth, S.; Juffermans, N.P.; Brohi, K.; Cohen, M.; Johansson, P.I.; Roislien, J.; Eken, T.; Naess, P.A.; Gaarder, C. Prevalence, predictors and outcome of hypofibrinogenaemia in trauma: A multicentre observational study. *Crit. Care* **2014**, *18*, R52. [CrossRef] [PubMed]
60. Foldesi, M.; Merkei, Z.; Ferenci, T.; Nardai, G. Fibrinogen level at hospital admission after multiple injury correlates with BMI and is negatively associated with the need for transfusion and early multiple organ failure. *Injury* **2021**, *52* (Suppl. 1), S15–S20. [CrossRef]
61. Agren, A.; Wikman, A.T.; Ostlund, A.; Edgren, G. TEG(R) Functional Fibrinogen Analysis May Overestimate Fibrinogen Levels. *Anesth. Analg.* **2014**, *118*, 933–935. [CrossRef]
62. Castellano, G.; Woltman, A.M.; Nauta, A.J.; Roos, A.; Trouw, L.A.; Seelen, M.A.; Schena, F.P.; Daha, M.R.; van Kooten, C. Maturation of dendritic cells abrogates C1q production in vivo and in vitro. *Blood* **2004**, *103*, 3813–3820. [CrossRef]
63. Davis, P.K.; Musunuru, H.; Walsh, M.; Cassady, R.; Yount, R.; Losiniecki, A.; Moore, E.E.; Wohlauer, M.V.; Howard, J.; Ploplis, V.A.; et al. Platelet dysfunction is an early marker for traumatic brain injury-induced coagulopathy. *Neurocrit. Care* **2013**, *18*, 201–208. [CrossRef]
64. Chapin, J.C.; Hajjar, K.A. Fibrinolysis and the control of blood coagulation. *Blood Rev.* **2015**, *29*, 17–24. [CrossRef]
65. Moore, H.B.; Moore, E.E.; Gonzalez, E.; Chapman, M.P.; Chin, T.L.; Silliman, C.C.; Banerjee, A.; Sauaia, A. Hyperfibrinolysis, physiologic fibrinolysis, and fibrinolysis shutdown: The spectrum of postinjury fibrinolysis and relevance to antifibrinolytic therapy. *J. Trauma Acute Care Surg.* **2014**, *77*, 811–817; discussion 817. [CrossRef] [PubMed]
66. Moore, H.B.; Moore, E.E.; Lawson, P.J.; Gonzalez, E.; Fragoso, M.; Morton, A.P.; Gamboni, F.; Chapman, M.P.; Sauaia, A.; Banerjee, A.; et al. Fibrinolysis shutdown phenotype masks changes in rodent coagulation in tissue injury versus hemorrhagic shock. *Surgery* **2015**, *158*, 386–392. [CrossRef] [PubMed]
67. Liras, I.N.; Cotton, B.A.; Cardenas, J.C.; Harting, M.T. Prevalence and impact of admission hyperfibrinolysis in severely injured pediatric trauma patients. *Surgery* **2015**, *158*, 812–818. [CrossRef] [PubMed]
68. Cotton, B.A.; Harvin, J.A.; Kostousouv, V.; Minei, K.M.; Radwan, Z.A.; Schochl, H.; Wade, C.E.; Holcomb, J.B.; Matijevic, N. Hyperfibrinolysis at admission is an uncommon but highly lethal event associated with shock and prehospital fluid administration. *J. Trauma Acute Care Surg.* **2012**, *73*, 365–370. [CrossRef] [PubMed]
69. Blackbourne, L.H.; Baer, D.G.; Cestero, R.F.; Inaba, K.; Rasmussen, T.E. Exsanguination shock: The next frontier in prevention of battlefield mortality. *J. Trauma* **2011**, *71*, S1–S3. [CrossRef] [PubMed]
70. Brohi, K.; Cohen, M.J.; Ganter, M.T.; Schultz, M.J.; Levi, M.; Mackersie, R.C.; Pittet, J.F. Acute coagulopathy of trauma: Hypoperfusion induces systemic anticoagulation and hyperfibrinolysis. *J. Trauma* **2008**, *64*, 1211–1217. [CrossRef]
71. Morton, A.P.; Moore, E.E.; Wohlauer, M.V.; Lo, K.; Silliman, C.C.; Burlew, C.C.; Banerjee, A. Revisiting early postinjury mortality: Are they bleeding because they are dying or dying because they are bleeding? *J. Surg. Res.* **2013**, *179*, 5–9. [CrossRef]
72. Schochl, H.; Cadamuro, J.; Seidl, S.; Franz, A.; Solomon, C.; Schlimp, C.J.; Ziegler, B. Hyperfibrinolysis is common in out-of-hospital cardiac arrest: Results from a prospective observational thromboelastometry study. *Resuscitation* **2013**, *84*, 454–459. [CrossRef]
73. Chapman, M.P.; Moore, E.E.; Moore, H.B.; Gonzalez, E.; Gamboni, F.; Chandler, J.G.; Mitra, S.; Ghasabyan, A.; Chin, T.L.; Sauaia, A.; et al. Overwhelming tPA release, not PAI-1 degradation, is responsible for hyperfibrinolysis in severely injured trauma patients. *J. Trauma Acute Care Surg.* **2016**, *80*, 16. [CrossRef]
74. Brohi, K.; Cohen, M.J.; Davenport, R.A. Acute coagulopathy of trauma: Mechanism, identification and effect. *Curr. Opin. Crit. Care* **2007**, *13*, 680–685. [CrossRef]
75. Madurska, M.J.; Sachse, K.A.; Jansen, J.O.; Rasmussen, T.E.; Morrison, J.J. Fibrinolysis in trauma: A review. *Eur. J. Trauma Emerg. Surg.* **2018**, *44*, 35–44. [CrossRef]

76. Meizoso, J.P.; Dudaryk, R.; Mulder, M.B.; Ray, J.J.; Karcutskie, C.A.; Eidelson, S.A.; Namias, N.; Schulman, C.I.; Proctor, K.G. Increased risk of fibrinolysis shutdown among severely injured trauma patients receiving tranexamic acid. *J. Trauma Acute Care Surg.* **2018**, *84*, 426–432. [CrossRef]
77. Moore, H.B.; Moore, E.E.; Neal, M.D.; Sheppard, F.R.; Kornblith, L.Z.; Draxler, D.F.; Walsh, M.; Medcalf, R.L.; Cohen, M.J.; Cotton, B.A.; et al. Fibrinolysis Shutdown in Trauma: Historical Review and Clinical Implications. *Anesth. Analg.* **2019**, *129*, 762–773. [CrossRef]
78. Gando, S. Microvascular thrombosis and multiple organ dysfunction syndrome. *Crit. Care Med.* **2010**, *38*, S35–S42. [CrossRef]
79. Pfeiler, S.; Massberg, S.; Engelmann, B. Biological basis and pathological relevance of microvascular thrombosis. *Thromb. Res.* **2014**, *133* (Suppl. 1), S35–S37. [CrossRef]
80. Tsikouris, J.P.; Suarez, J.A.; Meyerrose, G.E. Plasminogen activator inhibitor-1: Physiologic role, regulation, and the influence of common pharmacologic agents. *J. Clin. Pharmacol.* **2002**, *42*, 1187–1199. [CrossRef]
81. Carroll, S.L.; Dye, D.W.; Smedley, W.A.; Stephens, S.W.; Reiff, D.A.; Kerby, J.D.; Holcomb, J.B.; Jansen, J.O. Early and prehospital trauma deaths: Who might benefit from advanced resuscitative care? *J. Trauma Acute Care Surg.* **2020**, *88*, 776–782. [CrossRef]
82. Geeraedts, L.M., Jr.; Kaasjager, H.A.; van Vugt, A.B.; Frolke, J.P. Exsanguination in trauma: A review of diagnostics and treatment options. *Injury* **2009**, *40*, 11–20. [CrossRef]
83. Clarke, J.R.; Trooskin, S.Z.; Doshi, P.J.; Greenwald, L.; Mode, C.J. Time to laparotomy for intra-abdominal bleeding from trauma does affect survival for delays up to 90 minutes. *J. Trauma* **2002**, *52*, 420–425. [CrossRef] [PubMed]
84. Berkeveld, E.; Popal, Z.; Schober, P.; Zuidema, W.P.; Bloemers, F.W.; Giannakopoulos, G.F. Prehospital time and mortality in polytrauma patients: A retrospective analysis. *BMC Emerg. Med.* **2021**, *21*, 78. [CrossRef] [PubMed]
85. Elkbuli, A.; Dowd, B.; Sanchez, C.; Shaikh, S.; Sutherland, M.; McKenney, M. Emergency Medical Service Transport Time and Trauma Outcomes at an Urban Level 1 Trauma Center: Evaluation of Prehospital Emergency Medical Service Response. *Am. Surg.* **2021**, 3134820988827. [CrossRef]
86. Chen, X.; Gestring, M.L.; Rosengart, M.R.; Billiar, T.R.; Peitzman, A.B.; Sperry, J.L.; Brown, J.B. Speed is not everything: Identifying patients who may benefit from helicopter transport despite faster ground transport. *J. Trauma Acute Care Surg.* **2018**, *84*, 549–557. [CrossRef]
87. Choi, J.; Carlos, G.; Nassar, A.K.; Knowlton, L.M.; Spain, D.A. The impact of trauma systems on patient outcomes. *Curr. Probl. Surg.* **2021**, *58*, 100840. [CrossRef]
88. Schroder, H.; Beckers, S.K.; Ogrodzki, K.; Borgs, C.; Ziemann, S.; Follmann, A.; Rossaint, R.; Felzen, M. Tele-EMS physicians improve life-threatening conditions during prehospital emergency missions. *Sci. Rep.* **2021**, *11*, 14366. [CrossRef]
89. Zhu, C.S.; Cobb, D.; Jonas, R.B.; Pokorny, D.; Rani, M.; Cotner-Pouncy, T.; Oliver, J.; Cap, A.; Cestero, R.; Nicholson, S.E.; et al. Shock index and pulse pressure as triggers for massive transfusion. *J. Trauma Acute Care Surg.* **2019**, *87*, S159–S164. [CrossRef]
90. Sperry, J.L.; Guyette, F.X.; Brown, J.B.; Yazer, M.H.; Triulzi, D.J.; Early-Young, B.J.; Adams, P.W.; Daley, B.J.; Miller, R.S.; Harbrecht, B.G.; et al. Prehospital Plasma during Air Medical Transport in Trauma Patients at Risk for Hemorrhagic Shock. *N. Engl. J. Med.* **2018**, *379*, 315–326. [CrossRef]
91. Pusateri, A.E.; Moore, E.E.; Moore, H.B.; Le, T.D.; Guyette, F.X.; Chapman, M.P.; Sauaia, A.; Ghasabyan, A.; Chandler, J.; McVaney, K.; et al. Association of Prehospital Plasma Transfusion With Survival in Trauma Patients With Hemorrhagic Shock When Transport Times Are Longer Than 20 Minutes: A Post Hoc Analysis of the PAMPer and COMBAT Clinical Trials. *JAMA Surg.* **2020**, *155*, e195085. [CrossRef]
92. Braverman, M.A.; Smith, A.; Pokorny, D.; Axtman, B.; Shahan, C.P.; Barry, L.; Corral, H.; Jonas, R.B.; Shiels, M.; Schaefer, R.; et al. Prehospital whole blood reduces early mortality in patients with hemorrhagic shock. *Transfusion* **2021**, *61* (Suppl. 1), S15–S21. [CrossRef] [PubMed]
93. Shakur, H.; Roberts, I.; Bautista, R.; Caballero, J.; Coats, T.; Dewan, Y.; El-Sayed, H.; Gogichaishvili, T.; Gupta, S.; Herrera, J.; et al. Effects of tranexamic acid on death, vascular occlusive events, and blood transfusion in trauma patients with significant haemorrhage (CRASH-2): A randomised, placebo-controlled trial. *Lancet* **2010**, *376*, 23–32. [CrossRef] [PubMed]
94. Napolitano, L.M.; Cohen, M.J.; Cotton, B.A.; Schreiber, M.A.; Moore, E.E. Tranexamic acid in trauma: How should we use it? *J. Trauma Acute Care Surg.* **2013**, *74*, 1575–1586. [CrossRef] [PubMed]
95. Binz, S.; McCollester, J.; Thomas, S.; Miller, J.; Pohlman, T.; Waxman, D.; Shariff, F.; Tracy, R.; Walsh, M. CRASH-2 Study of Tranexamic Acid to Treat Bleeding in Trauma Patients: A Controversy Fueled by Science and Social Media. *J. Blood Transfus.* **2015**, *2015*, 874920. [CrossRef]
96. Imach, S.; Wafaisade, A.; Lefering, R.; Bohmer, A.; Schieren, M.; Suarez, V.; Frohlich, M.; TraumaRegister, D.G.U. The impact of prehospital tranexamic acid on mortality and transfusion requirements: Match-pair analysis from the nationwide German TraumaRegister DGU(R). *Crit. Care* **2021**, *25*, 277. [CrossRef]
97. Wafaisade, A.; Lefering, R.; Bouillon, B.; Bohmer, A.B.; Gassler, M.; Ruppert, M.; TraumaRegister, D.G.U. Prehospital administration of tranexamic acid in trauma patients. *Crit. Care* **2016**, *20*, 143. [CrossRef]
98. Moore, H.B.; Moore, E.E.; Huebner, B.R.; Stettler, G.R.; Nunns, G.R.; Einersen, P.M.; Silliman, C.C.; Sauaia, A. Tranexamic acid is associated with increased mortality in patients with physiological fibrinolysis. *J. Surg. Res.* **2017**, *220*, 438–443. [CrossRef]
99. Diebel, M.E.; Martin, J.V.; Liberati, D.M.; Diebel, L.N. The temporal response and mechanism of action of tranexamic acid in endothelial glycocalyx degradation. *J. Trauma Acute Care Surg.* **2018**, *84*, 75–80. [CrossRef]

100. Duque, P.; Gonzalez-Zarco, L.; Martinez, R.; Gago, S.; Varela, J.A. Tranexamic acid use in severely injured patients, is it always appropriate? *Rev. Esp. Anestesiol. Reanim. (Engl. Ed.)* **2021**, *68*, 301–303. [CrossRef]
101. Jenkins, D.H.; Rappold, J.F.; Badloe, J.F.; Berseus, O.; Blackbourne, L.; Brohi, K.H.; Butler, F.K.; Cap, A.P.; Cohen, M.J.; Davenport, R.; et al. Trauma hemostasis and oxygenation research position paper on remote damage control resuscitation: Definitions, current practice, and knowledge gaps. *Shock* **2014**, *41* (Suppl. 1), 3–12. [CrossRef]
102. Kheirbek, T.; Martin, T.J.; Cao, J.; Hall, B.M.; Lueckel, S.; Adams, C.A. Prehospital shock index outperforms hypotension alone in predicting significant injury in trauma patients. *Trauma Surg. Acute Care Open* **2021**, *6*, e000712. [CrossRef]
103. Schroll, R.; Swift, D.; Tatum, D.; Couch, S.; Heaney, J.B.; Llado-Farrulla, M.; Zucker, S.; Gill, F.; Brown, G.; Buffin, N.; et al. Accuracy of shock index versus ABC score to predict need for massive transfusion in trauma patients. *Injury* **2018**, *49*, 15–19. [CrossRef]
104. Liu, Y.C.; Liu, J.H.; Fang, Z.A.; Shan, G.L.; Xu, J.; Qi, Z.W.; Zhu, H.D.; Wang, Z.; Yu, X.Z. Modified shock index and mortality rate of emergency patients. *World J. Emerg. Med.* **2012**, *3*, 114–117. [CrossRef]
105. Campbell, R.; Ardagh, M.W.; Than, M. Validation of the pulse rate over pressure evaluation index as a detector of early occult hemorrhage: A prospective observational study. *J. Trauma Acute Care Surg.* **2012**, *73*, 286–288. [CrossRef] [PubMed]
106. Savage, S.A.; Sumislawski, J.J.; Zarzaur, B.L.; Dutton, W.P.; Croce, M.A.; Fabian, T.C. The new metric to define large-volume hemorrhage: Results of a prospective study of the critical administration threshold. *J. Trauma Acute Care Surg.* **2015**, *78*, 224–229; discussion 229–230. [CrossRef] [PubMed]
107. Shih, A.W.; Al Khan, S.; Wang, A.Y.; Dawe, P.; Young, P.Y.; Greene, A.; Hudoba, M.; Vu, E. Systematic reviews of scores and predictors to trigger activation of massive transfusion protocols. *J. Trauma Acute Care Surg.* **2019**, *87*, 717–729. [CrossRef] [PubMed]
108. Hu, P.; Uhlich, R.; Black, J.; Jansen, J.O.; Kerby, J.; Holcomb, J.B. A new definition for massive transfusion in the modern era of whole blood resuscitation. *Transfusion* **2021**, *61* (Suppl. 1), S252–S263. [CrossRef] [PubMed]
109. Arakaki, L.S.L.; Bulger, E.M.; Ciesielski, W.A.; Carlbom, D.J.; Fisk, D.M.; Sheehan, K.L.; Asplund, K.M.; Schenkman, K.A. Muscle Oxygenation as an Early Predictor of Shock Severity in Trauma Patients. *Shock* **2017**, *47*, 599–605. [CrossRef] [PubMed]
110. Schenkman, K.A.; Carlbom, D.J.; Bulger, E.M.; Ciesielski, W.A.; Fisk, D.M.; Sheehan, K.L.; Asplund, K.M.; Shaver, J.M.; Arakaki, L.S.L. Muscle oxygenation as an indicator of shock severity in patients with suspected severe sepsis or septic shock. *PLoS ONE* **2017**, *12*, e0182351. [CrossRef] [PubMed]
111. Schenkman, K.A.; Hawkins, D.S.; Ciesielski, W.A.; Delaney, M.; Arakaki, L.S. Non-invasive assessment of muscle oxygenation may aid in optimising transfusion threshold decisions in ambulatory paediatric patients. *Transfus. Med.* **2017**, *27*, 25–29. [CrossRef]
112. Arakaki, L.S.; Schenkman, K.A.; Ciesielski, W.A.; Shaver, J.M. Muscle oxygenation measurement in humans by noninvasive optical spectroscopy and Locally Weighted Regression. *Anal. Chim. Acta* **2013**, *785*, 27–33. [CrossRef] [PubMed]
113. Moore, E.E.; Moore, H.B.; Kornblith, L.Z.; Neal, M.D.; Hoffman, M.; Mutch, N.J.; Schochl, H.; Hunt, B.J.; Sauaia, A. Trauma-induced coagulopathy. *Nat. Rev. Dis. Prim.* **2021**, *7*, 30. [CrossRef] [PubMed]
114. Holcomb, J.B.; Jenkins, D.; Rhee, P.; Johannigman, J.; Mahoney, P.; Mehta, S.; Cox, E.D.; Gehrke, M.J.; Beilman, G.J.; Schreiber, M.; et al. Damage control resuscitation: Directly addressing the early coagulopathy of trauma. *J. Trauma* **2007**, *62*, 307–310. [CrossRef]
115. Van, P.Y.; Holcomb, J.B.; Schreiber, M.A. Novel concep.pts for damage control resuscitation in trauma. *Curr. Opin. Crit. Care* **2017**, *23*, 498–502. [CrossRef]
116. Moore, F.D. Should blood be whole or in parts? *N. Engl. J. Med.* **1969**, *280*, 327–328. [CrossRef]
117. Yazer, M.H.; Spinella, P.C.; Anto, V.; Dunbar, N.M. Survey of group A plasma and low-titer group O whole blood use in trauma resuscitation at adult civilian level 1 trauma centers in the US. *Transfusion* **2021**, *61*, 1757–1763. [CrossRef] [PubMed]
118. Troughton, M.; Young, P.P. Conservation of Rh negative Low Titer O Whole Blood (LTOWB) and the need for a national conversation to define its use in trauma transfusion protocols. *Transfusion* **2021**, *61*, 1966–1971. [CrossRef] [PubMed]
119. Malkin, M.; Nevo, A.; Brundage, S.I.; Schreiber, M. Effectiveness and safety of whole blood compared to balanced blood components in resuscitation of hemorrhaging trauma patients—A systematic review. *Injury* **2021**, *52*, 182–188. [CrossRef] [PubMed]
120. Shea, S.M.; Staudt, A.M.; Thomas, K.A.; Schuerer, D.; Mielke, J.E.; Folkerts, D.; Lowder, E.; Martin, C.; Bochicchio, G.V.; Spinella, P.C. The use of low-titer group O whole blood is independently associated with improved survival compared to component therapy in adults with severe traumatic hemorrhage. *Transfusion* **2020**, *60* (Suppl. 3), S2–S9. [CrossRef]
121. Clements, T.; McCoy, C.; Assen, S.; Cardenas, J.; Wade, C.; Meyer, D.; Cotton, B.A. The prehospital use of younger age whole blood is associated with an improved arrival coagulation profile. *J. Trauma Acute Care Surg.* **2021**, *90*, 607–614. [CrossRef]
122. Fadeyi, E.A.; Saha, A.K.; Naal, T.; Martin, H.; Fenu, E.; Simmons, J.H.; Jones, M.R.; Pomper, G.J. A comparison between leukocyte reduced low titer whole blood vs non-leukocyte reduced low titer whole blood for massive transfusion activation. *Transfusion* **2020**, *60*, 2834–2840. [CrossRef] [PubMed]
123. Salamea-Molina, J.C.; Himmler, A.N.; Valencia-Angel, L.I.; Ordonez, C.A.; Parra, M.W.; Caicedo, Y.; Guzman-Rodriguez, M.; Orlas, C.; Granados, M.; Macia, C.; et al. Whole blood for blood loss: Hemostatic resuscitation in damage control. *Colomb. Med. (Cali)* **2020**, *51*, e4044511. [CrossRef]
124. Yazer, M.H.; Triulzi, D.J.; Sperry, J.L.; Seheult, J.N. Rate of RhD-alloimmunization after the transfusion of multiple RhD-positive primary red blood cell-containing products. *Transfusion* **2021**, *61* (Suppl. 1), S150–S158. [CrossRef]

125. Shackelford, S.A.; Gurney, J.M.; Taylor, A.L.; Keenan, S.; Corley, J.B.; Cunningham, C.W.; Drew, B.G.; Jensen, S.D.; Kotwal, R.S.; Montgomery, H.R.; et al. Joint Trauma System, Defense Committee on Trauma, and Armed Services Blood Program consensus statement on whole blood. *Transfusion* **2021**, *61* (Suppl. 1), S333–S335. [CrossRef]
126. Williams, J.; Merutka, N.; Meyer, D.; Bai, Y.; Prater, S.; Cabrera, R.; Holcomb, J.B.; Wade, C.E.; Love, J.D.; Cotton, B.A. Safety profile and impact of low-titer group O whole blood for emergency use in trauma. *J. Trauma Acute Care Surg.* **2020**, *88*, 87–93. [CrossRef]
127. Yazer, M.H.; Freeman, A.; Harrold, I.M.; Anto, V.; Neal, M.D.; Triulzi, D.J.; Sperry, J.L.; Seheult, J.N. Injured recipients of low-titer group O whole blood have similar clinical outcomes compared to recipients of conventional component therapy: A single-center, retrospective study. *Transfusion* **2021**, *61*, 1710–1720. [CrossRef]
128. Seheult, J.N.; Anto, V.; Alarcon, L.H.; Sperry, J.L.; Triulzi, D.J.; Yazer, M.H. Clinical outcomes among low-titer group O whole blood recipients compared to recipients of conventional components in civilian trauma resuscitation. *Transfusion* **2018**, *58*, 1838–1845. [CrossRef] [PubMed]
129. Cruciani, M.; Franchini, M.; Mengoli, C.; Marano, G.; Pati, I.; Masiello, F.; Veropalumbo, E.; Pupella, S.; Vaglio, S.; Agostini, V.; et al. The use of whole blood in traumatic bleeding: A systematic review. *Intern. Emerg. Med.* **2021**, *16*, 209–220. [CrossRef]
130. Holcomb, J.B.; Tilley, B.C.; Baraniuk, S.; Fox, E.E.; Wade, C.E.; Podbielski, J.M.; del Junco, D.J.; Brasel, K.J.; Bulger, E.M.; Callcut, R.A.; et al. Transfusion of plasma, platelets, and red blood cells in a 1:1:1 vs. a 1:1:2 ratio and mortality in patients with severe trauma: The PROPPR randomized clinical trial. *JAMA* **2015**, *313*, 471–482. [CrossRef] [PubMed]
131. Kemp Bohan, P.M.; McCarthy, P.M.; Wall, M.E.; Adams, A.M.; Chick, R.C.; Forcum, J.E.; Radowsky, J.S.; How, R.A.; Sams, V.G. Safety and efficacy of low-titer O whole blood resuscitation in a civilian level I trauma center. *J. Trauma Acute Care Surg.* **2021**, *91*, S162–S168. [CrossRef]
132. Levy, J.H.; Neal, M.D.; Herman, J.H. Bacterial contamination of platelets for transfusion: Strategies for prevention. *Crit. Care* **2018**, *22*, 271. [CrossRef] [PubMed]
133. Devine, D.V.; Serrano, K. The platelet storage lesion. *Clin. Lab. Med.* **2010**, *30*, 475–487. [CrossRef] [PubMed]
134. Becker, G.A.; Tuccelli, M.; Kunicki, T.; Chalos, M.K.; Aster, R.H. Studies of platelet concentrates stored at 22 C nad 4 C. *Transfusion* **1973**, *13*, 61–68. [CrossRef] [PubMed]
135. Reddoch, K.M.; Pidcoke, H.F.; Montgomery, R.K.; Fedyk, C.G.; Aden, J.K.; Ramasubramanian, A.K.; Cap, A.P. Hemostatic function of apheresis platelets stored at 4 °C and 22 °C. *Shock* **2014**, *41* (Suppl. 1), 54–61. [CrossRef]
136. Murphy, S.; Gardner, F.H. Effect of storage temperature on maintenance of platelet viability–deleterious effect of refrigerated storage. *N. Engl. J. Med.* **1969**, *280*, 1094–1098. [CrossRef]
137. Milford, E.M.; Reade, M.C. Comprehensive review of platelet storage methods for use in the treatment of active hemorrhage. *Transfusion* **2016**, *56* (Suppl. 2), S140–S148. [CrossRef]
138. Pidcoke, H.F.; Spinella, P.C.; Ramasubramanian, A.K.; Strandenes, G.; Hervig, T.; Ness, P.M.; Cap, A.P. Refrigerated platelets for the treatment of acute bleeding: A review of the literature and reexamination of current standards. *Shock* **2014**, *41* (Suppl. 1), 51–53. [CrossRef]
139. Li, Y.; Xiong, Y.; Wang, R.; Tang, F.; Wang, X. Blood banking-induced alteration of red blood cell oxygen release ability. *Blood Transfus.* **2016**, *14*, 238–244. [CrossRef]
140. Tinmouth, A.; Fergusson, D.; Yee, I.C.; Hebert, P.C.; ABLE Investigators and the Canadian Critical Care Trials Group. Clinical consequences of red cell storage in the critically ill. *Transfusion* **2006**, *46*, 2014–2027. [CrossRef]
141. Fabron, A., Jr.; Lopes, L.B.; Bordin, J.O. Transfusion-related acute lung injury. *J. Bras. Pneumol.* **2007**, *33*, 206–212. [CrossRef]
142. Sparrow, R.L. Red blood cell storage duration and trauma. *Transfus Med. Rev.* **2015**, *29*, 120–126. [CrossRef]
143. Stan, A.; Zsigmond, E. The restoration in vivo of 2,3-diphosphoglycerate (2,3-DPG) in stored red cells, after transfusion. The levels of red cells 2,3-DPG. *Rom. J. Intern. Med.* **2009**, *47*, 173–177.
144. Sowers, N.; Froese, P.C.; Erdogan, M.; Green, R.S. Impact of the age of stored blood on trauma patient mortality: A systematic review. *Can. J. Surg.* **2015**, *58*, 335–342. [CrossRef]
145. Jones, A.R.; Patel, R.P.; Marques, M.B.; Donnelly, J.P.; Griffin, R.L.; Pittet, J.F.; Kerby, J.D.; Stephens, S.W.; DeSantis, S.M.; Hess, J.R.; et al. Older Blood Is Associated With Increased Mortality and Adverse Events in Massively Transfused Trauma Patients: Secondary Analysis of the PROPPR Trial. *Ann. Emerg. Med.* **2019**, *73*, 650–661. [CrossRef]
146. Remy, K.E.; Sun, J.; Wang, D.; Welsh, J.; Solomon, S.B.; Klein, H.G.; Natanson, C.; Cortes-Puch, I. Transfusion of recently donated (fresh) red blood cells (RBCs) does not improve survival in comparison with current practice, while safety of the oldest stored units is yet to be established: A meta-analysis. *Vox Sang.* **2016**, *111*, 43–54. [CrossRef]
147. Milford, E.M.; Reade, M.C. Resuscitation Fluid Choices to Preserve the Endothelial Glycocalyx. *Crit. Care* **2019**, *23*, 77. [CrossRef] [PubMed]
148. Cardigan, R.; Green, L. Thawed and liquid plasma–what do we know? *Vox Sang.* **2015**, *109*, 1–10. [CrossRef] [PubMed]
149. Sheffield, W.P.; Bhakta, V.; Mastronardi, C.; Ramirez-Arcos, S.; Howe, D.; Jenkins, C. Changes in coagulation factor activity and content of di(2-ethylhexyl)phthalate in frozen plasma units during refrigerated storage for up to five days after thawing. *Transfusion* **2012**, *52*, 493–502. [CrossRef] [PubMed]
150. Alhumaidan, H.; Cheves, T.; Holme, S.; Sweeney, J. Stability of coagulation factors in plasma prepared after a 24-hour room temperature hold. *Transfusion* **2010**, *50*, 1934–1942. [CrossRef]

151. Chhibber, V.; Greene, M.; Vauthrin, M.; Bailey, J.; Weinstein, R. Is group A thawed plasma suitable as the first option for emergency release transfusion? (CME). *Transfusion* **2014**, *54*, 1751–1755. [CrossRef] [PubMed]
152. Cooling, L. Going from A to B: The safety of incompatible group A plasma for emergency release in trauma and massive transfusion patients. *Transfusion* **2014**, *54*, 1695–1697. [CrossRef] [PubMed]
153. Mehr, C.R.; Gupta, R.; von Recklinghausen, F.M.; Szczepiorkowski, Z.M.; Dunbar, N.M. Balancing risk and benefit: Maintenance of a thawed Group A plasma inventory for trauma patients requiring massive transfusion. *J. Trauma Acute Care Surg* **2013**, *74*, 1425–1431. [CrossRef]
154. Meledeo, M.A.; Peltier, G.C.; McIntosh, C.S.; Bynum, J.A.; Corley, J.B.; Cap, A.P. Coagulation function of never frozen liquid plasma stored for 40 days. *Transfusion* **2021**, *61* (Suppl. 1), S111–S118. [CrossRef] [PubMed]
155. Mok, G.; Hoang, R.; Khan, M.W.; Pannell, D.; Peng, H.; Tien, H.; Nathens, A.; Callum, J.; Karkouti, K.; Beckett, A.; et al. Freeze-dried plasma for major trauma—Systematic review and meta-analysis. *J. Trauma Acute Care Surg.* **2021**, *90*, 589–602. [CrossRef]
156. Pusateri, A.E.; Given, M.B.; Schreiber, M.A.; Spinella, P.C.; Pati, S.; Kozar, R.A.; Khan, A.; Dacorta, J.A.; Kupferer, K.R.; Prat, N.; et al. Dried plasma: State of the science and recent developments. *Transfusion* **2016**, *56* (Suppl. 2), S128–S139. [CrossRef]
157. Sailliol, A.; Martinaud, C.; Cap, A.P.; Civadier, C.; Clavier, B.; Deshayes, A.V.; Mendes, A.C.; Pouget, T.; Demazeau, N.; Chueca, M.; et al. The evolving role of lyophilized plasma in remote damage control resuscitation in the French Armed Forces Health Service. *Transfusion* **2013**, *53* (Suppl. 1), 65S–71S. [CrossRef]
158. Shlaifer, A.; Siman-Tov, M.; Radomislensky, I.; Peleg, K.; Shina, A.; Baruch, E.N.; Glassberg, E.; Yitzhak, A.; ITG*. Prehospital administration of freeze-dried plasma, is it the solution for trauma casualties? *J. Trauma Acute Care Surg.* **2017**, *83*, 675–682. [CrossRef]
159. Winearls, J.; Campbell, D.; Hurn, C.; Furyk, J.; Ryan, G.; Trout, M.; Walsham, J.; Holley, A.; Shuttleworth, M.; Dyer, W.; et al. Fibrinogen in traumatic haemorrhage: A narrative review. *Injury* **2017**, *48*, 230–242. [CrossRef]
160. Winearls, J.; Wullschleger, M.; Wake, E.; Hurn, C.; Furyk, J.; Ryan, G.; Trout, M.; Walsham, J.; Holley, A.; Cohen, J.; et al. Fibrinogen Early In Severe Trauma studY (FEISTY): Study protocol for a randomised controlled trial. *Trials* **2017**, *18*, 241. [CrossRef]
161. Hayes, T. Dysfibrinogenemia and Thrombosis. *Arch. Pathol. Lab. Med.* **2002**, *126*, 1387–1390. [CrossRef]
162. Meyer, M.A.; Ostrowski, S.R.; Sorensen, A.M.; Meyer, A.S.; Holcomb, J.B.; Wade, C.E.; Johansson, P.I.; Stensballe, J. Fibrinogen in trauma, an evaluation of thrombelastography and rotational thromboelastometry fibrinogen assays. *J. Surg. Res.* **2015**, *194*, 581–590. [CrossRef]
163. Holcomb, J.B.; Fox, E.E.; Zhang, X.; White, N.; Wade, C.E.; Cotton, B.A.; Del Junco, D.J.; Bulger, E.M.; Cohen, M.J.; Schreiber, M.A.; et al. Cryoprecipitate Use in the Prospective Observational Multicenter Major Trauma Transfusion study (PROMMTT). *J. Trauma Acute Care Surg.* **2013**, *75*, S31–S39. [CrossRef]
164. Barry, M.; Trivedi, A.; Miyazawa, B.Y.; Vivona, L.R.; Khakoo, M.; Zhang, H.; Pathipati, P.; Bagri, A.; Gatmaitan, M.G.; Kozar, R.; et al. Cryoprecipitate attenuates the endotheliopathy of trauma in mice subjected to hemorrhagic shock and trauma. *J. Trauma Acute Care Surg.* **2021**, *90*, 1022–1031. [CrossRef]
165. Bugaev, N.; Como, J.J.; Golani, G.; Freeman, J.J.; Sawhney, J.S.; Vatsaas, C.J.; Yorkgitis, B.K.; Kreiner, L.A.; Garcia, N.M.; Aziz, H.A.; et al. Thromboelastography and rotational thromboelastometry in bleeding patients with coagulopathy: Practice management guideline from the Eastern Association for the Surgery of Trauma. *J. Trauma Acute Care Surg.* **2020**, *89*, 999–1017. [CrossRef]
166. Einersen, P.M.; Moore, E.E.; Chapman, M.P.; Moore, H.B.; Gonzalez, E.; Silliman, C.C.; Banerjee, A.; Sauaia, A. Rapid thrombelastography thresholds for goal-directed resuscitation of patients at risk for massive transfusion. *J. Trauma Acute Care Surg.* **2017**, *82*, 114–119. [CrossRef]
167. Sharp, G.; Young, C.J. Point-of-care viscoelastic assay devices (rotational thromboelastometry and thromboelastography): A primer for surgeons. *ANZ J. Surg.* **2019**, *89*, 291–295. [CrossRef]
168. Brill, J.B.; Cotton, B.A.; Brenner, M.; Duchesne, J.; Ferrada, P.; Horer, T.; Kauvar, D.; Khan, M.; Roberts, D.; Ordonez, C.; et al. The Role of TEG and ROTEM in Damage Control Resuscitation. *Shock* **2021**. [CrossRef] [PubMed]
169. Gall, L.S.; Vulliamy, P.; Gillespie, S.; Jones, T.F.; Pierre, R.S.J.; Breukers, S.E.; Gaarder, C.; Juffermans, N.P.; Maegele, M.; Stensballe, J.; et al. The S100A10 Pathway Mediates an Occult Hyperfibrinolytic Subtype in Trauma Patients. *Ann. Surg.* **2019**, *269*, 1184–1191. [CrossRef] [PubMed]
170. Curry, N.S.; Davenport, R.; Pavord, S.; Mallett, S.V.; Kitchen, D.; Klein, A.A.; Maybury, H.; Collins, P.W.; Laffan, M. The use of viscoelastic haemostatic assays in the management of major bleeding: A British Society for Haematology Guideline. *Br. J. Haematol.* **2018**, *182*, 789–806. [CrossRef] [PubMed]
171. Roullet, S.; de Maistre, E.; Ickx, B.; Blais, N.; Susen, S.; Faraoni, D.; Garrigue, D.; Bonhomme, F.; Godier, A.; Lasne, D.; et al. Position of the French Working Group on Perioperative Haemostasis (GIHP) on viscoelastic tests: What role for which indication in bleeding situations? *Anaesth. Crit. Care Pain Med.* **2019**, *38*, 539–548. [CrossRef]
172. CRASH-2 Collaborators; Roberts, I.; Shakur, H.; Afolabi, A.; Brohi, K.; Coats, T.; Dewan, Y.; Gando, S.; Guyatt, G.; Hunt, B.J.; et al. The importance of early treatment with tranexamic acid in bleeding trauma patients: An exploratory analysis of the CRASH-2 randomised controlled trial. *Lancet* **2011**, *377*, 1096–1101.e1–2. [CrossRef]

173. Myers, S.P.; Kutcher, M.E.; Rosengart, M.R.; Sperry, J.L.; Peitzman, A.B.; Brown, J.B.; Neal, M.D. Tranexamic acid administration is associated with an increased risk of posttraumatic venous thromboembolism. *J. Trauma Acute Care Surg.* **2019**, *86*, 20–27. [CrossRef]
174. Moore, E.E.; Moore, H.B.; Gonzalez, E.; Chapman, M.P.; Hansen, K.C.; Sauaia, A.; Silliman, C.C.; Banerjee, A. Postinjury fibrinolysis shutdown: Rationale for selective tranexamic acid. *J. Trauma Acute Care Surg.* **2015**, *78*, S65–S69. [CrossRef]
175. Barrett, C.D.; Moore, H.B.; Vigneshwar, N.; Dhara, S.; Chandler, J.; Chapman, M.P.; Sauaia, A.; Moore, E.E.; Yaffe, M.B. Plasmin thrombelastography rapidly identifies trauma patients at risk for massive transfusion, mortality, and hyperfibrinolysis: A diagnostic tool to resolve an international debate on tranexamic acid? *J. Trauma Acute Care Surg.* **2020**, *89*, 991–998. [CrossRef] [PubMed]
176. Khan, M.; Jehan, F.; Bulger, E.M.; O'Keeffe, T.; Holcomb, J.B.; Wade, C.E.; Schreiber, M.A.; Joseph, B.; Group, P.S. Severely injured trauma patients with admission hyperfibrinolysis: Is there a role of tranexamic acid? Findings from the PROPPR trial. *J. Trauma Acute Care Surg.* **2018**, *85*, 851–857. [CrossRef]
177. Selby, R. "TEG talk": Expanding clinical roles for thromboelastography and rotational thromboelastometry. *Hematol. Am. Soc. Hematol. Educ. Program.* **2020**, *2020*, 67–75. [CrossRef]
178. British Committee for Standards in Haematology Writing Group; Stainsby, D.; MacLennan, S.; Thomas, D.; Isaac, J.; Hamilton, P.J. Guidelines on the management of massive blood loss. *Br. J. Haematol.* **2006**, *135*, 634–641. [CrossRef] [PubMed]
179. Hiippala, S.T.; Myllyla, G.J.; Vahtera, E.M. Hemostatic factors and replacement of major blood loss with plasma-poor red cell concentrates. *Anesth. Analg.* **1995**, *81*, 360–365. [PubMed]
180. Inaba, K.; Branco, B.C.; Rhee, P.; Blackbourne, L.H.; Holcomb, J.B.; Teixeira, P.G.; Shulman, I.; Nelson, J.; Demetriades, D. Impact of plasma transfusion in trauma patients who do not require massive transfusion. *J. Am. Coll. Surg.* **2010**, *210*, 957–965. [CrossRef] [PubMed]
181. McQuilten, Z.K.; Wood, E.M.; Bailey, M.; Cameron, P.A.; Cooper, D.J. Fibrinogen is an independent predictor of mortality in major trauma patients: A five-year statewide cohort study. *Injury* **2017**, *48*, 1074–1081. [CrossRef] [PubMed]
182. Nakamura, Y.; Ishikura, H.; Kushimoto, S.; Kiyomi, F.; Kato, H.; Sasaki, J.; Ogura, H.; Matsuoka, T.; Uejima, T.; Morimura, N.; et al. Fibrinogen level on admission is a predictor for massive transfusion in patients with severe blunt trauma: Analyses of a retrospective multicentre observational study. *Injury* **2017**, *48*, 674–679. [CrossRef] [PubMed]
183. Innerhofer, P.; Fries, D.; Mittermayr, M.; Innerhofer, N.; von Langen, D.; Hell, T.; Gruber, G.; Schmid, S.; Friesenecker, B.; Lorenz, I.H.; et al. Reversal of trauma-induced coagulopathy using first-line coagulation factor concentrates or fresh frozen plasma (RETIC): A single-centre, parallel-group, open-label, randomised trial. *Lancet Haematol.* **2017**. [CrossRef]
184. Nascimento, B.; Callum, J.; Tien, H.; Peng, H.; Rizoli, S.; Karanicolas, P.; Alam, A.; Xiong, W.; Selby, R.; Garzon, A.M.; et al. Fibrinogen in the initial resuscitation of severe trauma (FiiRST): A randomized feasibility trial. *Br. J. Anaesth.* **2016**, *117*, 775–782. [CrossRef] [PubMed]
185. Schochl, H.; Nienaber, U.; Maegele, M.; Hochleitner, G.; Primavesi, F.; Steitz, B.; Arndt, C.; Hanke, A.; Voelckel, W.; Solomon, C. Transfusion in trauma: Thromboelastometry-guided coagulation factor concentrate-based therapy versus standard fresh frozen plasma-based therapy. *Crit. Care* **2011**, *15*, R83. [CrossRef]
186. Yamamoto, K.; Yamaguchi, A.; Sawano, M.; Matsuda, M.; Anan, M.; Inokuchi, K.; Sugiyama, S. Pre-emptive administration of fibrinogen concentrate contributes to improved prognosis in patients with severe trauma. *Trauma Surg. Acute Care Open* **2016**, *1*, e000037. [CrossRef]
187. Simurda, T.; Stanciakova, L.; Stasko, J.; Dobrotova, M.; Kubisz, P. Yes or no for secondary prophylaxis in afibrinogenemia? *Blood Coagul. Fibrinolysis* **2015**, *26*, 978–980. [CrossRef]
188. Su, Y.; Chen, Y.; Zhang, W.; Liu, L.; Cao, X.; Wu, J. Platelet factor 4 and beta-thromboglobulin mRNAs in circulating microparticles of trauma patients as diagnostic markers for deep vein thrombosis. *J. Thromb. Thrombolysis* **2020**, *50*, 525–532. [CrossRef] [PubMed]
189. Neisser-Svae, A.; Hegener, O.; Gorlinger, K. Differences in the biochemical composition of three plasma derived human fibrinogen concentrates. *Thromb. Res.* **2021**, *205*, 44–46. [CrossRef]
190. Schlimp, C.J.; Cadamuro, J.; Solomon, C.; Redl, H.; Schochl, H. The effect of fibrinogen concentrate and factor XIII on thromboelastometry in 33% diluted blood with albumin, gelatine, hydroxyethyl starch or saline in vitro. *Blood Transfus.* **2013**, *11*, 510–517. [CrossRef]
191. Nagashima, F.; Inoue, S.; Koami, H.; Miike, T.; Sakamoto, Y.; Kai, K. High-dose Factor XIII administration induces effective hemostasis for trauma-associated coagulopathy (TAC) both in vitro and in rat hemorrhagic shock in vivo models. *J. Trauma Acute Care Surg.* **2018**, *85*, 588–597. [CrossRef] [PubMed]
192. Perner, A.; Haase, N.; Wiis, J.; White, J.O.; Delaney, A. Central venous oxygen saturation for the diagnosis of low cardiac output in septic shock patients. *Acta Anaesthesiol. Scand.* **2010**, *54*, 98–102. [CrossRef]
193. Reinhart, K.; Bloos, F. The value of venous oximetry. *Curr. Opin. Crit. Care* **2005**, *11*, 259–263. [CrossRef]
194. Reinhart, K.; Kuhn, H.J.; Hartog, C.; Bredle, D.L. Continuous central venous and pulmonary artery oxygen saturation monitoring in the critically ill. *Intensive Care Med.* **2004**, *30*, 1572–1578. [CrossRef]
195. Edwards, J.D.; Mayall, R.M. Importance of the sampling site for measurement of mixed venous oxygen saturation in shock. *Crit. Care Med.* **1998**, *26*, 1356–1360. [CrossRef]
196. Martin, C.; Auffray, J.P.; Badetti, C.; Perrin, G.; Papazian, L.; Gouin, F. Monitoring of central venous oxygen saturation versus mixed venous oxygen saturation in critically ill patients. *Intensive Care Med.* **1992**, *18*, 101–104. [CrossRef]

197. Pope, J.V.; Jones, A.E.; Gaieski, D.F.; Arnold, R.C.; Trzeciak, S.; Shapiro, N.I.; Emergency Medicine Shock Research Network (EMShockNet) Investigators. Multicenter study of central venous oxygen saturation (ScvO(2)) as a predictor of mortality in patients with sepsis. *Ann. Emerg. Med.* **2010**, *55*, 40–46 e41. [CrossRef]
198. Mallat, J.; Lazkani, A.; Lemyze, M.; Pepy, F.; Meddour, M.; Gasan, G.; Temime, J.; Vangrunderbeeck, N.; Tronchon, L.; Thevenin, D. Repeatability of blood gas parameters, PCO2 gap, and PCO2 gap to arterial-to-venous oxygen content difference in critically ill adult patients. *Medicine (Baltimore)* **2015**, *94*, e415. [CrossRef]
199. Mallat, J.; Lemyze, M.; Tronchon, L.; Vallet, B.; Thevenin, D. Use of venous-to-arterial carbon dioxide tension difference to guide resuscitation therapy in septic shock. *World J. Crit. Care Med.* **2016**, *5*, 47–56. [CrossRef]
200. Vallet, B.; Pinsky, M.R.; Cecconi, M. Resuscitation of patients with septic shock: Please "mind the gap"! *Intensive Care Med.* **2013**, *39*, 1653–1655. [CrossRef]
201. Pohlman, T.H.; Walsh, M.; Aversa, J.; Hutchison, E.M.; Olsen, K.P.; Lawrence Reed, R. Damage control resuscitation. *Blood Rev.* **2015**, *29*, 251–262. [CrossRef]
202. Gutterman, D.D.; Chabowski, D.S.; Kadlec, A.O.; Durand, M.J.; Freed, J.K.; Ait-Aissa, K.; Beyer, A.M. The Human Microcirculation: Regulation of Flow and Beyond. *Circ. Res.* **2016**, *118*, 157–172. [CrossRef]

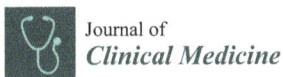

Article

Application of Pelvic Circumferential Compression Devices in Pelvic Ring Fractures—Are Guidelines Followed in Daily Practice?

Valerie Kuner [1,*], Nicole van Veelen [1], Stephanie Studer [2], Bryan Van de Wall [1], Jürgen Fornaro [3], Michael Stickel [4], Matthias Knobe [1], Reto Babst [5], Frank J.P. Beeres [1] and Björn-Christian Link [1]

1. Department of Orthopaedic and Trauma Surgery, Cantonal Hospital Lucerne, 6000 Luzern, Switzerland; Nicole.vanVeelen@luks.ch (N.v.V.); Bryan.VandeWall@luks.ch (B.V.d.W.); Matthias.Knobe@luks.ch (M.K.); Frank.Beeres@luks.ch (F.J.P.B.); Bjoern-Christian.Link@luks.ch (B.-C.L.)
2. Medical Faculty, University of Zurich, 8091 Zurich, Switzerland; StephanieStuder@gmx.ch
3. Department of Radiology, Cantonal Hospital Lucerne, 6000 Luzern, Switzerland; Juergen.Fornaro@luks.ch
4. Department of Emergency Care, Cantonal Hospital Lucerne, 6000 Luzern, Switzerland; Michael.Stickel@icloud.com
5. Department of Health Science and Medicine, University of Lucerne, 6002 Luzern, Switzerland; Reto.Babst@luks.ch
* Correspondence: Valerie.Kuner@googlemail.com

Abstract: Early administration of a pelvic circumferential compression device (PCCD) is recommended for suspected pelvic trauma. This study was conducted to evaluate the prevalence of PCCD in patients with pelvic fractures assigned to the resuscitation room (RR) of a Level I trauma center. Furthermore, correct application of the PCCD as well as associated injuries with potential clinical sequelae were assessed. All patients with pelvic fractures assigned to the RR of a level one trauma center between 2016 and 2017 were evaluated retrospectively. Presence and position of the PCCD on the initial trauma scan were assessed and rated. Associated injuries with potential adverse effects on clinical outcome were analysed. Seventy-seven patients were included, of which 26 (34%) had a PCCD in place. Eighteen (23%) patients had an unstable fracture pattern of whom ten (56%) had received a PCCD. The PCCD was correctly placed in four (15%) cases, acceptable in 12 (46%) and incorrectly in ten (39%). Of all patients with pelvic fractures (n = 77, 100%) treated in the RR, only one third (n = 26, 34%) had a PCCD. In addition, 39% of PCCDs were positioned incorrectly. Of the patients with unstable pelvic fractures (n = 18, 100%), more than half either did not receive any PCCD (n = 8, 44%) or had one which was inadequately positioned (n = 2, 11 %). These results underline that preclinical and clinical education programs on PCCD indication and application should be critically reassessed.

Keywords: pelvic ring fracture; PCCD; position; associated injuries

1. Introduction

About 20% of polytrauma patients have a pelvic injury [1], with an estimated incidence of about 23 per 100,000 persons per year [2,3]. The examination of pelvic stability is part of the primary survey of trauma patients as an unstable pelvic ring fracture may result in severe intra- or retroperitoneal bleeding [4–6]. If, based on the mechanism of injury or clinical findings, an unstable pelvic ring injury is suspected, current guidelines recommend applying a pelvic circumferential compression device (PCCD) [4,7,8] to minimize the risk of intrapelvic haemorrhage and promote coagulation by realigning the pelvic ring and therefore reducing the pelvic volume [6,9–12]. A further option to reduce anterior diastasis is simple internal rotation of the lower extremities, which can be held by tape as reported by Gardner et al. However, this technique is problematic if the lower limbs are unstable due to long bone fractures [13–15]. Ideally, the PCCD is applied in the preclinical setting directly at the site of the accident. Typically, it is left in place until either the injury is ruled out or treatment is initiated [16,17]. The PCCD should be positioned over the greater trochanters to allow for optimal transmission of forces via the proximal femur to the pelvis to reduce anterior diastasis [18,19]. Potential disadvantages of PCCDs such as skin necrosis and nerve lesions have been described in case reports [20–26].

This study aimed to evaluate the prevalence and quality of PCCD application in pelvic fractures of patients assigned to the resuscitation room (RR) in a level I trauma center in Switzerland as well as to assess potential adverse effects in relation to associated injuries using a PCCD.

The hypothesis of this study is that the majority of patients with pelvic fractures treated in the resuscitation room at this level I trauma center have a correctly positioned PCCD in place and few adverse effects occur.

2. Materials and Methods

This article was written in accordance with the STROBE statement [27]. The study was approved by the Ethics Committee of Northwest- and Central Switzerland (project ID 2018-00411). The need for informed consent was waived.

2.1. Study Design, Setting and Participants

The imaging and electronic patient records of all consecutive patients treated in the RR of a level one trauma center in Switzerland were evaluated retrospectively for the years 2016 and 2017. Resuscitation room management at this trauma center follows a defined algorithm, which is based on the Advanced Trauma Life Support (ATLS) algorithm [7,28,29] and has been adjusted according to the Whitebook Medical Care of the Severely Injured of the German Society for Trauma Surgery [30]. If hemodynamically stable, all patients receive a whole-body computer tomography (CT) after the primary survey has been completed. All patients with a traumatic pelvic fracture diagnosed in the whole-body CT were included in this study. Fragility and subacute fractures were excluded. Fractures obtained from low-energy trauma such as a fall from standing height were defined as fragility fractures [31]. In fragility fractures the ligament structures remain intact, so there is no major bleeding and therefore no role for PCCDs. Subacute fractures were defined as fractures with visible callus formation with or without previous documentation of the fracture.

2.2. Data Measurement and Variables

Demographic data of each patient were collected from the electronic medical records (Medfolio, Nexus AG, Donaueschingen, Germany) as well as the Swiss Trauma Register (STR) and the register of the German Society for Trauma Surgery (DGU). In these registers there are six possible trauma mechanisms to allocate the case to: car, motorcycle, cyclist, pedestrian, fall from height or other (such as explosion or blow). Any fall that was from higher than standing height was defined as a fall from height. The New Injury Severity Score (NISS) total was compiled and divided into groups <16 and ≥16 points on the NISS scale [32–34]. To be able to classify the fractures and evaluate the positioning of the PCCD patients had to have had a CT. Hemodynamically unstable patients, who required immediate intervention prior to CT imaging were therefore excluded.

Images were viewed using the Picture Archiving and Communication System (Phönix-PACS GmbH, Freiburg i.Br, Germany). All fractures were classified according to the modified Tile AO classification by an orthopaedic resident and revised by a fellowship-trained pelvic surgeon [35,36]. Unstable fractures were defined as Tile B1, B3, C1, C2 or C3. Stable fractures were defined as Tile A1, A2, A3 and B2. Type B2 fractures (ipsilateral internal rotation injury) were classified as stable fractures, as these fractures are caused by an internal rotation force and the volume of the pelvis is not enlarged by the injury. Further, it is assumed that the anatomy of these fractures is restored by the elastic recoil of the pelvis [35]. For these reasons, such injuries do not benefit from the use of a PCCD. Fractures that could not be classified according to Tile, such as acetabular fractures classified according to Judet and Letournel [37] and sacral fractures according to Denis [38] I-III plus sacral transversal, sacral U- and H-shaped fractures, were rated as stable fracture patterns, since these do not benefit from the use of a PCCD. Further, it was assessed whether the fracture involved the neuroforamina.

In the catchment area of this trauma center two different types of PCCD, the T-POD™ (Cybertech Medical, Laverne, CA, USA) and the SAM Pelvic-sling II™ (SAM Medical Products, Tualatin, OR, USA) are in use [39,40].

Presence upon arrival in the emergency room (yes or no), type (the T-POD lap loop or the SAM Pelvic-sling II) and position of a PCCD were assessed on the CT scans. The position of the PCCD was rated as 'correct' if it covered both greater trochanters completely, 'acceptable' if the PCCD partly covered the greater trochanters and ´incorrect´ if the PCCD did not cover the greater trochanters at all (Figure 1) [18,19].

All associated injuries based on the CT findings like presence of bladder injury, neuroforaminal fracture involvement, vascular injury, pelvic hematoma and based on medical records of presence of neurogenic bladder disorder, posttraumatic peripheral neurologic injury of the lower extremities and skin necrosis were recorded.

Bladder injury, neurogenic bladder disorder, neuroforaminal fracture involvement with simultaneous posttraumatic peripheral neurologic injury of the lower extremities and vascular injury were defined as associated injuries which could be aggravated by the application of a PCCD.

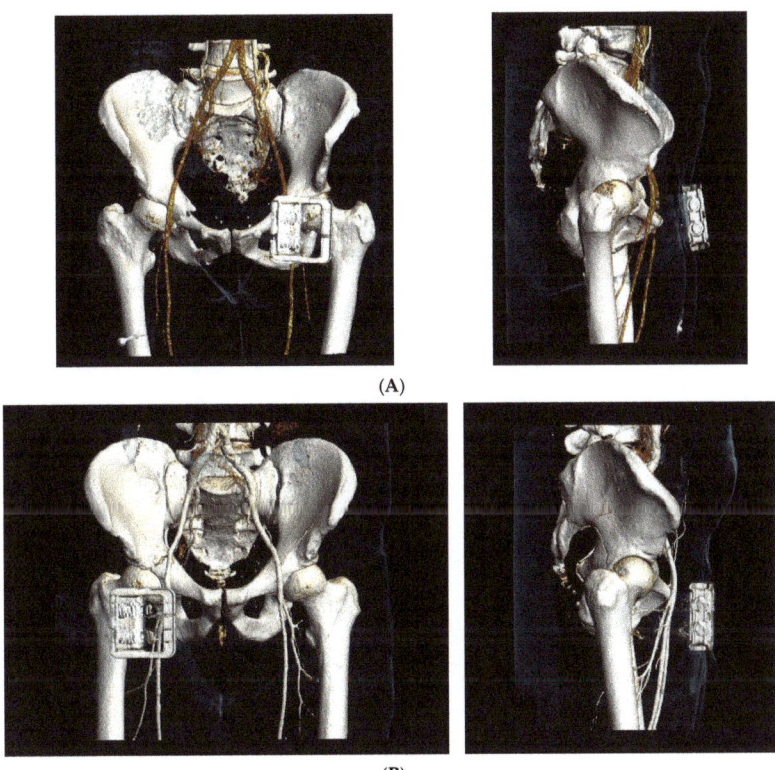

Figure 1. *Cont.*

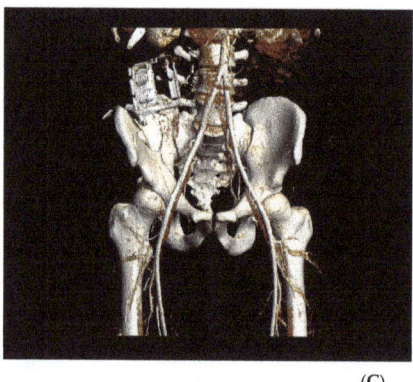
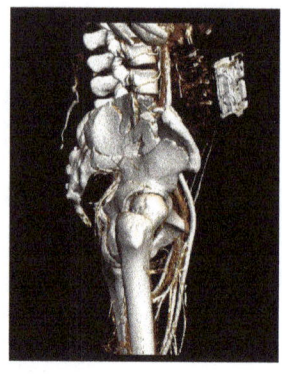

(C)

Figure 1. Pelvic circumferential compression device (PCCD) positioning (example of the SAM Pelvicsling II). (**A**) Correct positioning of a PCCD at the level of the trochanters; (**B**) Acceptable positioning of a PCCD with partial coverage of the trochanters; (**C**) Incorrect positioning of a PCCD without any covering of the trochanters.

2.3. Statistical Methods

The data collected were analysed using SPSS (IBM® SPSS® Statistics 24, IBM, Armonk, NY, USA). Mean values, medians, standard deviation and percentages were calculated. The Fisher exact test was used for the statistical analysis of associated injuries and PCCD presence (significance level $p < 0.05$). Subgroup analysis was tempted stratified for fracture stability by using the Fisher exact test. The Chi- Square Test was used to analyze the relationship between the positioning of PCCD and the associated injuries (significance level $p < 0.05$).

3. Results

A total of 730 patients were admitted to the RR during the study period. Eighty-two (11%) had a pelvic fracture. All patients were hemodynamically stable enough to receive a CT prior to any intervention. Four patients with a fragility fracture and one patient with a subacute pubic fracture were excluded leaving a total of 77 patients (Figure 2). The demographic data are summarized in Table 1. All patients sustained their injuries by blunt trauma.

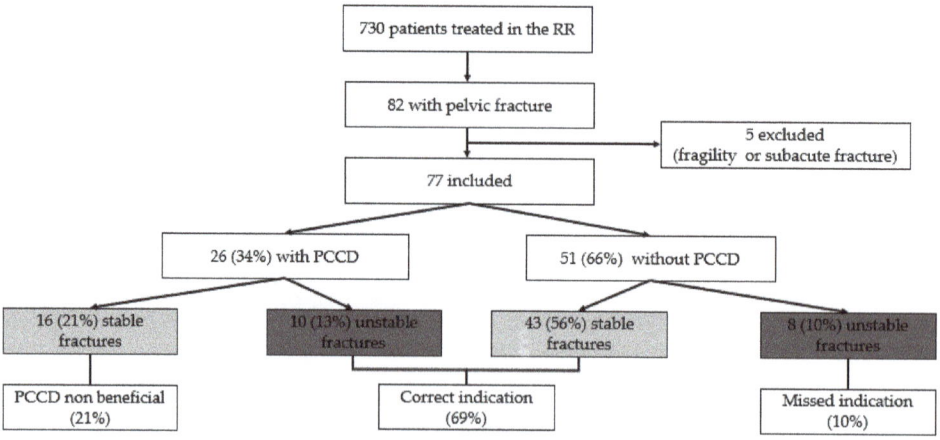

Figure 2. Included patients, prevalence of a PCCD and indication for PCCD.

Table 1. Demographic data.

Demographic Data	N	Mean
Sex		
Male	49 (64%)	
Female	28 (36%)	
Age		50 years (range 14–93, SD ± 21.2)
Trauma mechanism		
Blunt	77 (100%)	
Type of accident		
Car	6 (8%)	
Motorcycle	13 (17%)	
Cyclist	6 (8%)	
Pedestrian	8 (10%)	
Fall from height	36 (47%)	
Other (like blow, explosion)	8 (10%)	
NISS		20 (range 4–66, SD ± 16)
NISS≥/<16		
≥16	54 (70%)	
<16	23 (30%)	
Intensive medical treatment		
Yes	40 (52%)	
No	37 (48%)	
Survivors	71 (92%)	
Death	6 (8%)	
Length of hospital stay (days)		11 (0–98 days, SD ± 14)

Twenty-six (34%) patients had a PCCD in place at the time of the CT examination (Figure 2). Out of these, 24 PCCDs had been placed preclinically, for the remaining two no reliable documentation on the time of application was found. Eighteen (69%) patients had the T-POD device and eight (31%) the SAM pelvic sling II in place.

Fracture classification according to Tile is listed in Table 2. There were no C1 fractures in the cohort. Fifty-eight (75%) patients could be classified according to Tile. The remaining 25% had acetabular or sacral fractures which could not be classified according to Tile and were therefore assigned to the stable fracture patterns (Table 2).

Table 2. Prevalence of fractures and pelvic circumferential compression device (PCCD).

Fracture Type	Total $n = 77$	PCCD Placed $n = 26$	PCCD Not Placed $n = 51$
Pelvic ring fractures according to Tile stable and unstable	58 (75%)		
A1	2 (3%)	0	2
A2	16 (21%)	4	12
A3	2 (3%)	1	1
B1	5 (6%)	2[1]	3[2]
B2	20 (26%)	5	15
B3	8 (10%)	5[1]	3[2]
C1	0 (0%)	0	0
C2	2 (3%)	2[1]	0
C3	3 (4%)	1[1]	2[2]
acetabular fracture	17 (22%)	6	11
isolated sacral fracture	2 (3%)	0	2
additional femoral neck fracture	3 (in 1 bilateral)	1	2
additional Pipkin fracture	2	2	0

[1] Ten (13%) correct indications for PCCD. [2] Eight (10%) unstable fractures, indication for PCCD.

Eighteen (23%) patients had an unstable fracture pattern, of which ten (56%) received a PCCD, while 16 (27%) of the patients with a stable fracture had one applied. This leaves a total of 51 patients without PCCD, 43 (73%) of the patients with stable fractures, and eight (44%) of those with unstable fractures.

In total ten (13%) patients correctly received a PCCD based on the fracture pattern, eight (10%) should have received a PCCD, 43 (56%) did not get a PCCD since there was no indication for application and 16 (21%) received a PCCD although indication was not given (Figure 2).

The position of the PCCD was correct in four (15%) cases, acceptable in 12 (46%) and incorrect in ten (39%) (Table 3). Regarding the ten patients with unstable fractures, PCCD position was correct in one patient, acceptable in seven patients and inadequate in two (Table 3).

Table 3. PCCD positioning.

Position of PCCD	Unstable Factures $n = 10$	Stable Fractures $n = 16$
correct	1 (10%)	3 (19%)
acceptable	7 (70%)	5 (31%)
incorrect	2 (20%)	8 (50%)

The type of PCCD and the respective positioning are listed in (Table 4).

Table 4. PCCD type (T-POD or SAM Pelvic Sling) in unstable fractures.

Position of T-POD ($n = 7$)		Position of SAM Pelvic Sling ($n = 3$)	
correct	1 (14%)	correct	0
acceptable	5 (71%)	acceptable	2 (67%)
incorrect	1 (14%)	incorrect	1 (33%)

The associated injuries are listed in Table 5. One patient had two associated injuries (neurogenic bladder disorder and neuroforaminal fracture involvement with simultaneous posttraumatic peripheral neurologic injury of the lower extremities). In this collective no PCCD related adverse effects such as skin necrosis were registered.

Patients with applied PCCD showed a significantly higher rate of associated injuries like bladder injury ($n = 3$), neurogenic bladder disorder ($n = 3$), neuroforaminal fracture involvement with simultaneous posttraumatic peripheral neurologic injury of the lower extremities ($n = 1$), traumatic vascular injury ($n = 7$) than patients without PCCD according to the Fisher exact test ($p = 0.0075$) (Table 6).

Within the group of PCCD patients, the subgroup analysis stratified for fracture stability showed no significant difference regarding the incidence of associated injuries for unstable fracture patterns (Fisher exact test $p = 0.3137$) (Table 6), while there was a significant association in the stable fracture group (Fisher exact test $p = 0.0278$) (Table 6).

There was a statistically significant relationship between the positioning of PCCD and the occurrence of associated injuries according to the Chi-Square Test ($X2(1, N = 77) = 5.0667$, $p < 0.05$) (Table 7).

Table 5. Associated injuries of pelvic fracture.

Associated Injury	n = 77	Fracture Type
Bladder injury	3 (4%)	B1
		B2 + Denis I + acetabular anterior wall
		acetabular anterior column, posterior hemitransverse
Neurogenic bladder disorder	3 (4%)	B2 + sacrum fracture H- type
		C3 + sacrum fracture H- type + acetabular anterior column [1]
		acetabular anterior column
Neuroforaminal fracture involvement	14 (18%)	A3 + transverse sacrum fracture
		B2 + Denis II
		B2 + Denis II
		B2 + Denis II
		B2 + Denis II
		B2 + Denis II
		B2 + Denis III
		B2 + sacrum fracture H- type
		B3 + transverse sacrum fracture
		B3 + sacrum fracture U- type
		C2 + Denis II
		C3 + sacrum fracture H- type
		Denis II + acetabular anterior colum with hemitransverse
		Denis II + acetabular 2 colum fracture
Nerve lesion of the lower extremities	4 (5%)	C3 + sacrum fracture H- type
		sacrum fracture H- type
		acetabular transverse fracture
		acetabular 2 colum fracture
Neuroforaminal fracture involvement + posttraumatic peripheral neurologic injury of the lower extremities	1 (1%)	C3 + sacrum fracture H- type + acetabular anterior column [1]
Traumatic vascular injury	7 (9%)	A3 + transverse sacrum fracture
		B1
		B1
		B2 + Denis II
		B2 + Denis III
		C2 + Denis II
		acetabular transverse fracture

Table 5. Cont.

Associated Injury	n = 77	Fracture Type
Pelvic hematoma	19 (25%)	A2
		A2
		A2 + Denis I
		A3 + transverse sacrum fracture
		B1 + Denis I
		B2 + Denis I
		B2 + Denis I
		B2 + Denis I
		B2 + Denis II
		B2 + sacrum fracture H- type
		B2 + acetabular anterior wall
		B3
		B3 + Denis I
		B3 + Denis I
		C2 + Denis I
		C3 + sacrum fracture H- type + acetabular anterior colum
		acetabular anterior colum with hemitransverse
		acetabular 2 colum fracture
		left acetabular transverse + posterior wall, right acetabular posterior wall

[1] One patient showed two associated injuries.

Table 6. Contingency table of all documented associated injuries in relation to applied PCCD. (**a**) Contingency table of all documented associated injuries in patients with unstable fractures in relation to applied PCCD. (**b**) Contingency table of all documented associated injuries in patients with stable fractures in relation to applied PCCD.

	PCCD	No PCCD	
Associated injury	9 (69 %)	4 (31%)	13
No associated injury	17 (27 %)	47 (73%)	64
	26	51	77

(**a**)

	PCCD	No PCCD	
Associated injury	4 (80%)	1 (20%)	5
No associated injury	6 (46%)	7 (54%)	13
	10	8	18

(**b**)

	PCCD	No PCCD	
Associated injury	5 (62.5%)	3 (37.5%)	8
No associated injury	11 (22%)	40 (78%)	51
	16	43	59

The Fisher exact test statistic value is 0.0075. The result is significant at $p < 0.05$. (**a**) The Fisher exact test statistic value is 0.3137. The result is not significant at $p < 0.05$. (**b**) The Fisher exact test statistic value is 0.0278. The result is significant at $p < 0.05$.

Table 7. Contingency table of all documented associated injuries in relation to the position of the applied PCCD.

	PCCD Correct or PCCD Acceptable	PCCD Incorrect or No PCCD	
Associated injury	6 (43%)	8 (57%)	14
No associated injury	10 (16%)	53 (84%)	63
	16	61	77

The chi-square statistic is 5.0667. The p-value is 0.02439. Significant at $p < 0.05$.

4. Discussion

In this retrospective study comprising of 77 patients with a pelvic fracture only one third (26/77; 34%) had a PCCD applied. The position of the PCCD was correct in four (15%) cases, acceptable in 12 (46%) and incorrect in ten (39%).

Several recent studies are in accordance with these findings that only a minority of patients with pelvic ring fractures are preclinically treated with a PCCD [41–44]. The largest cohort so far is described by another Swiss study overlooking a period of 6 years that found a PCCD applied in only 552/2366 (23%) of the cases [45]. Also in a recent study of Vaidya et al. one third of patients with unstable pelvic fractures did not receive a PCCD [41]. In this study, the rate was even higher with 44% (8/18).

According to studies that mainly examined external rotation injuries and the reduction of symphyseal diastasis by PCCD, the PCCD needs to be positioned over the greater trochanters for optimal efficiency [18,19,46]. Retrospective studies which analysed the position of the PCCD in relation to the trochanters have shown that the position is incorrect in up to 50% [18,47–50].

In this cohort, 39% had incorrect positioning. Williamson et al. found a similar sub-optimal placing of PCCD in 43.5%, 39.7% were placed superior and 3.8% inferior to the greater trochanter line [48]. Other studies demonstrate a PCCD misalignment of up to 50% [49,50].

Of the 10 patients with an unstable fracture and a PCCD seven (70%) received the T-POD and three (30%) the SAM pelvic sling II. No superiority of one PCCD model over the other could be found by Knops et al. [51]. This study cohort was too small to evaluate the superiority of one type of device over the other.

The retrospective observational design and the relatively small size of the study population limit the conclusive strength of this study. The small number of patients who received a PCCD does not allow for statistical evaluation regarding the type of PCCD applied and limited the statistical power of subanalysis regarding a connection between PCCD positioning and potential adverse effects on associated injuries. The correction for other confounders was not possible due to the low sample size, therefore, it was chosen to only stratify for stable and unstable fractures. A low rate of accurate indication and correct PCCD application has been reported by several authors [18,41–45,47–50].

The evaluation of pelvic ring stability at the site of an accident is often hampered by several factors such as patient consciousness, environmental circumstances and clothing. These inherent factors seem to limit the accuracy of the clinical evaluation of pelvic stability. Studies assessing these difficulties concluded that since clinical stability testing of the pelvis showed low sensitivity [46–48], the accident mechanism was a more relevant factor influencing the decision on whether or not a PCCD is indicated [52–54]. However, the trauma mechanism might be unclear in a substantial proportion of cases emphasising the challenges encountered in the field. The classification into stable fractures, for which the PCCD is not beneficial, and unstable fractures, for which the indication is given, was used for retrospective analysis. This classification was based on the review of CT images of the fractures, which is naturally impossible for preclinical staff who must rely on clinical signs and the mechanism of injury to judge the stability of a pelvic injury. It does however, highlight the fact that unstable pelvic fractures were undersupplied with PCCDs in this study population and that there is room for improvement.

The low rate of correctly positioned PCCD could be addressed by sensitising and instructing paramedics and RR personnel on accurate identification of anatomical landmarks. Williamson et al. defined the correct position of the PCCD as a position between the tip of the greater trochanter and the inferior border of the lesser trochanter. He found a significantly higher risk for misplacement of the PCCD if the distance between those anatomic landmarks was small (<8.9 cm) and in females [48]. Due to smaller body size in females the palpable bony mass of the greater trochanter is also smaller. This might cause additional problems in positioning the PCCD correctly. Familiarization with different PCCD models through training seems to be an additional factor [44,55], as different types of PCCDs will require knowledge for their correct positioning in relation to palpable landmarks. Obesity or secondary dislocation during patient transport of the PCCD are also factors that can hamper correct positioning.

The accident kinematics as well as the preclinical assessment and initial clinical examination should trigger the suspicion of a pelvic ring injury [4,7]. If an unstable pelvic ring injury is suspected, stabilization using a PCCD is an effective temporary measure in an emergency situation [4,7,26]. Additional advantages of a PCCD are pain control, haemorrhage control [39,56], reduced transfusion requirement [12,57], reduction in the length of hospitalization [12,57] and decreased mortality [12]. PCCDs are non-invasive and can be applied rapidly on the scene of an accident [40].

In the preclinical phase, the PCCD is the gold standard for pelvic stabilization. The stabilization of pelvic fractures with severe and persistent hemodynamic instability can be achieved by invasive procedures in the RR such as the C-clamp [58–60] for pelvic ring lesions of type C and by external fixation [61–64] for the B-type [65,66]. PCCDs show an equivalence to invasive procedures like the C-clamp, which requires more user knowledge, time, training and equipment [67]. It also provides comparable stability to invasive procedures such as the external fixators [68]. However, in contrast to the PCCD, the c-clamp and external fixator can be used for definitive treatment.

In respect to the fracture pattern, to our knowledge there is no evidence in the literature that compression of internal rotation injuries or acetabular fractures with a PCCD may cause adverse effects [10,11,42,51]. However, known potential disadvantages of PCCD application are pressure decubitus or aggravating nerve compression with long lasting application, as described in case reports and studies that analyze pressure measurement on models or healthy subjects [22,69–72]. No skin necrosis complication occurred in this patient population. Due to short transport distances and prompt patient care in the catchment area of central Switzerland the paramedic should not hesitate to apply a PCCD because of potential risk of skin necrosis. However, the current study found more potential aggravation of associated injuries with PCCD application (Table 6). Despite these differences being statistically significant, the total number of patients included in this study population was relatively low, prohibiting the ability to draw a sound conclusion. It however demonstrates the need for further investigation into this topic.

Interestingly, this potential aggravation of associated injuries was statistically significant for stable fractures (Table 6), but not for unstable fractures (Table 6) in the subgroup analysis. The definition of a stable (A1-3, B2) and unstable (B1, B3, C1-3) fracture chosen for this study may be a potential confounder in this sub-analysis. It was assumed that the anatomy in B2 fractures is restored by the elastic recoil of the pelvis near to normal so it does not benefit from the use of a PCCD. The compressive effect of a PCCD, however, may reproduce or even aggravate the initial accident mechanism, therefore potentially leading to further injuries. Out of the five patients with stable fractures who received a PCCD and had associated injuries two were B2 fractures. Both of these cases had a vascular injury. The other three were two A2 and one A3 fracture. Further studies are needed to address risk factors in terms of PCCD effects. These could give rise to balance potential life- saving benefits against potential adverse events [26].

Conversely, the rate of PCCD in patients with pelvic fractures in general and specifically in patients with unstable pelvic ring fractures is rather low. Naturally, there seems to be room for improvement in education. In Central Switzerland, paramedics receive lessons on how to correctly apply a PCCD as part of their training, this includes an instructional video and a handout. Qualified paramedics must complete a total of 40 h of mandatory annual training which includes the application of PCCDs. In the latest (10th) edition of the ATLS Student Manual, for the first time a video on PCCD application including anatomic landmark instructions is linked to the App [7]. These educational efforts underline the observed knowledge gap regarding the indication for and correct application of PCCDs. Perhaps more practical training with instruction of additional palpable anatomic landmarks besides the level of the trochanters such as the relation of the upper belt border to the anterior superior iliac spine is needed to avoid grossly incorrect PCCD positioning and could increase the rate of correct PCCD applications.

5. Conclusions

Only one third (34%) of patients with pelvic fractures assigned to the RR had a PCCD placed. Moreover, of these, 39% were applied incorrectly. These results, in accordance with similar results from the recent literature, clearly demonstrate the need for focused preclinical and clinical education programs on when and how to apply a PCCD.

The observed rate of potential aggravated adverse effects of PCCD's seems to be higher in the treated group irrespective of the fracture pattern. Higher patient numbers are needed to balance the live saving benefits of PCCD's against potential adverse effects of its application.

In the meantime, the PCCD remains the gold standard, however by rising the awareness of correct indication and positioning in the catchment area of this level I trauma center potential adverse effects could likely be minimised and benefits increased.

Author Contributions: Conceptualization and Methodology, V.K., F.J.P.B. and R.B.; Software, Medfolio (Nexus AG, Donaueschingen, Germany) and Picture Archiving and Communication System (Phönix-PACS GmbH, Freiburg i.Br, Germany) and SPSS (IBM® SPSS® Statistics 24); formal analysis and investigation, V.K., S.S., B.-C.L., M.S. and J.F.; data curation, V.K.; Writing—original draft preparation, V.K., N.v.V., R.B. and B.-C.L.; Writing—review and editing, all authors; visualisation, V.K., R.B. and B.-C.L.; Supervision, R.B., F.J.P.B. and B.-C.L. All authors have read and agreed to the published version of the manuscript.

Funding: This research received no external funding.

Institutional Review Board Statement: The study was conducted according to the guidelines of the Declaration of Helsinki, and approved by the Ethics Committee of Northwest- and Central Switzerland (project ID 2018-00411).

Informed Consent Statement: Patient consent was waived. No consent could be obtained for the injury patterns examined prior to data collection. This fact was explicitly communicated to the ethics committee. The ethics committee granted permission to carry out the study and to publish the study.

Data Availability Statement: The data presented in this study are available on request from the corresponding author. The data are not publicly available due to privacy reasons.

Conflicts of Interest: The authors declare no conflict of interest.

References

1. Freitas, C.D.; Garotti, J.E.R.; Nieto, J.; Guimarães, R.P.; Ono, N.K.; Honda, E.; Polesello, G.C. There Have Been Changes in the Incidence and Epidemiology of Pelvic Ring Fractures in Recent Decades? *Rev. Bras. Ortop.* **2013**, *48*, 475–481. [CrossRef]
2. Toimela, J.; Brinck, T.; Handolin, L. Evolution of High-Energy Pelvic Trauma in Southern Finland: A 12-Year Experience from a Tertiary Trauma Centre. *Eur. J. Trauma Emerg. Surg.* **2019**. [CrossRef]
3. Wong, J.M.-L.; Bucknill, A. Fractures of the Pelvic Ring. *Injury* **2017**, *48*, 795–802. [CrossRef] [PubMed]
4. Polytrauma Guideline Update Group. Level 3 Guideline on the Treatment of Patients with Severe/Multiple Injuries. *Eur. J. Trauma Emerg. Surg.* **2018**, *44*, 3–271. [CrossRef]
5. Hemorrhage in Major Pelvic Fractures. Available online: https://europepmc.org/article/med/3046004 (accessed on 14 June 2020).
6. Ben-Menachem, Y.; Coldwell, D.M.; Young, J.W.; Burgess, A.R. Hemorrhage Associated with Pelvic Fractures: Causes, Diagnosis, and Emergent Management. *Am. J. Roentgenol.* **1991**, *157*, 1005–1014. [CrossRef] [PubMed]

7. ATLS 10th Edition Offers New Insights into Managing Trauma Patients. Available online: https://bulletin.facs.org/2018/06/atls-10th-edition-offers-new-insights-into-managing-trauma-patients/ (accessed on 11 April 2020).
8. Coccolini, F.; Stahel, P.F.; Montori, G.; Biffl, W.; Horer, T.M.; Catena, F.; Kluger, Y.; Moore, E.E.; Peitzman, A.B.; Ivatury, R.; et al. Pelvic Trauma: WSES Classification and Guidelines. *World J. Emerg. Surg.* **2017**, *12*, 5. [CrossRef]
9. Bottlang, M.; Krieg, J.C.; Mohr, M.; Simpson, T.S.; Madey, S.M. Emergent Management of Pelvic Ring Fractures with Use of Circumferential Compression. *JBJS* **2002**, *84*, S43. [CrossRef] [PubMed]
10. DeAngelis, N.A.; Wixted, J.J.; Drew, J.; Eskander, M.S.; Eskander, J.P.; French, B.G. Use of the Trauma Pelvic Orthotic Device (T-POD) for Provisional Stabilisation of Anterior-Posterior Compression Type Pelvic Fractures: A Cadaveric Study. *Injury* **2008**, *39*, 903–906. [CrossRef]
11. Krieg, J.C.; Mohr, M.; Ellis, T.J.; Simpson, T.S.; Madey, S.M.; Bottlang, M. Emergent Stabilization of Pelvic Ring Injuries by Controlled Circumferential Compression: A Clinical Trial. *J. Trauma Acute Care Surg.* **2005**, *59*, 659–664. [CrossRef]
12. Croce, M.A.; Magnotti, L.J.; Savage, S.A.; Wood, G.W.; Fabian, T.C. Emergent Pelvic Fixation in Patients with Exsanguinating Pelvic Fractures. *J. Am. Coll. Surg.* **2007**, *204*, 935–939; discussion 940–942. [CrossRef]
13. Gardner, M.J.; Parada, S.; Chip Routt, M.L. Internal Rotation and Taping of the Lower Extremities for Closed Pelvic Reduction. *J. Orthop. Trauma* **2009**, *23*, 361–364. [CrossRef] [PubMed]
14. Gänsslen, A.; Lindahl, J.; Füchtmeier, B. Emergency Stabilization: Pelvic Binder. In *Pelvic Ring Fractures*; Gänsslen, A., Lindahl, J., Grechenig, S., Füchtmeier, B., Eds.; Springer International Publishing: Cham, Germany, 2021; pp. 135–140, ISBN 978-3-030-54730-1.
15. Littlejohn, L.; Bennett, B.L.; Drew, B. Application of Current Hemorrhage Control Techniques for Backcountry Care: Part Two, Hemostatic Dressings and Other Adjuncts. *Wilderness Environ. Med.* **2015**, *26*, 246–254. [CrossRef]
16. Severe Pelvic Injury with Pelvic Mass Hemorrhage: Determining Severity of Hemorrhage and Clinical Experience with Emergency Stabilization. Available online: https://europepmc.org/article/med/9005750 (accessed on 12 April 2020).
17. Burkhardt, M.; Culemann, U.; Seekamp, A.; Pohlemann, T. Strategies for surgical treatment of multiple trauma including pelvic fracture. Review of the literature. *Unfallchirurg* **2005**, *108*, 812, 814–820. [CrossRef]
18. Bonner, T.J.; Eardley, W.G.P.; Newell, N.; Masouros, S.; Matthews, J.J.; Gibb, I.; Clasper, J.C. Accurate Placement of a Pelvic Binder Improves Reduction of Unstable Fractures of the Pelvic Ring. *J. Bone Jt. Surg. Br.* **2011**, *93*, 1524–1528. [CrossRef]
19. Bottlang, M.; Simpson, T.; Sigg, J.; Krieg, J.C.; Madey, S.M.; Long, W.B. Noninvasive Reduction of Open-Book Pelvic Fractures by Circumferential Compression. *J. Orthop. Trauma* **2002**, *16*, 367–373. [CrossRef] [PubMed]
20. Suzuki, T.; Kurozumi, T.; Watanabe, Y.; Ito, K.; Tsunoyama, T.; Sakamoto, T. Potentially Serious Adverse Effects from Application of a Circumferential Compression Device for Pelvic Fracture: A Report of Three Cases. *Trauma Case Rep.* **2020**, *26*. [CrossRef]
21. Schaller, T.M.; Sims, S.; Maxian, T. Skin Breakdown Following Circumferential Pelvic Antishock Sheeting: A Case Report. *J. Orthop. Trauma* **2005**, *19*, 661–665. [CrossRef] [PubMed]
22. Krieg, J.C.; Mohr, M.; Mirza, A.J.; Bottlang, M. Pelvic Circumferential Compression in the Presence of Soft-Tissue Injuries: A Case Report. *J. Trauma* **2005**, *59*, 470–472. [CrossRef]
23. Mason, L.W.; Boyce, D.E.; Pallister, I. Catastrophic Myonecrosis Following Circumferential Pelvic Binding after Massive Crush Injury: A Case Report. *Inj. Extra* **2009**, *40*, 84–86. [CrossRef]
24. Shank, J.R.; Morgan, S.J.; Smith, W.R.; Meyer, F.N. Bilateral Peroneal Nerve Palsy Following Emergent Stabilization of a Pelvic Ring Injury. *J. Orthop. Trauma* **2003**, *17*, 67–70. [CrossRef]
25. Garner, A.A.; Hsu, J.; McShane, A.; Sroor, A. Hemodynamic Deterioration in Lateral Compression Pelvic Fracture After Prehospital Pelvic Circumferential Compression Device Application. *Air Med. J.* **2017**, *36*, 272–274. [CrossRef] [PubMed]
26. Bakhshayesh, P.; Boutefnouchet, T.; Tötterman, A. Effectiveness of Non Invasive External Pelvic Compression: A Systematic Review of the Literature. *Scand. J. Trauma, Resusc. Emerg. Med.* **2016**, *24*, 73. [CrossRef] [PubMed]
27. STROBE Statement: Home. Available online: https://www.strobe-statement.org/index.php?id=strobe-home (accessed on 14 June 2020).
28. Olson, C.J.; Arthur, M.; Mullins, R.J.; Rowland, D.; Hedges, J.R.; Mann, N.C. Influence of Trauma System Implementation on Process of Care Delivered to Seriously Injured Patients in Rural Trauma Centers. *Surgery* **2001**, *130*, 273–279. [CrossRef]
29. van Olden, G.D.J.; Dik Meeuwis, J.; Bolhuis, H.W.; Boxma, H.; Goris, R.J.A. Clinical Impact of Advanced Trauma Life Support. *Am. J. Emerg. Med.* **2004**, *22*, 522–525. [CrossRef]
30. Siebert, H. White book of severely injured—Care of the DGU. Recommendations on structure, organization and provision of hospital equipment for care of severely injured in the Federal Republic of Germany. *Unfallchirurg* **2006**, *109*, 815–820. [CrossRef]
31. Rommens, P.M.; Hofmann, A. Comprehensive Classification of Fragility Fractures of the Pelvic Ring: Recommendations for Surgical Treatment. *Injury* **2013**, *44*, 1733–1744. [CrossRef]
32. Osler, T.; Baker, S.P.; Long, W. A Modification of the Injury Severity Score That Both Improves Accuracy and Simplifies Scoring. *J. Trauma Acute Care Surg.* **1997**, *43*, 922–926. [CrossRef]
33. Lavoie, A.; Moore, L.; LeSage, N.; Liberman, M.; Sampalis, J.S. The New Injury Severity Score: A More Accurate Predictor of In-Hospital Mortality than the Injury Severity Score. *J. Trauma Acute Care Surg.* **2004**, *56*, 1312–1320. [CrossRef]
34. Ringdal, K.G.; Coats, T.J.; Lefering, R.; Di Bartolomeo, S.; Steen, P.A.; Røise, O.; Handolin, L.; Lossius, H.M. Utstein TCD expert panel. The Utstein Template for Uniform Reporting of Data Following Major Trauma: A Joint Revision by SCANTEM, TARN, DGU-TR and RITG. *Scand. J. Trauma Resusc. Emerg. Med.* **2008**, *16*, 7. [CrossRef] [PubMed]
35. Tile, M. Pelvic Ring Fractures: Should They Be Fixed? *J. Bone Jt. Surg. Br.* **1988**, *70*, 1–12. [CrossRef] [PubMed]

36. Tile, M. Null Acute Pelvic Fractures: I. Causation and Classification. *J. Am. Acad. Orthop. Surg.* **1996**, *4*, 143–151. [CrossRef]
37. Judet, R.; Judet, J.; Letournel, E. Fractures of the acetabulum: Classification and surgical approaches for open reduction. Preliminary report. *J. Bone Jt. Surg. Am.* **1964**, *46*, 1615–1646. [CrossRef]
38. Sacral Fractures: An Important Problem. Retrospective Analysis of 236 Cases. Available online: https://europepmc.org/article/med/3338224 (accessed on 15 April 2020).
39. Tan, E.C.T.H.; van Stigt, S.F.L.; van Vugt, A.B. Effect of a New Pelvic Stabilizer (T-POD®) on Reduction of Pelvic Volume and Haemodynamic Stability in Unstable Pelvic Fractures. *Injury* **2010**, *41*, 1239–1243. [CrossRef] [PubMed]
40. Bryson, D.J.; Davidson, R.; Mackenzie, R. Pelvic Circumferential Compression Devices (PCCDs): A Best Evidence Equipment Review. *Eur. J. Trauma Emerg. Surg.* **2012**, *38*, 439–442. [CrossRef] [PubMed]
41. Vaidya, R.; Roth, M.; Zarling, B.; Zhang, S.; Walsh, C.; Macsuga, J.; Swartz, J. Application of Circumferential Compression Device (Binder) in Pelvic Injuries: Room for Improvement. *West. J. Emerg. Med.* **2016**, *17*, 766–774. [CrossRef]
42. Toth, L.; King, K.L.; McGrath, B.; Balogh, Z.J. Efficacy and Safety of Emergency Non-Invasive Pelvic Ring Stabilisation. *Injury* **2012**, *43*, 1330–1334. [CrossRef] [PubMed]
43. Bakhshayesh, P.; Heljesten, S.; Weidenhielm, L.; Enocson, A. Experience and Availability of Pelvic Binders at Swedish Trauma Units; A Nationwide Survey. *Bull. Emerg. Trauma* **2018**, *6*, 221–225. [CrossRef]
44. Jain, S.; Bleibleh, S.; Marciniak, J.; Pace, A. A National Survey of United Kingdom Trauma Units on the Use of Pelvic Binders. *Int. Orthop.* **2013**, *37*, 1335–1339. [CrossRef] [PubMed]
45. Zingg, T.; Piaget-Rossel, R.; Steppacher, J.; Carron, P.-N.; Dami, F.; Borens, O.; Albrecht, R.; Darioli, V.; Taffé, P.; Maudet, L.; et al. Prehospital Use of Pelvic Circumferential Compression Devices in a Physician-Based Emergency Medical Service: A 6-Year Retrospective Cohort Study. *Sci. Rep.* **2020**, *10*, 5106. [CrossRef]
46. Prasarn, M.L.; Small, J.; Conrad, B.; Horodyski, N.; Horodyski, M.; Rechtine, G.R. Does Application Position of the T-POD Affect Stability of Pelvic Fractures? *J. Orthop. Trauma* **2013**, *27*, 262–266. [CrossRef]
47. Wincheringer, D.; Langheinrich, A.; Schmidt-Horlohé, K.; Wohlrath, B.; Schröder, A.; Hoffmann, R.; Schweigkofler, U. *Analyse der Positionierung von Beckengurten in der Notfallversorgung von Instabilen Beckenfrakturen*; German Medical Science GMS Publishing House: Düsseldorf, Germany, 2015; pp. 29–1344.
48. Williamson, F.; Coulthard, L.G.; Hacking, C.; Martin-Dines, P. Identifying Risk Factors for Suboptimal Pelvic Binder Placement in Major Trauma. *Injury* **2020**. [CrossRef] [PubMed]
49. Naseem, H.; Nesbitt, P.; Sprott, D.; Clayson, A. An Assessment of Pelvic Binder Placement at a UK Major Trauma Centre. *Annals* **2017**, *100*, 101–105. [CrossRef]
50. Henning, S.; Norris, R.; Hill, C.E. Pelvic Binder Placement in a Regional Trauma Centre. *J. Paramed. Pract.* **2018**, *10*, 463–467. [CrossRef]
51. Knops, S.P.; Schep, N.W.L.; Spoor, C.W.; van Riel, M.P.J.M.; Spanjersberg, W.R.; Kleinrensink, G.J.; van Lieshout, E.M.M.; Patka, P.; Schipper, I.B. Comparison of Three Different Pelvic Circumferential Compression Devices: A Biomechanical Cadaver Study. *JBJS* **2011**, *93*, 230–240. [CrossRef]
52. How (Un)Useful Is the Pelvic Ring Stability Examination in Blunt Trauma Patients: Journal of Trauma and Acute Care Surgery. Available online: https://journals.lww.com/jtrauma/Fulltext/2009/03000/How__Un_Useful_is_the_Pelvic_Ring_Stability.34.aspx (accessed on 21 April 2020).
53. Schweigkofler, U.; Wohlrath, B.; Trentsch, H.; Greipel, J.; Tamimi, N.; Hoffmann, R.; Wincheringer, D. Diagnostics and Early Treatment in Prehospital and Emergency-Room Phase in Suspicious Pelvic Ring Fractures. *Eur. J. Trauma Emerg. Surg.* **2018**, *44*, 747–752. [CrossRef] [PubMed]
54. Significance of Physical Examination and Radiography of the Pelvis during Treatment in the Shock Emergency Room. Available online: https://europepmc.org/article/med/12955235 (accessed on 21 April 2020).
55. Magner, A.; Smith, N.; Douglin, T. Application of Pelvic Binders by Student Paramedics: An Observational Cohort Study. *J. Paramed. Pract.* **2019**, *11*, 526–531. [CrossRef]
56. Importance of the Correct Placement of the Pelvic Binder for Stabilisation of Haemodynamically Compromised Patients. Available online: https://europepmc.org/article/med/23296559 (accessed on 19 April 2020).
57. Fu, C.-Y.; Wu, Y.-T.; Liao, C.-H.; Kang, S.-C.; Wang, S.-Y.; Hsu, Y.-P.; Lin, B.-C.; Yuan, K.-C.; Kuo, I.-M.; Ouyang, C.-H. Pelvic Circumferential Compression Devices Benefit Patients with Pelvic Fractures Who Need Transfers. *Am. J. Emerg. Med.* **2013**, *31*, 1432–1436. [CrossRef]
58. Ganz, R.; Rj, K.; Rp, J.; Küffer, J. The Antishock Pelvic Clamp. *Clin. Orthop. Relat. Res.* **1991**, 71–78. [CrossRef]
59. Pohlemann, T.; Culemann, U.; Tosounidis, G.; Kristen, A. Application of the pelvic C-clamp. *Unfallchirurg* **2004**, *107*, 1185–1191. [CrossRef]
60. Tiemann, A.H.; Böhme, J.; Josten, C. Use of the pelvic clamp in polytraumatised patients with unstable disruption of the posterior pelvic ring. Modified technique—risks—problems. *Orthopade* **2006**, *35*, 1225–1236. [CrossRef]
61. Kellam, J.F. The Role of External Fixation in Pelvic Disruptions. *Clin. Orthop. Relat. Res.* **1989**, *241*, 66–82. [CrossRef]
62. Broos, P.; Vanderschot, P.; Craninx, L.; Reynders, P.; Rommens, P. Internal hemorrhages associated with fractures of the pelvic girdle. Importance of early stabilization using an external fixator. *Acta Orthop. Belg.* **1993**, *59*, 130–138. [PubMed]
63. Gänsslen, A.; Pohlemann, T.; Krettek, C. A simple supraacetabular external fixation for pelvic ring fractures. *Oper. Orthop. Traumatol.* **2005**, *17*, 296–312. [CrossRef] [PubMed]

64. Kim, W.Y.; Hearn, T.C.; Seleem, O.; Mahalingam, E.; Stephen, D.; Tile, M. Effect of Pin Location on Stability of Pelvic External Fixation. *Clin. Orthop. Relat. Res.* **1999**, 237–244. [CrossRef]
65. Rommens, P.M.; Hofmann, A.; Hessmann, M.H. Management of Acute Hemorrhage in Pelvic Trauma: An Overview. *Eur. J. Trauma* **2010**, *36*, 91–99. [CrossRef] [PubMed]
66. Schmal, H.; Larsen, M.S.; Stuby, F.; Strohm, P.C.; Reising, K.; Burri, K.G. Effectiveness and Complications of Primary C-Clamp Stabilization or External Fixation for Unstable Pelvic Fractures. *Injury* **2019**, *50*, 1959–1965. [CrossRef] [PubMed]
67. Audretsch, C.K.; Mader, D.; Bahrs, C.; Trulson, A.; Höch, A.; Herath, S.C.; Küper, M.A. Comparison of Pelvic C-Clamp and Pelvic Binder for Emergency Stabilization and Bleeding Control in Type-C Pelvic Ring Fractures. *Sci. Rep.* **2021**, *11*. [CrossRef]
68. Zeckey, C.; Cavalcanti Kußmaul, A.; Suero, E.M.; Kammerlander, C.; Greiner, A.; Woiczinski, M.; Braun, C.; Flatz, W.; Boecker, W.; Becker, C.A. The T-Pod Is as Stable as Supraacetabular Fixation Using 1 or 2 Schanz Screws in Partially Unstable Pelvic Fractures: A Biomechanical Study. *Eur. J. Med. Res.* **2020**, *25*. [CrossRef]
69. Spanjersberg, W.R.; Knops, S.P.; Schep, N.W.L.; van Lieshout, E.M.M.; Patka, P.; Schipper, I.B. Effectiveness and Complications of Pelvic Circumferential Compression Devices in Patients with Unstable Pelvic Fractures: A Systematic Review of Literature. *Injury* **2009**, *40*, 1031–1035. [CrossRef]
70. Jowett, A.J.L.; Bowyer, G.W. Pressure Characteristics of Pelvic Binders. *Injury* **2007**, *38*, 118–121. [CrossRef]
71. Knops, S.P.; van Riel, M.P.J.M.; Goossens, R.H.M.; van Lieshout, E.M.M.; Patka, P.; Schipper, I.B. Measurements of the Exerted Pressure by Pelvic Circumferential Compression Devices. *Open Orthop. J.* **2010**, *4*, 101–106. [CrossRef] [PubMed]
72. Knops, S.P.; Van Lieshout, E.M.M.; Spanjersberg, W.R.; Patka, P.; Schipper, I.B. Randomised Clinical Trial Comparing Pressure Characteristics of Pelvic Circumferential Compression Devices in Healthy Volunteers. *Injury* **2011**, *42*, 1020–1026. [CrossRef] [PubMed]

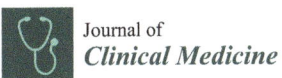

Article

Epidemiologic, Postmortem Computed Tomography-Morphologic and Biomechanical Analysis of the Effects of Non-Invasive External Pelvic Stabilizers in Genuine Unstable Pelvic Injuries

Christian Kleber [1,*], Mirja Haussmann [2], Michael Hetz [1], Michael Tsokos [3] and Claas T. Buschmann [3,4]

1. University Center of Orthopaedic, Trauma and Plastic Surgery, University Hospital Carl Gustav Carus, 01307 Dresden, Germany; Michael.Hetz@uniklinikum-dresden.de
2. Department of Anesthesiology and Operative Intensive Care Medicine, Charité-Universitätsmedizin, 10117 Berlin, Germany; mirja.haussmann@charite.de
3. Institute of Legal Medicine and Forensic Sciences, Charité-Universitätsmedizin, 10117 Berlin, Germany; michael.tsokos@charite.de (M.T.); Claas.Buschmann@uksh.de (C.T.B.)
4. Institute of Legal Medicine and Forensic Sciences, UKSH Universitätsklinikum Schleswig-Holstein, 24105 Kiel, Germany
* Correspondence: Christian.Kleber@uniklinikum-dresden.de; Tel.: +49-351-4583071

Citation: Kleber, C.; Haussmann, M.; Hetz, M.; Tsokos, M.; Buschmann, C.T. Epidemiologic, Postmortem Computed Tomography-Morphologic and Biomechanical Analysis of the Effects of Non-Invasive External Pelvic Stabilizers in Genuine Unstable Pelvic Injuries. *J. Clin. Med.* **2021**, *10*, 4348. https://doi.org/10.3390/jcm10194348

Academic Editor: Roman Pfeifer

Received: 30 July 2021
Accepted: 23 September 2021
Published: 24 September 2021

Publisher's Note: MDPI stays neutral with regard to jurisdictional claims in published maps and institutional affiliations.

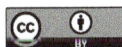

Copyright: © 2021 by the authors. Licensee MDPI, Basel, Switzerland. This article is an open access article distributed under the terms and conditions of the Creative Commons Attribution (CC BY) license (https://creativecommons.org/licenses/by/4.0/).

Abstract: Unstable pelvic injuries are rare (3–8% of all fractures) but are associated with a mortality of up to 30%. An effective way to treat venous and cancellous sources of bleeding prehospital is to reduce intrapelvic volume with external noninvasive pelvic stabilizers. Scientifically reliable data regarding pelvic volume reduction and applicable pressure are lacking. Epidemiologic data were collected, and multiple post-mortem CT scans and biomechanical measurements were performed on real, unstable pelvic injuries. Unstable pelvic injury was shown to be the leading source of bleeding in only 19%. All external non-invasive pelvic stabilizers achieved intrapelvic volume reduction; the T-POD® succeeded best on average (333 ± 234 cm^3), but with higher average peak traction (110 N). The reduction results of the VBM® pneumatic pelvic sling consistently showed significantly better results at a pressure of 200 mmHg than at 100 mmHg at similar peak traction forces. All pelvic stabilizers exhibited the highest peak tensile force shortly after application. Unstable pelvic injuries must be considered as an indicator of serious concomitant injuries. Stabilization should be performed prehospital with specific pelvic stabilizers, such as the T-POD® or the VBM® pneumatic pelvic sling. We recommend adjusting the pressure recommendation of the VBM® pneumatic pelvic sling to 200 mmHg.

Keywords: trauma; non-invasive external pelvic stabilizers; bleeding; pelvic fractures; post mortem analysis; biomechanical force; pneumatic pelvic sling VBM®; T-POD®; cloth sling; SAM Sling®

1. Introduction

With a proportion of 2–8%, pelvic fractures represent a rare injury. They occur most frequently in the 2nd and 3rd life decades [1] and are often the result of high-energy trauma, thus appearing in up to 20% of polytrauma patients [1,2]. Complex pelvic ring fractures are associated with a mortality rate of 5–42% [3–5]. In many cases, the high energy trauma causes extra and intrapelvic concomitant injuries, which can be life threatening [1,6]. Despite achieving improved survival rates in recent years, the mortality of open pelvic fractures is reported at up to 70% [1,7–9]. The immediate risk to life is linked to the possible occurrence of refractory hemorrhagic shock, with associated major coagulation disorders [3,8,10].

The pelvic ring is anatomically connected to many blood vessels [10]. Three main sources of hemorrhage are described. These include arterial bleeding from the great arterial pelvic vessels, the venous vascular system, and exposed cancellous fracture surfaces of the posterior pelvic ring [8,11–13]. Auto tamponade is unlikely due to torn retroperitoneal structures with potentially massive intrapelvic or retroperitoneal blood loss, which may lead to exsanguination [1,8]. It is important for modern priority-guided trauma management to detect the leading injury and source of immediate life threat ("treat first what kills first"). Therefore, in the first part of this study we analyzed the epidemiology of genuine pelvic injuries referring to the cause of death and primary bleeding source. The application of external non-invasive external pelvic stabilization is recommended in several guidelines and is nearly the only measure to treat unstable pelvic injuries in a prehospital setting [11,14,15].

A theoretical way to minimize bleeding, especially venous and spongy sources, is to reduce the intrapelvic volume with the approximate reduction of the fracture ends and closure of the anterior/posterior pelvic ring using external noninvasive pelvic stabilizers [13,16]. This hypothesis is based on clinical experience and two studies. Tan et al. revealed improved blood pressure in a small case series after the application of external non-invasive pelvic stabilization [17]. Grimm et al. showed increased retroperitoneal pressure in an artificial cadaver pelvic injury model via closed reduction with an external fixation of the pelvic ring and an infusion of the retroperitoneum [18]. Furthermore, several studies reveal the biomechanical impact of external non-invasive pelvic stabilization in artificial models of pelvic injuries [4,19–21]; however, the proof to reduced intrapelvine volume in unstable pelvic injuries is still missing.

Therefore, in the second part of this study, we analyzed for the first time the effects of different external noninvasive pelvic stabilizers on intrapelvic volume in real pelvic injuries using a postmortem CT scan and compared their effects on pelvic biomechanics.

2. Materials and Methods

This study is divided into a retrospective case series to collect epidemiologic data and a prospective intervention study to analyze the effect and biomechanical properties of external noninvasive pelvic stabilizers (Ethics Vote EA1/250/11). Substantial elements of this script are based on the dissertation by Dr. Haussmann [22].

In the retrospective part, all cases of deceased patients with mechanically unstable pelvic injuries in the archives of the Institute of Legal Medicine and Forensic Sciences, Charité-Universitätsmedizin, Berlin, were analyzed (n = 91). The survey period was 3 January 2012 to 30 September 2013. In addition to age and sex, accident mechanism, preclinical measures, and the place of death were investigated. Furthermore, the autopsy protocols were used to ascertain the cause of death, the leading bleeding source, and vascular injury in the abdominal and pelvic regions. Peripelvic bleeding was defined as bleeding sources around the bony pelvis, including vessel branches of the internal/external iliac vessels, muscles, soft tissue, and skin.

The second prospective interventional part of the study with the application of external pelvic stabilization and CT-guided measurements were performed from 3 January 2012 to 30 September 2013 (n = 36).

The inclusion criteria for both subprojects were legally authorized autopsy, death after traumatic injury, pelvic instability in physical examination, minimum age of 18 years, preserved integrity of the peripelvic soft tissues, and the absence of osteosynthetic treatment. Exclusion criteria were the emergency operations and invasive pelvic stabilization. The external pelvic stabilization devices tested were the following:

- The pneumatic pelvic sling Standard® (100 and 200 mmHg; VBM Medizintechnik GmbH, Sulz, Germany)
- T-POD® (Pyng Medical, Richmond, ON, Canada)
- Conventional cloth sling (bed sheet)
- SAM Pelvic Sling II® (SAM Medical Products, Wilsonville, OR, USA)

All devices were applied according to the study of Bottlang et al. at the level of the greater trochanters [4].

The breaking of rigor mortis was followed by the placement of the three devices for provisional external pelvic stabilization for the respective computed tomographic documentation of the compression effect of the fractured pelvis. The cranial limit of the scan area was chosen for these scans at the level of the third lumbar vertebrae and caudally at the level of the middle of the femur. A native image of the selected scan area was taken immediately prior to application of the corresponding device in each case to ensure a direct before and after comparison. All CT scans of the pelvic region were taken with a slice thickness of 0.5 mm (Activion 16; Toshiba).

To measure the traction forces, the different devices were prepared and a tension spring (Kraftaufnehmer OCDZ 0-3000N; Wazau Mess- und Prüfsysteme GmbH) was integrated (Figure 1).

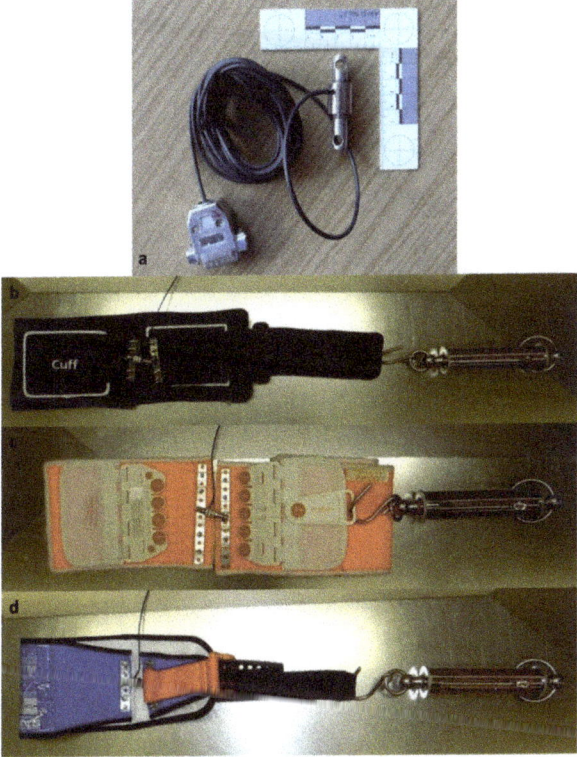

Figure 1. Used devices: (**a**) Newtonmeter; (**b**) Pneumatic pelvic sling VBM® prepared with Newtonmeter and tension spring; (**c**) T-POD® prepared with Newtonmeter and tension spring; (**d**) SAM Sling® prepared with Newtonmeter and tension spring (source: Haussmann [22], modified).

The calibration of the equipment was performed by a biomechanist of the Julius-Wolff-Institute of the Charité—Universitätsmedizin.

The documentation of the applied traction forces with the pelvic sling in place during the performance of CT scans was performed at four defined time points: 45 s (t1), 80 s (t2), and 120 s (t3). The maximum achieved traction force (Fmax)—independent of the time point—was also recorded.

Before and after application of the respective pelvic stabilization device, the volumetry of the pelvic ring, area of the pelvic entrance plane, distances between the centers of both femoral heads, the Köhler's tear figures, the sacroiliac joints ventrally and dorsally, and the distance/width of the symphysis were measured. The program OsiriX® (vers. 4.1, Pixmeo, Bernex, Switzerland) was used for image analysis.

For the volumetrics, the pelvis was primarily standardized in all three planes and distances were defined as follows (Figure 2):

- cranial to caudal: the junction between lumbar vertebrae 4 and 5 to the caudal end of the ischiatic tuber
- the area of pelvic entrance plane: the transverse plane between the lower edge of sacral vertebra 1 and the upper edge of the symphysis
- the symphysis width: the point of greatest distance between the pubic bones
- the femoral head distance: the distance between the centers of the femoral heads (in frontal plane)
- the distance between the Köhler's tear figures: the shortest distance between the most caudal poles (in frontal plane)
- the distance between the sacroiliac joints (SIJ): the ventral portions of the SIJ space, and for the dorsal distance, the most dorsal bony border of the Os ileum.

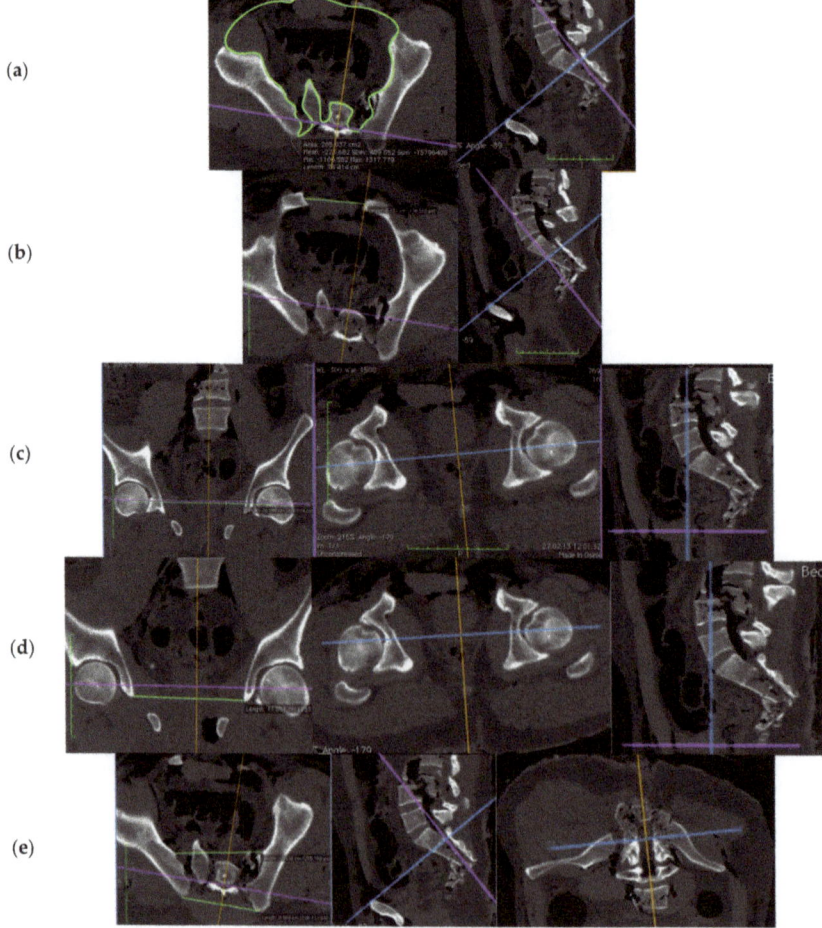

Figure 2. Representation of the different measurement planes and distances using OsiriX®: (**a**) pelvic entrance plane; (**b**) symphyseal width; (**c**) femoral head distance; (**d**) distance of Köhler's tear figures; (**e**) ventral and dorsal distance between sacroiliac joints (source: Haussmann [22], modified).

Data processing was performed using IBM SPSS Statistics 22® (IBM Corporation Armonk, NY, USA) and Microsoft Office Excel 2007® (Microsoft Corporation, Redmond, WA, USA). The Wilcoxon and Kolmogorov tests were applied for non-normally distributed variables and a paired t-test for normally distributed variables. The significance was assumed at a $p < 0.05$.

CT scans were again taken in the identical, standardized sequence on a total of six patients with mechanically unstable pelvic findings in the external cadaveric examination. In addition, the measurements were now supplemented by the application of the SAM Sling®.

All four pelvic slings were prepared with tension springs for the CT scans to document the acting tension forces after proper application.

3. Results

3.1. Epidemiological Data

Epidemiologic data was analyzed for 91 casualties, 36 from the prospective interventional study collective, and 55 patients after file review in the archives of the Institute of Legal and Forensic Medicine, Charité-Universitätsmedizin, Berlin.

The mean age of the 91 patients was 49 ± 19 years (range 18 to 92). 67 of the patients were male. 13% (n = 12) of deaths were caused by a traffic accident, in 23% (n = 21) by train rollover trauma, and in 64% (n = 58) by a fall from a substantial height. 79 patients (87%) died prehospital, and 12 patients (13%) died in the hospital (Figure 3).

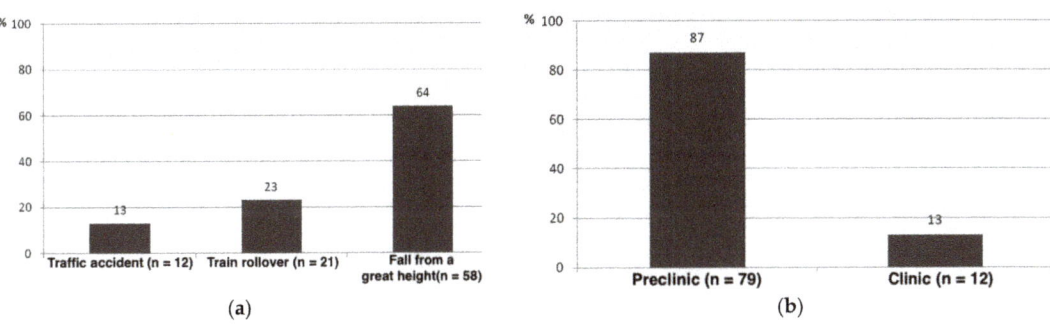

Figure 3. Distribution of accident mechanisms and localization of death (n = 91): (**a**) Most patients died as a result of a fall from a great height, followed by train rollovers and traffic accidents. (**b**) Majority of patients died in the prehospital setting (source: Haussmann [22], modified).

The leading sources of bleeding were thoracic, followed by peripelvic bleeding, hemorrhage of the liver, aortic rupture, and destruction of the heart. External sources of bleeding—due to transfemoral amputation—occurred in only one case. In 34% of the patients, a clear assignment of the main source of bleeding was not possible during autopsy due to multiple injuries (Figure 4).

As shown in Figure 4, thoracic concomitant injuries led the way, followed by peripelvic injuries and traumatic brain injury (Figure 5).

The cause of death was mainly multiple trauma (93%, n = 85). In 6% of the cases (n = 5), death occurred by exsanguination. In one patient (1%), traumatic brain injury was the cause of death.

Based on our postmortem CT scans, pelvic ring injuries were classified according to AO. Type C pelvic injuries were the most common in the studied population, and their distribution is shown in Figure 6.

Type B pelvic injuries were not detected in the studied collective. One patient with a type A pelvic injury was included in the study because of the clinical impression of the unstable pelvis during clinical stability testing for Ala fracture. A postmortem CT analysis revealed that it was a type A injury.

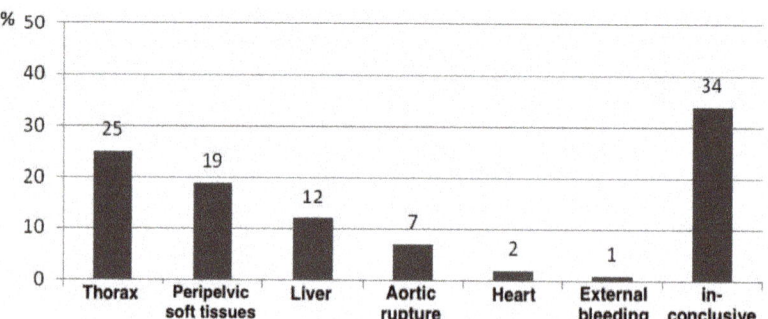

Figure 4. Overview of the main sources of hemorrhage in the examined collective: thoracic (25%, n = 23), followed by peripelvic (19%, n = 17) bleeding, hemorrhage of the liver (12%, n = 11), aortic rupture (7%, n = 6), and destruction of the heart (2%, n = 2). External sources of bleeding—due to transfemoral amputation—occurred in only one case (1%, n = 1). In 34% (n = 31) of the patients, a clear assignment of the main source of bleeding was not possible during autopsy due to multiple injuries. (Source: Haussmann [22], modified).

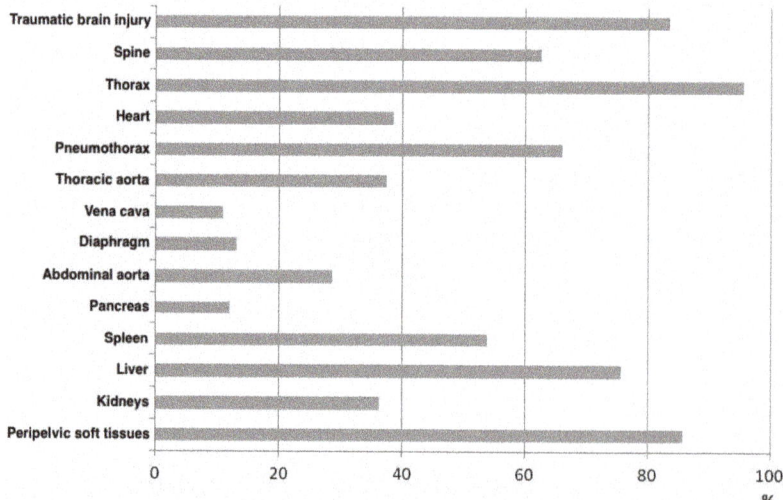

Figure 5. Summary of injury distribution in deceased patients with unstable pelvic injury: almost all patients showed thoracic injuries (96%, n = 87): 66% of patients (n = 60) had pneumothorax, 39% (n = 35) cardiac injury. Traumatic brain injury was documented in 84% (n = 76). Injuries to the spine in 63% (n = 57). 76% of patients (n = 69) showed injury to the liver, 54% (n = 49) to the spleen. Renal and pancreatic injuries were less frequent with 36% (n = 33) and 12% (n = 11), respectively. Diaphragmatic ruptures as a sign of extensive two-cavity trauma were detected in 13% of the collective (n = 12). In 37% of patients (n = 34), an injury to the aorta was found, in 29% (n = 26) of the thoracic aorta. In contrast, the superior or inferior vena cava was injured in 11% (n = 10). Peripelvic soft tissue damage was evident in 86% of the studied collective (n = 78). In 11% of the population (n = 10), the condition of the peripelvic soft tissues was not documented in the autopsy protocols (source: Haussmann [22], modified).

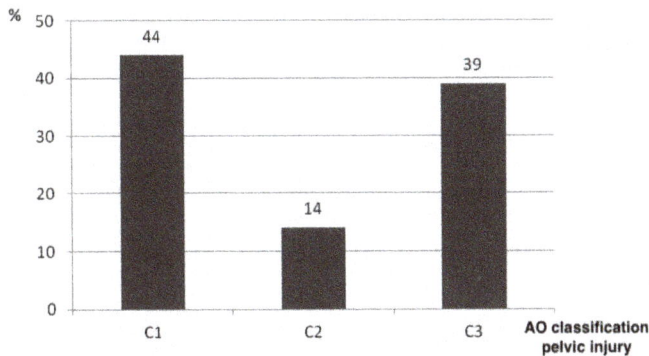

Figure 6. Distribution of type C pelvic injuries of the studied collective. Leading were type-C1 injuries, followed by type-C3 pelvic injuries (source: Haussmann [22], modified).

3.2. Effects on Pelvic Bioarchitecture of External, Non-Invasive Pelvic Stabilizers

The following results refer to the CT scans of the study population. Table 1 serves as a summary of the average intrapelvic volume reduction results of the external noninvasive pelvic stabilizers tested:

Table 1. Overview of the reduction results based on the mean values and standard deviation in direct comparison of the tested pelvic stabilizers to the native scans (PS1 = pneumatic pelvic sling VBM® with applied pressure of 100 mmHg; PS2 = pneumatic pelvic sling VBM® with applied pressure of 200 mmHg, TP = T-POD®; TS = cloth sling, SAM = SAM Sling®; SD = standard deviation; * $p < 0.001$; source: Haussmann [22], modified).

	Reduction of Intrapelvic Volume (cm³ ± SD)	Reduction Area Pelvic Entrance Level (cm ± SD)	Reduction Symphysis Width (cm ± SD)	Reduction Femoral Head Distance (cm ± SD)	Reduction Distance Köhler's Tear Figure (cm ± SD)	Reduction SIJ Distance Ventral (cm ± SD)	Reduction SIJ Distance Dorsal (cm ± SD)
PS1	268 * ± 185	34 * ± 29	1.1 ± 1.9	2.5 ± 1.3	2 ± 1.2	1.2 ± 0.9	0.8 ± 2
PS2	306 * ± 176	35 * ± 29	1.2 ± 2	2.9 ± 1.4	2.3 ± 1.2	1.4 ± 1	0.5 ± 1.3
TP	333 * ± 234	28 * ± 24	1.1 ± 1.8	2.1 ± 1.4	1.6 ± 1.1	1.1 ± 0.9	0.36 ± 1
TS	186 * ± 222	18 * ± 18	0.6 ± 1	1.1 ± 1	0.9 ± 0.8	0.7 ± 0.6	0.4 ± 1
SAM	184 ± 114	14 ± 8	0.06 ± 0.1	1.1 ± 0.5	0.9 ± 0.6	0.5 ± 0.4	-

All applied external non-invasive pelvic stabilizers were able to achieve a reduction of the area in the pelvic entrance plane, symphysis width, reduction of the femoral head distance, and reduction of the distance of the Köhler's tear figure, reduction of the ventral and dorsal distance of the ileosacral joint.

With regard to the reduction of intrapelvic volume (PV), the pneumatic pelvic sling VBM® with an applied pressure of 200 mmHg showed the best results (for detailed data please see Tables 1 and 2). This was followed in descending order by the VBM® at 100 mmHg the T-POD® and the cloth sling.

The results of the area reduction of the pelvic entrance level (PA) are, in descending order: pneumatic VBM® pelvic sling with 200 mmHg pressure, followed by the same with 100 mmHg, T-POD® and the cloth sling.

The comparison of the cloth sling with the pneumatic VBM® pelvic sling at an applied pressure of 100 mmHg showed significantly lower reduction results, regarding the reduction of symphysis width (SW).

Regarding femoral head distance (FH), the VBM® pneumatic pelvic sling at 200 mmHg also achieved the best reduction results. This was followed by VBM® at 100 mmHg, T-POD® ($p = 0.001$), and the cloth sling.

Table 2. Overview of the reduction results based on the mean values and standard deviation in direct comparison of the tested pelvic stabilizers to the native scans (PS1 = pneumatic pelvic sling VBM® with applied pressure of 100 mmHg; PS2 = pneumatic pelvic sling VBM® with applied pressure of 200 mmHg, TP = T-POD®; TS = cloth sling; SD = standard deviation; source: Haussmann [22], modified).

	PS1	PS2	TP	TS
P1	x			
P2	PV ($p = 0.002$) PA ($p < 0.001$) FH ($p < 0.001$) KT ($p < 0.001$) SIJv ($p < 0.001$)	x		
TP	KT ($p < 0.05$)	PA ($p = 0.004$) FH ($p = 0.001$) KT ($p = 0.001$) SIJv ($p < 0.05$)	x	
TS	PV ($p = 0.01$) PA ($p < 0.001$) SW ($p < 0.005$) FH ($p < 0.001$) KT ($p < 0.001$) SIJv ($p < 0.001$)	PV ($p < 0.001$) PA ($p < 0.001$) FH ($p < 0.001$) KT ($p < 0.001$) SIJv ($p < 0.001$)	PV ($p < 0.001$) PA ($p < 0.001$) FH ($p < 0.001$) KT ($p < 0.001$) SIJv ($p < 0.001$)	x

The reduction of the distance between Köhler's tear figures (KT) was again significantly better achieved by the pneumatic pelvic sling VBM® with 200 mmHg than with an applied pressure of 100 mmHg. The T-POD® followed. The cloth sling achieved significantly lower results.

Reduction of ventral ileosacral joint distance (SIJv) with the VBM® pneumatic pelvic sling at 200 mmHg also produced the best results, followed by 100 mmHg, T-POD®, and the cloth sling.

A comparison of the reduction in dorsal ileosacral joint (SIJd) distance among the pelvic stabilizers showed no significant differences.

3.3. Biomechanical Force Measurement of the Acting Tensile Forces after Pelvic Stabilizer Device

The average peak tensile force achieved by the VBM® pneumatic pelvic sling with a pressure of 100 mmHg was 73.4 ± 33.1 N. However, at already 45 s after application, the acting tensile forces were reduced to 54.9 ± 28.6 N, after 80 s to 49.4 ± 27.6 N and after 120 s to 46.4 ± 33.1 N. The average peak tensile force achieved at 200 mmHg was 81.5 ± 37.7 N. Here, too, the tensile forces decreased rapidly, as shown in Table 3.

Table 3. Mean values of the acting tensile forces of the five measurements with each of the four pelvic slings (PS1 = pneumatic sling VBM® with pressure of 100 mmHg, PS2 = pneumatic sling VBM® with pressure of 200 mmHg; TP = T-POD®; CS = cloth sling; SAM = SAM Sling®) at the defined time points (Fmax = maximum force; t1 = 45 sec after application; t2 = 80 sec after application; t3 = 120 s after application; source: Haussmann [22], modified)).

	PS1	PS2	TP	CS	SAM
Fmax [N]	73.4	81.5	109.9	105.2	132.3
t1 [N]	54.9	69	43.8	−4.4	30.6
t2 [N]	49.4	65.5	41.6	−4	29
t3 [N]	46.4	63.2	40.1	−4	27.9

The peak tensile force of 109.9 ± 40.5 N achieved by T-POD® was also reached immediately after application. Here, too, there was a decrease in the acting forces during the defined measurement times, which was more noticeable than in the case of the VBM® pneumatic pelvic sling (Table 3).

The peak tensile force of the cloth sling was on average 105.2 ± 72.6 N. It was noticeable that although there was a rapid reduction in the tensile force after the cloth loop was applied, the other measured values determined over time remained relatively stable.

The SAM Sling® was able to achieve high peak tensile forces, which—analogous to the other pelvic stabilizers tested—became apparent shortly after installation. The rapid decrease in the acting tensile forces was disproportionately strong: After only 45 s, an average of 30.6 ± 25.5 N was recorded. After 80 s, the average values were 29 ± 25.2 N and after 120 s 27.9 ± 24.9 N.

The peak force was reached immediately after application for all pelvic stabilizers. The measured tensile forces decreased rapidly over time for all external, non-invasive pelvic stabilizers. This was most evident with the cloth sling and the SAM Sling®. The VBM® pneumatic pelvic sling was able to demonstrate the lowest loss of traction over time at an applied pressure of 200 mmHg.

4. Discussion

To our knowledge, this work is the first to describe the biomechanical effects of noninvasive external pelvic stabilizers on the bony structures and intrapelvic volume of pelvic ring injuries. In addition, an epidemiologic analysis of concomitant injuries and autopsy results is performed.

4.1. Epidemiology of Pelvic Trauma

The epidemiologic results of this study are consistent with those reported by other authors. The majority of our collective was male (67%). In international study collectives, the polytrauma patient is male in approximately 70% of cases and has an average age of 38 to 47 years [23–25]. The determined mean age of 49 years may be due to demographic trends.

In our collective, metropolitan-specific trauma mechanisms emerged with predominantly falls from heights (64%), followed by train rollover trauma (23%) and traffic accidents (13%).

In contrast, data from recent years show that high-altitude falls account for an average of only 20–25% of trauma patient deaths [26,27]. Traffic accidents, to which rollover traumas from trains have often been added, are shown to cause death more frequently, up to 72%, especially in less densely populated areas [27,28].

Parreira et al. illustrated that, for a study population of 103 patients with unstable pelvic injuries, traffic accidents lead with 79% and falls from greater heights with only 17% [29]. These results were confirmed in further studies of patients with unstable pelvic fractures for both the Asian and Australian regions [30,31]. In a previous work, we were able to show already, in a 2010 study collective of trauma-related deaths that falls from heights appear as a frequent death-causing mechanism typical for Berlin [32].

However, our collective included only patients who died in the trauma setting; accordingly, a higher overall injury severity can be assumed. In a large proportion of our patient population (60%, n = 55), death occurred immediately as a result of the accidental event or shortly thereafter (before arrival of the emergency medical services). Consecutively, it can be assumed that the trauma mechanisms identified are causative for the higher overall injury severity in the collective evident in the autopsies.

The majority of patients in the studied collective (87%) died in the prehospital period, which can also be explained by the trauma severity and the high proportion of patients already with certain signs of death showing on finding. In an international comparison, the data on prehospital mortality of trauma patients show a wide range of 41–85% [27,32–35], which also seems to depend on the localization of the accident. While 72% of patients in rural areas died at the scene of the accident, only 41% did so in urban settings [35].

4.2. "Treat First What Kills First" in Pelvic Trauma

The patient collective with unstable pelvic injuries additionally showed very high incidences of injuries to or in the thorax (96%), peripelvic soft tissue injuries (86%), and traumatic brain injury (84%). However, unstable pelvic injury was shown to be the leading source of bleeding in only 19%; thoracic injuries were shown to be the main source of bleeding in our collective (25%).

This represents essential information, which has enormous influence on the prioritization of emergency and surgical management in patients with unstable pelvic injury. Several retrospective studies were found to be congruent with our findings: both Parreira et al. and Poole et al. postulated that although unstable pelvic injury carries a tremendous risk for the development of hemorrhagic shock, the outcome of patients is essentially dependent on concomitant injuries [29,36]. Poole et al. showed that of the 236 patients studied, 18 died, seven because of hemorrhagic shock [36]. However, only one patient was shown to have a pelvic major source of bleeding, whereas the remaining six patients died from extrapelvic major sources of bleeding [36].

For example, in our collective, 12% of patients showed injury to the liver alone as the leading major source of bleeding. Therefore, unstable pelvic injury should always be considered as an indicator of severe internal injury and bleeding until proven otherwise. Consequently, in the case of abdominal major sources of bleeding, for example, due to severe liver injury, clear preference should be given to laparotomy. These findings should be considered in ATLS/ETC concepts and applied to trauma management.

However, it should be kept in mind that in case of a necessary packing of the abdominal cavity in case of surgically uncontrollable bleeding, e.g., from the hepatic stromal area, the surgically stabilized pelvis is a better abutment.

4.3. Reproducibility of Genuine Pelvic Trauma with Artificial Pelvic Trauma Models

The case of misinterpretation of a type A fracture of the Ala ossis ileum as unstable pelvic injury shows some limitations of physical examination to determine pelvic ring instability. The definite diagnosis of a type B or type C pelvic ring injury is only possible by radiological imaging [37]. With a sensitivity of up to 93% [38,39], the result of the physical examination should nevertheless be relied upon and, if there is the slightest suspicion of an unstable pelvic injury, the stabilization of the pelvis by an external, noninvasive pelvic stabilizer should already be performed preclinically. The use of a pelvic stabilizer is indicated in cases of mechanically unstable pelvic ring fractures and simultaneous hemodynamic instability. If the pelvis is mechanically stable during the manual examination, pelvic instability is unlikely. If hemodynamics does not stabilize after application, arterial intrapelvic and extrapelvic sources of bleeding must be sought [40].

It is interesting to note that all other patients in our study collective had only Pennal and Tile type C unstable pelvic fractures. Type B fractures were not observed in our collective. The high applied forces during trauma will be causative for this. This fact should be further investigated and, if necessary, lead to a reevaluation of the artificial model and its applicability mostly using artificial type B injuries.

4.4. Effect of External Pelvic Stabilization in Real Pelvic Trauma

The results obtained with this study represent the first quantitative data on the effectiveness of external pelvic stabilizers in reducing various parameters of the pelvic area in non-artificial unstable pelvic injuries.

Most of the data published are studies of cadavers with artificially induced pelvic fractures and single case reports [19,20,41–47]. For the first time, we can present data on quantitative changes in intrapelvic volume, pelvic entrance area, and acting traction forces after the application of external noninvasive pelvic stabilizers to unstable pelvic injuries in real injured patients using computed tomographic imaging and biomechanical measurements.

All external non-invasive pelvic stabilizers achieved a reduction of intrapelvic volume. Therefore, if an unstable pelvic injury is suspected, an external, non-invasive pelvic stabilizer should be applied already in a prehospital setting. The T-POD® succeeded best on average (333 ± 234 cm³) but with higher average peak traction force (110 N) compared to the tested devices in this study. The reduction results of the VBM® pneumatic pelvic sling consistently showed significantly better results at an applied pressure of 200 mmHg than at 100 mmHg, with negligible differences in traction force (peak traction force 82 vs. 73 N). In terms of reduction of area in the pelvic entrance plane, the VBM® pneumatic pelvic sling demonstrated the greatest reduction effects in our study at 200 mmHg.

Since the peak traction forces differed only minimally at both pressures, as a result of this study, the recommendation for the adjustment of the recommended pressure level on the manometer of the VBM® pneumatic pelvic sling was adjusted to 200 mmHg by the manufacturer.

The distances between the femoral head and Köhler's tear figures showed excellent reduction results. In particular, the VBM® pneumatic pelvic sling was able to significantly reduce these parameters.

All pelvic stabilizers succeeded in reducing the symphysis width.

The results regarding the femoral head distance confirmed in each case the results of the area reduction in the pelvic entrance plane. Thus, for clinical practice, femoral head distance can be used as a simple surrogate parameter to control a sufficient reduction of the pelvis by means of pelvic overview imaging in pelvic ring fractures.

The comparison of reduction of the pelvic inlet area and the distances between the femoral heads and the Köhler's tear figures showed almost congruent results with mostly significantly better results of the pneumatic pelvic sling VBM®. Thus, these parameters are shown to be suitable as a measure for assessing the reduction of the anterior pelvic ring.

The relatively small reduction of the dorsal SIJ distance in combination with the predominantly good and congruent reduction results of the parameters of the ventral pelvic ring (femoral head distance, distance between the Köhler's tear figures, and symphysis width) suggests that external, non-invasive pelvic stabilizers ostensibly influence the ventral pelvic ring.

Assessing the reduction of dorsal SIJ distances for the effectiveness of external noninvasive pelvic stabilizers is severely limited. It can be speculated that especially instabilities in the area of the ventral pelvis can be sufficiently reduced by the application of an external, non-invasive pelvic stabilizer.

Stabilization by means of a conventional sling already has reducing effects. The lack of a pneumatic sling VBM®, T-POD®, SAM Sling®, or other devices designed for this purpose on emergency vehicles or rescue helicopters, should not and must not be considered as an argument against pelvic stabilization already performed prehospital.

Knops et al. demonstrated with their study that the T-POD® required the lowest traction forces compared to the SAM Sling® and the Pelvic Binder for a sufficient reduction of the symphysis width with an average of 43 N [20]. In our study, the T-POD® also required significantly lower peak traction forces than the SAM Sling® (130 N) with an average of 110 N. However, these were still well above the maximum force determined for the VBM® pneumatic pelvic sling (73 and 82 N at 100 and 200 mmHg, respectively).

The characteristic of reaching the highest peak force immediately after application was shared by all four tested external non-invasive pelvic stabilizers. However, our study revealed that the measured tensile forces then decreased rapidly during the time course. This effect was most evident with the cloth sling and the SAM Sling®. For example, the SAM Sling® showed a reduction in tensile forces of almost 80% after just two minutes. Knotting in the ventral pelvis or the nature of the material with consecutive loss of pressure is the main limitation of the use of a cloth sling. The results (high maximum force, rapid loss of force) can be well explained by the narrow design of the cloth sling: The cloth sling shows a width of only a few centimeters in the anterior region—if applied correctly—due to the ventral knotting technique. Interestingly, the high maximum tensile force measured did not have a higher reductive effect on the quality or effectiveness of the reduction of intrapelvic volume or pelvic entrance area. Our study was able to show that the reduction results of the cloth sling were significantly worse than those of the specific pelvic stabilizers. DeAngelis et al. demonstrated a significantly better reduction in symphysis width with the T-POD® compared to the cloth sling [19]. Our results correspond to previously published international literature: Knops et al. showed in their cadaver study that the SAM Sling® required significantly higher traction forces compared to the T-POD® and the Pelvic Binder for sufficient fracture reduction in type B as well as type C pelvic injuries (average 112 N vs. 43 N and 60 N, respectively), whereas the T-POD® succeeded in this reduction already at one third of the traction force [20].

Nevertheless, pelvic stabilization using a cloth sling should not be omitted, as it has proven beneficial effects on fracture reduction and presumably also on patient hemodynamics. If it is possible to use a specific device designed for pelvic stabilization, such as a pneumatic pelvic sling or the T-POD®, this should be preferred in any case.

All pelvic stabilizers exhibited the highest peak tensile force shortly after application, with rapid decreases in tensile forces over time (two minutes). This was most evident with SAM Sling® and cloth Sling.

Causes of pressure loss are likely to be pressure distribution in soft tissue, redistribution of interstitial and lymphatic fluid and blood into venous capacity vessels, and reduction of the pelvic injury.

As can be seen from the data in Table 3 and Figure 7, the forces generated by T-POD® and SAM Sling® were only initially the greatest and then quickly decreased. The pneumatic sling VBM®, on the other hand, was able to maintain the initially generated forces over a longer period of time. This could be an explanation for the better radiological reduction results.

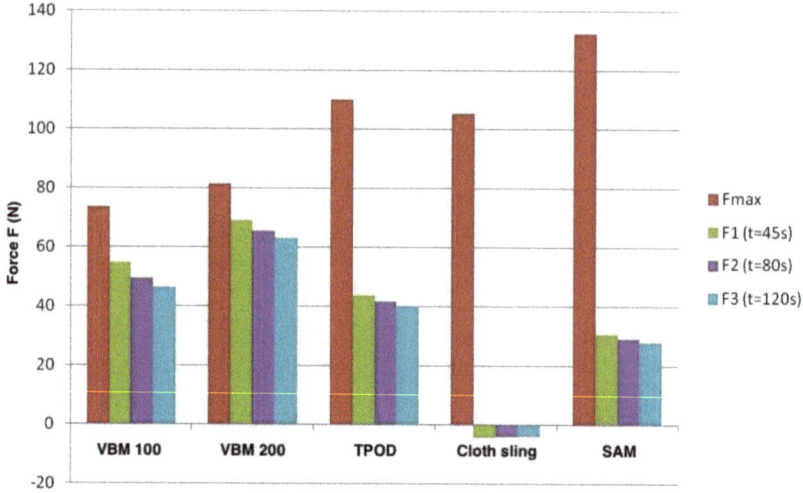

Figure 7. Kinetics of the pelvic stabilizers. Maximum and mean forces achieved at the various predefined times after application of the respective pelvic sling: The SAM Sling® was able to achieve the highest peak tensile forces, but that these fell rapidly and disproportionately. The most constant tensile force of all pelvic slings at the time points examined was demonstrated by the VBM® pneumatic pelvic sling with an applied pressure of 200 mmHg (source: Haussmann [22], modified).

In terms of intrapelvic volume reduction, the VBM® pneumatic pelvic sling showed a similar volume reduction compared to the T-POD® and predominantly achieved the best results in a comparison of all pelvic stabilizers, despite initially lower force application. Its advantage could be the arrangement of the pneumatic pads, which, when correctly placed, are each placed dorsolaterally on the pelvis. This achieves the compression of both pelvic sides, which could lead to more effective reduction results than purely circumferential application of force to the pelvis.

The T-POD®, on the other hand, achieved comparable reduction results, but required a significantly higher maximum force to do so. Over time, however, the reduction in intrapelvic volume is maintained, even under lower pressures.

This could be explained by the vector of the force but also by the amount of the initial applied pressure, which leads to an initial reduction. The lower forces over time could be sufficient to ensure the retention.

Critically, the exact time points of application of the external pelvic stabilizers after fracture or until the CT scan were not part of the data collection. Also, the experimental design could influence the results in that the VBM® pneumatic pelvic sling was applied prior to the T-POD®. It remains unclear to what extent some residual retention is maintained on the cadavers due, for example, to rigor mortis.

Bony fractures, possibly also with existing osteoporotic bone structure, were not observed after application of the various devices.

For clinical handling, a readjustment of the pelvic stabilizers may therefore be necessary. The pressure manometer of the VBM® pneumatic pelvic sling has the advantage that the user can measure the pressure and easily readjust.

5. Conclusions

Unstable pelvic injuries must be seen predominantly as an indicator of serious, especially thoracic and abdominal, concomitant injuries. In only a fifth of the analyzed cases, the pelvic injury was the leading bleeding source. This has a direct impact on clinical management and prioritization of emergency surgery within multiple trauma management.

Stabilization of unstable pelvic injuries should be performed as soon as possible using specific pelvic stabilizers, such as a T-POD® or pneumatic pelvic sling VBM®. A cloth sling should be used only in the absence of specific external pelvic stabilizers. To achieve optimal reduction results using a pneumatic pelvic sling VBM®, we advocate an adjustment of the recommended pressure application to 200 mmHg. The extent to which regular readjustment of the pelvic stabilizers is required should be further investigated in future studies.

The specific external, non-invasive pelvic stabilizers pneumatic pelvic sling VBM® and T-POD® could, for the most part, show significantly better reduction results compared to the conventional cloth sling. Therefore, the provision of these specific pelvic stabilizers should be demanded. The DIN standard for the equipment of rescue devices should be adapted.

Author Contributions: Conceptualization, C.K., M.H. (Mirja Haussmann), M.T. and C.T.B.; Formal analysis, C.K., M.H. (Michael Hetz), M.T. and C.T.B.; Investigation, C.K., M.H. (Mirja Haussmann). and M.H. (Michael Hetz); Methodology, M.H. (Mirja Haussmann), M.T. and C.T.B.; Resources, C.T.B.; Supervision, C.K.; Visualization, C.K. and M.H. (Michael Hetz); Writing—original draft, M.H. (Mirja Haussmann) and M.H. (Michael Hetz); Writing—review and editing, C.K., M.T., M.H. (Michael Hetz) and C.T.B. All authors have read and agreed to the published version of the manuscript.

Funding: This research received no external funding.

Institutional Review Board Statement: The study was conducted according to the guidelines of the Declaration of Helsinki and approved by the Ethics Committee of Charité-Universitätsmedizin, Berlin, Germany (ethical vote EA1/250/11).

Informed Consent Statement: Not applicable.

Acknowledgments: We would like to thank J. E. Ode for the calibration of the used equipment.

Conflicts of Interest: The authors declare no conflict of interest.

Limitations: Regarding the results of the SAM Sling® data collection, we explicitly point out the small number of cases used to investigate its properties compared to the other devices. Due to this methodological deficiency, we therefore distance ourselves from a recommendation of a model.

References

1. Esmer, E.; Derst, P.; Schulz, M.; Siekmann, H.; Delank, K.S.; das TraumaRegister DGU®. Einfluss der externen Beckenstabilisierung bei hämodynamisch instabilen Beckenfrakturen. *Unfallchirurg* **2017**, *120*, 312–319. [CrossRef]
2. Gänsslen, A.; Giannoudis, P.; Pape, H.-C. Hemorrhage in Pelvic Fracture: Who Needs Angiography? *Curr. Opin. Crit. Care* **2003**, *9*, 515–523. [CrossRef] [PubMed]
3. Scaglione, M.; Parchi, P.; Digrandi, G.; Latessa, M.; Guido, G. External Fixation in Pelvic Fractures. *Musculoskelet. Surg.* **2010**, *94*, 63–70. [CrossRef]
4. Bottlang, M.; Simpson, T.; Sigg, J.; Krieg, J.C.; Madey, S.M.; Long, W.B. Noninvasive Reduction of Open-Book Pelvic Fractures by Circumferential Compression. *J. Orthop. Trauma* **2002**, *16*, 367–373. [CrossRef] [PubMed]
5. Fu, C.-Y.; Wu, Y.-T.; Liao, C.-H.; Kang, S.-C.; Wang, S.-Y.; Hsu, Y.-P.; Lin, B.-C.; Yuan, K.-C.; Kuo, I.-M.; Ouyang, C.-H. Pelvic Circumferential Compression Devices Benefit Patients with Pelvic Fractures Who Need Transfers. *Am. J. Emerg. Med.* **2013**, *31*, 1432–1436. [CrossRef]
6. Schmal, H.; Markmiller, M.; Mehlhorn, A.T.; Sudkamp, N.P. Epidemiology and Outcome of Complex Pelvic Injury. *Acta Orthop. Belg* **2005**, *71*, 7.
7. Bakhshayesh, P.; Boutefnouchet, T.; Tötterman, A. Effectiveness of Non Invasive External Pelvic Compression: A Systematic Review of the Literature. *Scand. J. Trauma Resusc. Emerg. Med.* **2016**, *24*, 73. [CrossRef]
8. Heetveld, M.J.; Harris, I.; Schlaphoff, G.; Sugrue, M. Guidelines for the Management of Haemodynamically Unstable Pelvic Fracture Patients. *ANZ J. Surg.* **2004**, *74*, 520–529. [CrossRef]
9. Caillot, M.; Hammad, E.; Le Baron, M.; Villes, V.; Leone, M.; Flecher, X. Pelvic Fracture in Multiple Trauma: A 67-Case Series. *Orthop. Traumatol. Surg. Res.* **2016**, *102*, 1013–1016. [CrossRef]
10. Geeraerts, T.; Chhor, V.; Cheisson, G.; Martin, L.; Bessoud, B.; Ozanne, A.; Duranteau, J. Clinical Review: Initial Management of Blunt Pelvic Trauma Patients with Haemodynamic Instability. *Crit. Care* **2007**, *11*, 204. [CrossRef]
11. Hak, D.J.; Smith, W.R.; Suzuki, T. Management of Hemorrhage in Life-Threatening Pelvic Fracture. *J. Am. Acad. Orthop. Surg.* **2009**, *17*, 447–457. [CrossRef]
12. Jang, J.Y.; Shim, H.; Jung, P.Y.; Kim, S.; Bae, K.S. Preperitoneal Pelvic Packing in Patients with Hemodynamic Instability Due to Severe Pelvic Fracture: Early Experience in a Korean Trauma Center. *Scand. J. Trauma Resusc. Emerg. Med.* **2016**, *24*, 3. [CrossRef]
13. Riepl, C.; Beck, A.; Kraus, M. Präklinisches Management von Beckenverletzungen. *Der Notarzt* **2012**, *28*, 125–136. [CrossRef]
14. Lee, C.; Porter, K. The Prehospital Management of Pelvic Fractures. *Emerg. Med. J.* **2007**, *24*, 130–133. [CrossRef] [PubMed]
15. Schweigkofler, U. Is There Any Benefit in the Pre-Hospital Application of Pelvic Binders in Patients with Suspected Pelvic Injuries? *Eur. J. Trauma Emerg. Surg.* **2021**, *47*, 493–498. [CrossRef] [PubMed]
16. Scott, I.; Porter, K.; Laird, C.; Greaves, I.; Bloch, M. The Prehospital Management of Pelvic Fractures: Initial Consensus Statement. *Emerg. Med. J.* **2013**, *30*, 1070–1072. [CrossRef] [PubMed]
17. Tan, E.C.T.H.; van Stigt, S.F.L.; van Vugt, A.B. Effect of a New Pelvic Stabilizer (T-POD®) on Reduction of Pelvic Volume and Haemodynamic Stability in Unstable Pelvic Fractures. *Injury* **2010**, *41*, 1239–1243. [CrossRef]
18. Grimm, M.R.; Vrahas, M.S.; Thomas, K.A. Pressure-Volume Characteristics of the Intact and Disrupted Pelvic Retroperitoneum. *J. Trauma Acute Care Surg.* **1998**, *44*, 454–459. [CrossRef]
19. DeAngelis, N.A.; Wixted, J.J.; Drew, J.; Eskander, M.S.; Eskander, J.P.; French, B.G. Use of the Trauma Pelvic Orthotic Device (T-POD) for Provisional Stabilisation of Anterior–Posterior Compression Type Pelvic Fractures: A Cadaveric Study. *Injury* **2008**, *39*, 903–906. [CrossRef] [PubMed]
20. Knops, S.P.; Schep, N.W.L.; Spoor, C.W.; van Riel, M.P.J.M.; Spanjersberg, W.R.; Kleinrensink, G.J.; van Lieshout, E.M.M.; Patka, P.; Schipper, I.B. Comparison of Three Different Pelvic Circumferential Compression Devices: A Biomechanical Cadaver Study. *JBJS* **2011**, *93*, 230–240. [CrossRef]
21. Krieg, J.; Mohr, M.; Ellis, T.; Simpson, T.; Madey, S.; Bottlang, M. Emergent Stabilization of Pelvic Ring Injuries by Controlled Circumferential Compression: A Clinical Trial. *J. Trauma Inj. Infect. Crit. Care* **2005**, *59*, 659–664. [CrossRef]
22. Haussmann, M.M. Epidemiologische, Postmortale Computertomographie—Morphologische Und Biomechanische Analyse Der Effekte Nicht-Invasiver Externer Beckenstabilisatoren Bei Reellen Instabilen Beckenverletzungen. Ph.D. Thesis, Universitätsmedizin Berlin, Berlin, Germany, 2018. [CrossRef]
23. Bardenheuer, M.; Obertacke, U.; Waydhas, C.; Nast-Kolb, D. Epidemiology of the severe multiple trauma-a prospective registration of preclinical and clinical supply. *J. Orthop. Trauma* **2000**, *14*, 453. [CrossRef]
24. Cothren, C.C.; Moore, E.E.; Hedegaard, H.B.; Meng, K. Epidemiology of Urban Trauma Deaths: A Comprehensive Reassessment 10 Years Later. *World J. Surg.* **2007**, *31*, 1507–1511. [CrossRef] [PubMed]
25. Siegmeth, A.; Müllner, T.; Kukla, C.; Vécsei, V. Begleitverletzungen beim schweren Beckentrauma. *Der Unfallchirurg* **2000**, *103*, 572–581. [CrossRef]
26. Søreide, K.; Krüger, A.J.; Vårdal, A.L.; Ellingsen, C.L.; Søreide, E.; Lossius, H.M. Epidemiology and Contemporary Patterns of Trauma Deaths: Changing Place, Similar Pace, Older Face. *World J. Surg.* **2007**, *31*, 2092–2103. [CrossRef]
27. Pang, J.-M.; Civil, I.; Ng, A.; Adams, D.; Koelmeyer, T. Is the Trimodal Pattern of Death after Trauma a Dated Concept in the 21st Century? Trauma Deaths in Auckland 2004. *Injury* **2008**, *39*, 102–106. [CrossRef]
28. Evans, J.A.; van Wessem, K.J.P.; McDougall, D.; Lee, K.A.; Lyons, T.; Balogh, Z.J. Epidemiology of Traumatic Deaths: Comprehensive Population-Based Assessment. *World J. Surg.* **2010**, *34*, 158–163. [CrossRef]

29. Gustavo Parreira, J.; Coimbra, R.; Rasslan, S.; Oliveira, A.; Fregoneze, M.; Mercadante, M. The Role of Associated Injuries on Outcome of Blunt Trauma Patients Sustaining Pelvic Fractures. *Injury* **2000**, *31*, 677–682. [CrossRef]
30. Dong, J.; Zhou, D. Management and Outcome of Open Pelvic Fractures: A Retrospective Study of 41 Cases. *Injury* **2011**, *42*, 1003–1007. [CrossRef]
31. Esser, M.; Gabbe, B.; de Steiger, R.; Bucknill, A.; Russ, M.; Cameron, P. Predictors of Mortality Following Severe Pelvic Ring Fracture: Results of a Population-Based Study. *Orthop. Proc.* **2012**, *94*, 133. [CrossRef]
32. Kleber, C.; Giesecke, M.T.; Tsokos, M.; Haas, N.P.; Schaser, K.D.; Stefan, P.; Buschmann, C.T. Overall Distribution of Trauma-Related Deaths in Berlin 2010: Advancement or Stagnation of German Trauma Management? *World J. Surg.* **2012**, *36*, 2125–2130. [CrossRef]
33. Sobrino, J.; Shafi, S. Timing and Causes of Death After Injuries. *Bayl. Univ. Med. Cent. Proc.* **2013**, *26*, 120–123. [CrossRef]
34. Wisborg, T.; Høylo, T.; Siem, G. Death after Injury in Rural Norway: High Rate of Mortality and Prehospital Death. *Acta Anaesthesiol. Scand.* **2003**, *47*, 153–156. [CrossRef] [PubMed]
35. Rogers, F.B.; Shackford, S.R.; Hoyt, D.B.; Camp, L.; Osler, T.M.; Mackersie, R.C.; Davis, J.W. Trauma Deaths in a Mature Urban vs. Rural Trauma System: A Comparison. *Arch. Surg.* **1997**, *132*, 376–382. [CrossRef] [PubMed]
36. Poole, G.V.; Ward, E.F.; Muakkassa, F.F.; Hsu, H.S.; Griswold, J.A.; Rhodes, R.S. Pelvic Fracture from Major Blunt Trauma. Outcome Is Determined by Associated Injuries. *Ann. Surg.* **1991**, *213*, 532–539. [CrossRef]
37. Ballard, R.B.; Rozycki, G.S.; Newman, P.G.; Cubillos, J.E.; Salomone, J.P.; Ingram, W.L.; Feliciano, D.V. An Algorithm to Reduce the Incidence of False-Negative FAST***Focused Assessment for the Sonographic Examination of the Trauma Patient. Examinations in Patients at High Risk for Occult Injury11No Competing Interests Declared. *J. Am. Coll. Surg.* **1999**, *189*, 145–150. [CrossRef]
38. Culemann, U.; Oestern, H.J.; Pohlemann, T. Aktuelle Behandlung der Beckenringfraktur. *Unfallchirurg* **2014**, *117*, 145–161. [CrossRef]
39. Sauerland, S.; Bouillon, B.; Rixen, D.; Raum, M.R.; Koy, T.; Neugebauer, E.A.M. The Reliability of Clinical Examination in Detecting Pelvic Fractures in Blunt Trauma Patients: A Meta-Analysis. *Arch. Orthop. Trauma Surg.* **2004**, *124*, 123–128. [CrossRef]
40. Arbeitsgruppe Trauma des Deutschen Rats für, Wiederbelebung; Roessler, M.S.; Buschmann, C.; Gliwitzky, B.; Hoedtke, J.; Kulla, M.; Wurmb, T.; Kleber, C. Externe, nichtinvasive Beckenstabilisatoren—Wann ist die Anlage indiziert?: Eine Empfehlung der Arbeitsgruppe Trauma des Deutschen Rats für Wiederbelebung. *Notf. Rett.* **2021**. [CrossRef]
41. Szalay, G.; Meyer, C.; Schaumberg, A.; Mann, V.; Weigand, M.A.; Schnettler, R. Stabilisierung instabiler Beckenfrakturen mittels pneumatischer Beckenschlinge im Schockraum. *Notf. Rett.* **2010**, *13*, 47–51. [CrossRef]
42. Simpson, T.; Krieg, J.C.; Heuer, F.; Bottlang, M. Stabilization of Pelvic Ring Disruptions with a Circumferential Sheet. *J. Trauma Acute Care Surg.* **2002**, *52*, 158–161. [CrossRef]
43. Warme, W.J.; Todd, M.S. The Circumferential Antishock Sheet. *Mil. Med.* **2002**, *167*, 438–441. [CrossRef]
44. Rudol, G.; Ramdass, S.; Mestha, P.; Doughan, S.; Skyrme, A. Major Pelvic Injury Complicated by Abdominal Compartment Syndrome. *Inj. Extra* **2006**, *8*, 299–301. [CrossRef]
45. Routt, C.M.L.J.; Falicov, A.; Woodhouse, E.; Schildhauer, T.A. Circumferential Pelvic Antishock Sheeting: A Temporary Resuscitation Aid. *J. Orthop. Trauma* **2002**, *16*, 45–48. [CrossRef] [PubMed]
46. Prasarn, M.L.; Conrad, B.; Small, J.; Horodyski, M.; Rechtine, G.R. Comparison of Circumferential Pelvic Sheeting versus the T-POD on Unstable Pelvic Injuries: A Cadaveric Study of Stability. *Injury* **2013**, *44*, 1756–1759. [CrossRef] [PubMed]
47. Bonner, T.J.; Eardley, W.G.P.; Newell, N.; Masouros, S.; Matthews, J.J.; Gibb, I.; Clasper, J.C. Accurate Placement of a Pelvic Binder Improves Reduction of Unstable Fractures of the Pelvic Ring. *J. Bone Jt. Surg. Br.* **2011**, *93*, 1524–1528. [CrossRef] [PubMed]

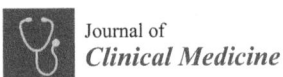

Article

Severe Traumatic Injury Induces Phenotypic and Functional Changes of Neutrophils and Monocytes

Andrea Janicova [1,2], Nils Becker [1,2,3], Baolin Xu [1], Marija Simic [1], Laurens Noack [1], Nils Wagner [2], Andreas J. Müller [4,5], Jessica Bertrand [6], Ingo Marzi [2] and Borna Relja [1,*]

1. Experimental Radiology, Department of Radiology and Nuclear Medicine, Otto-von-Guericke-University Magdeburg, Leipziger Straße 44, 39120 Magdeburg, Germany; andrea.janicova@med.ovgu.de (A.J.); nibecker@ukaachen.de (N.B.); xubaolin325@outlook.com (B.X.); marija.simic@med.ovgu.de (M.S.); laurens.noack@st.ovgu.de (L.N.)
2. Department of Trauma, Hand and Reconstructive Surgery, Goethe University, Theodor-Stern-Kai 7, 60590 Frankfurt am Main, Germany; nils.wagner@kgu.de (N.W.); ingo.marzi@kgu.de (I.M.)
3. Department of Trauma Surgery, Hospital of the RWTH University, Pauwelsstraße 30, 52074 Aachen, Germany
4. Institute of Molecular and Clinical Immunology, Health Campus Immunology Infectiology and Inflammation, Otto-von-Guericke-University Magdeburg, Leipziger Straße 44, 39120 Magdeburg, Germany; andreas.mueller@med.ovgu.de
5. Intravital Microscopy in Infection and Immunity, Helmholtz Centre for Infection Research, Inhoffenstraße 7, 38124 Braunschweig, Germany
6. Department of Orthopaedic Surgery, Otto-von-Guericke University Magdeburg, Leipziger Straße 44, 39120 Magdeburg, Germany; jessica.bertrand@med.ovgu.de
* Correspondence: borna.relja@med.ovgu.de; Tel.: +49-(0)391-6728242; Fax: +49-(0)391-6728248

Citation: Janicova, A.; Becker, N.; Xu, B.; Simic, M.; Noack, L.; Wagner, N.; Müller, A.J.; Bertrand, J.; Marzi, I.; Relja, B. Severe Traumatic Injury Induces Phenotypic and Functional Changes of Neutrophils and Monocytes. *J. Clin. Med.* 2021, 10, 4139. https://doi.org/10.3390/jcm10184139

Academic Editor: Roman Pfeifer

Received: 31 August 2021
Accepted: 11 September 2021
Published: 14 September 2021

Publisher's Note: MDPI stays neutral with regard to jurisdictional claims in published maps and institutional affiliations.

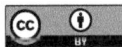

Copyright: © 2021 by the authors. Licensee MDPI, Basel, Switzerland. This article is an open access article distributed under the terms and conditions of the Creative Commons Attribution (CC BY) license (https://creativecommons.org/licenses/by/4.0/).

Abstract: Background: Severe traumatic injury has been associated with high susceptibility for the development of secondary complications caused by dysbalanced immune response. As the first line of the cellular immune response, neutrophils and monocytes recruited to the site of tissue damage and/or infection, are divided into three different subsets according to their CD16/CD62L and CD16/CD14 expression, respectively. Their differential functions have not yet been clearly understood. Thus, we evaluated the phenotypic changes of neutrophil and monocyte subsets among their functionality regarding oxidative burst and the phagocytic capacity in severely traumatized patients. Methods: Peripheral blood was withdrawn from severely injured trauma patients (TP; $n = 15$, ISS ≥ 16) within the first 12 h post-trauma and from healthy volunteers (HV; $n = 15$) and stimulated with fMLP and PMA. CD16^{dim}CD62L^{bright} (immature), CD16^{bright}CD62L^{bright} (mature) and CD16^{bright}CD62L^{dim} (CD62L^{low}) neutrophil subsets and CD14^{bright}CD16^{-} (classical), CD14^{bright}CD16^{+} (intermediate) and CD14^{dim}CD16^{+} (non-classical) monocyte subsets of HV and TP were either directly analyzed by flow cytometry or the examined subsets of HV were sorted first by fluorescence-activated cell sorting and subsequently analyzed. Subset-specific generation of reactive oxygen species (ROS) and of *E. coli* bioparticle phagocytosis were evaluated. Results: In TP, the counts of immature neutrophils were significantly increased vs. HV. The numbers of mature and CD62L^{dim} neutrophils remained unchanged but the production of ROS was significantly enhanced in TP vs. HV and the stimulation with fMLP significantly increased the generation of ROS in the mature and CD62L^{dim} neutrophils of HV. The counts of phagocyting neutrophils did not change but the mean phagocytic capacity showed an increasing trend in TP. In TP, the monocytes shifted toward the intermediate phenotype, whereas the classical and non-classical monocytes became less abundant. ROS generation was significantly increased in all monocyte subsets in TP vs. HV and PMA stimulation significantly increased those level in both, HV and TP. However, the PMA-induced mean ROS generation was significantly lower in intermediate monocytes of TP vs. HV. Sorting of monocyte and neutrophil subsets revealed a significant increase of ROS and decrease of phagocytic capacity vs. whole blood analysis. Conclusions: Neutrophils and monocytes display a phenotypic shift following severe injury. The increased functional abnormalities of certain subsets may contribute to the dysbalanced immune response and attenuate the antimicrobial function and thus, may represent a potential therapeutic target. Further studies on isolated subsets are necessary for evaluation of their physiological role after severe traumatic injury.

Keywords: traumatic injury; reactive oxygen species; phagocytosis; CD14; CD16; CD62L; fMLP; PMA

1. Introduction

Severe traumatic injury is with 5.8 million annual deaths one of the most common causes of death worldwide [1]. Although the survival rates have improved globally in the past decades due to advanced post-traumatic treatment, the development of immune-related secondary complications such as systemic inflammatory response syndrome, nosocomial infections, or sepsis, remains the major contributing factor in trauma-associated mortality [2–4]. Approximately 55% of polytrauma patients suffer from severe chest injury, leading to a direct lung tissue damage on the one hand and to activation of inflammatory response on the other hand, resulting in alveolocapillary membrane breakdown [5]. These patients are highly susceptible for disseminated intravascular coagulation, pneumonia, as well as acute lung injury, and its more severe form acute respiratory distress syndrome (ARDS) [5]. ARDS is associated with a dysregulated immune response, an overall mortality between 35% and 50%, and treatment of those patients is limited [6]. An excessive generation of ROS by the injured endothelium and epithelium as well as recruited leukocytes play a major role in ARDS progression and lung damage [7]. Moreover, a dysregulated immune response after trauma has been associated with post-traumatic phenotypical and functional aberrations of certain cells of the innate immune system such as neutrophils and monocytes [7–10].

Neutrophils and monocytes represent the first line of immune defense following an infection or a sterile injury [11,12]. Both are released from the bone marrow into the circulation and are recruited to sites of infection or tissue damage towards the pathogen-derived signaling molecules (pathogen-associated molecular patterns) or host-produced inflammatory signaling molecules (damage-associated molecular patterns), respectively [11,12]. The ability to recognize and eliminate bacteria and debris is critical for timely resolution of inflammation and recovery from the injury [13,14]. An impairment of phagocytic activity ex vivo has been observed in patients with community-acquired pneumonia [15], spinal cord injury [16] and traumatic brain injury [17,18] compared to healthy individuals. Moreover, neutrophil depletion impedes the clearance of the debris from necrotic sites in sterile hepatic injury, leading to impairment of regeneration and revascularization of the focal injury [10]. As some neutrophils in human peripheral neutrophil pool phagocyte their targets better than others [19], certain neutrophil populations may have differential functionality in this process.

Although the production of reactive oxygen species (ROS) is essential for the pathogen clearance, an exaggerated release of proteases and oxygen radicals may lead to collateral tissue damage and contribute to the development of secondary complications [20,21]. In the context of acute lung injury or its most severe form ARDS, excessive generation of ROS leads to the loss of junctional integrity of vascular microvessels, promoting the migration of polymorphonuclear leukocytes and the transition of fluids in the alveolar lumen, causing pulmonary edema [7].

Three different subsets of neutrophils were described according to their expression of the cluster of differentiation (CD)16 and CD62L expression [22]. $CD16^{dim}CD62L^{bright}$ subset shows the characteristics of immature neutrophils with banded nuclei, $CD16^{bright}CD62L^{bright}$ population represents the mature neutrophils with prototypically segmented nuclei, and $CD16^{bright}CD62L^{dim}$ neutrophils are characterized by hypersegmented nuclei. The latter have been shown to directly suppress lymphocyte proliferation by ROS release into the immunological synapse between neutrophil and T-cell, suggesting its immunosuppressive features [22]. Although all neutrophil subsets enter the circulation almost immediately after trauma, their precise post-traumatic function still remains elusive [8].

Similarly, three different subsets of monocyte can be distinguished according to their CD16 and CD14 surface expression [23,24]. Classical monocytes, characterized by

$CD16^-CD14^{bright}$ expression contribute to bacterial clearing and immune sensing, whereas non-classical $CD16^+CD14^{dim}$ monocytes patrol along the blood vessel walls [25]. Intermediate $CD16^+CD14^{bright}$ monocytes share particularly the functions of classical and non-classical subsets but have more pro-inflammatory features and have been linked to the regulation of apoptosis and transendothelial migration [23,24]. Following human experimental endotoxemia, all monocyte subsets are lost within one to two hours after lipopolysaccharide administration and recover from classical, over intermediate to non-classical monocytes within 8–24 h [9]. This clearly confirms the generally accepted theory, that monocyte subsets differentiate from classical to intermediate and non-classical monocytes in a dynamic process. There is no evidence about the subset dynamics including specific kinetics and functions following traumatic injury in humans.

Considering that a well-orchestrated immune response is essential for the initiation and subsequent resolution of inflammation and an adverse phenotype and functional transition of neutrophils and monocytes may negatively affect the post-traumatic outcome, we evaluated the phenotypic shift of neutrophils and monocytes as well as their phagocytic capacity and ROS production in the currently known subsets of those cell types.

We hypothesized that major traumatic injury shifts the cell subset ratios toward the pro-inflammatory phenotypes early after trauma and that along with this, the circulatory cells will exert modified functions regarding phagocytosis and oxidative burst.

2. Materials and Methods

2.1. Ethics

The current study was performed at the University Hospital of the Goethe-University Frankfurt in accordance with the Declaration of Helsinki and following the Strengthening the Reporting of Observational studies in Epidemiology-guidelines [26].

2.2. Patient Cohort

Fifteen healthy volunteers and 15 severely injured patients between 18 and 50 years of age were enrolled. Trauma patients with an injury severity score (ISS) $\geq$ 16 were included and the samples were collected and analyzed within the first 12 h post-injury. Exclusion criteria included an acute infection, pre-existing chronic inflammatory diseases, immunological disorders, human immunodeficiency virus infection, infectious hepatitis, immunosuppressive medication, and pregnancy.

2.3. Staining of Neutrophil and Monocyte Subsets for Flow Cytometry

The blood of trauma patients and healthy volunteers was withdrawn into Li-Heparin blood collection tube (Sarstedt, Nümbrecht, Germany), stored on ice and processed within 30 min. A total of 100 µL of heparinized blood was transferred into FACS tube (Corning, New York, NY, USA). For neutrophils, heparinized blood was stimulated with 1×10^{-3} mM N-formyl-methionyl-leucyl-phenylalanine (fMLP) on ice for 15 min. Subsequently, samples were washed with 2 mL ice-cold FACS buffer (0.5% bovine serum albumin in 1× phosphate-buffered saline (PBS) without Mg^{2+} and Ca^{2+}), gently vortexed, and centrifuged at 350× g and at 4 °C for 7 min. After the supernatant was discarded, 5 µL Alexa Fluor 647-conjugated anti-human CD16 antibody (clone 3G8; BD Biosciences, Franklin Lakes, NJ, USA) and 20 µL PE-conjugated anti-human CD62L antibody (clone SK11; BD Biosciences, USA) were added. For monocytes, heparinized blood was stimulated with 1×10^{-4} mM phorbol 12-myristate 13-acetate (PMA) on ice for 15 min. Subsequently, the samples were washed. 5 µL Alexa Fluor 647-conjugated anti-human CD16 antibody (clone 3G8; BD Biosciences, USA) and 5 µL PE-conjugated anti-human CD14 antibody (clone M5E2; BioLegend, San Diego, CA, USA) were added, all samples gently vortexed and incubated in the dark on ice for 30 min. Subsequently, the samples were washed. Then, the protocols for functional analyses regarding the phagocytic capacity (see Section 2.4) and ROS generation (see Section 2.5) followed as described below.

2.4. Analysis of Bacterial Intake by Neutrophils by Flow Cytometry

FITC-labeled *E. coli* bioparticles were reconstituted in 1× PBS without Mg^{2+} and Ca^{2+} according to the manufacturer's instructions (*Escherichia coli* (K-12 strain) BioParticles E-2861; Thermo Fisher Scientific, Waltham, MA, USA), aliquoted and stored at −20 °C and in dark until use. In the experiment, 10 bioparticles per leukocyte were added to the sample and incubated at 37 °C and 5% CO_2 for 60 min. Following "bacterial" loading, cells were washed with 2 mL ice-cold FACS buffer and centrifuged at 350× *g* and at 4 °C for 7 min. For red blood cells lysis, 2 mL cold lysis buffer were added, and the samples were incubated in the dark at 4 °C for 10 min. Washing step with 2 mL ice-cold FACS buffer was repeated. Cells were resuspended in 500 µL ice-cold FACS buffer and immediately evaluated by flow cytometry. Granulocytes were defined by gating the corresponding forward and side scatter scan. From each sample a minimum of 5.0×10^4 cells were measured, which were subsequently analyzed. The percentage of $CD16^{dim}CD62L^{bright}$ (immature), $CD16^{bright}CD62L^{bright}$ (mature) and $CD16^{bright}CD62L^{dim}$ (hypersegmented) neutrophils as well the percentage and mean fluorescent units of phagocytosis-positive out of the respective subsets were assessed by flow cytometric analyses using a BD FACSCanto 2™ and FACS DIVA™ software (BD Biosciences, USA).

2.5. Analysis of Reactive Oxygen Species Production in Neutrophils and Monocytes by Flow Cytometry

Totals of 90 µL warm PBS and 2 µL 100 µM CM-H $_2$DCFDA (Thermo Fisher Scientific, USA) were added to samples (see Section 2.3) and incubated at 37 °C and 5% CO_2 for 30 min. 2 mL warm RPMI 1640 medium (Gibco, Carlsbad, CA, USA), supplemented with 10% heat-inactivated fetal calf serum (Gibco, Carlsbad, CA, USA), 100 IU/mL penicillin (Gibco, USA), 10 µg/mL streptomycin (Gibco, Carlsbad, CA, USA) and 20 mM HEPES buffer (Sigma Aldrich, St. Lois, MO, USA) were added and samples were centrifuged at 350× *g* and at room temperature for 7 min. Supernatant was discarded and subsequently, 1 mL medium with supplements was added and the samples were incubated at 37 °C and 5% CO_2 for further 60 min. Following the recovery step, samples were centrifuged at 350× *g* and at room temperature for 7 min and the supernatant was discarded. For red blood cells lysis, 2 mL lysis buffer (0.155 M NH_4Cl, 0.01 M $KHCO_3$, 0.1 mM ethylenediaminetetraacetic acid in distilled water) were added and incubated in the dark at 4 °C for 10 min. Washing step with 2 mL ice-cold FACS buffer was repeated. Cells were resuspended in 500 µL ice-cold FACS buffer. Granulocyte and monocyte populations were defined by gating the corresponding forward and side scatter scan. Their ratio out of leukocyte population was assessed after excluding the cell debris. From each sample a minimum of 5.0×10^4 cells were measured, which were subsequently analyzed. For neutrophils, the percentage of $CD16^{dim}CD62L^{bright}$ (immature), $CD16^{bright}CD62L^{bright}$ (mature) and $CD16^{bright}CD62L^{dim}$ ($CD62L^{dim}$) neutrophils and for monocytes, the percentage of $CD14brightCD16^-$ (classical), $CD14^{bright}CD16^+$ (intermediate) and $CD14^{dim}CD16^+$ (non-classical) as well the percentage and mean fluorescent units of ROS-positive out of the respective subsets were assessed by flow cytometric analyses using a BD FACS Canto 2™ and FACS DIVA™ software (BD Biosciences, USA).

2.6. Fluorescence-Activated Cell Sorting of Neutrophil and Monocyte Subsets

For each neutrophil and monocyte subsets, the blood of healthy volunteers was freshly withdrawn into Li-Heparin blood collection tubes (Sarstedt, Germany), stored on ice and processed within 30 min. For each neutrophil subset, 200 µL of heparinized blood was transferred into FACS tube (Corning, USA). For neutrophils, 10 µL Alexa Fluor 647-conjugated anti-human CD16 antibody (clone 3G8; BD Biosciences, USA) and 40 µL PE-conjugated anti-human CD62L antibody (clone SK11; BD Biosciences, USA) were added. The sample was gently mixed and incubated in the dark and on ice for 30 min. For washing, 2 mL ice-cold FACS buffer were added, and samples were subsequently centrifuged at 350× *g* and at 4 °C for 7 min. The supernatant was discarded. For red blood cells lysis, 2 mL of cold red blood cell lysis buffer were added and incubated in the dark at 4 °C for 10 min. Washing step with 2 mL ice-cold FACS buffer was repeated. Cells were resuspended in 1000 µL ice-cold FACS buffer and immediately sorted by using BD FACSCalibur (BD Biosciences, USA).

For monocyte subsets, peripheral blood mononuclear cells (PBMCs) were isolated first by a density-gradient centrifugation (Biocoll separation solution, 1.077 g/mL density; Biochrom, Berlin, Germany). Here, 10 mL of Biocoll separation solution (room temperature) were carefully overlaid with 10 mL of at room temperature tempered heparinized blood and centrifuged at $800 \times g$ and at room temperature for 25 min. PBMCs in the interphase were transferred into FACS tube and washed with 3 mL ice-cold FACS buffer. Remaining red blood cells were lysed by 500 µL cold red blood cell lysis buffer at 4 °C for 10 min. After further washing step, PBMCs were resuspended in 200 µL ice-cold FACS buffer. Next, 20 µL Alexa Fluor 647-conjugated anti-human CD16 antibody (clone 3G8; BD Biosciences, USA) and 20 µL PE-conjugated anti-human CD14 antibody (clone M5E2; BioLegend, USA) were added. The sample was gently mixed and incubated in the dark and on ice for 30 min. Subsequently, cells were washed with 2 mL ice-cold FACS buffer and resuspended in 1000 µL ice-cold FACS buffer and immediately sorted by using BD FACSCalibur (BD Biosciences, USA).

Granulocyte and monocyte populations were defined by gating the corresponding forward and side scatter scan and the doublets were excluded. Neutrophil subsets were sorted as $CD16^{bright}CD62L^{bright}$ (mature) and $CD16^{bright}CD62L^{dim}$ ($CD62L^{dim}$) using BD FACSCalibur™ (BD Biosciences, USA). Monocyte subsets were sorted as $CD14^{bright}CD16^-$ (classical), $CD14^{bright}CD16^+$ (intermediate) and $CD14^{dim}CD16^+$ (non-classical). Cell number and cell viability of the sorted populations were determined by Türk's solution exclusion assay (Merck, Darmstadt, Germany). Sorted populations were reanalyzed and typically >95% pure. The generation of ROS (see Section 2.4; excluding the red blood cells lysis step) and the phagocytic capacity (see Section 2.5; excluding the red blood cells lysis step) were assessed.

2.7. Statistics

GraphPad Prism 5.0 software (GraphPad Software Inc., San Diego, CA, USA) was used to perform the statistical analysis. Data are given as mean ± standard error of the mean (SEM). The differences between the healthy volunteers and trauma patients were analyzed by Mann–Whitney U-test. The Kruskal–Wallis test with a Dunn's post hoc test was applied to compare the differences between the subsets. A p-value below 0.05 was considered statistically significant.

3. Results
3.1. Patient Cohort

Fifteen patients with severe trauma and 15 healthy volunteers were enrolled in this study. The mean age of the patients was 38.2 ± 4.99 years of age. Two thirds of patients were male. All patients were substantially injured with an ISS of 27.7 ± 2.27. The mean stay in the intensive care unit was 15.5 ± 4.15 days, and the total duration of the in-hospital stay was 29.0 ± 7.32 days. The mean time of artificial ventilation was 8.4 ± 2.97 days. No patients developed ARDS, sepsis, or died. One patient developed pneumonia two days after admission to emergency department. The mean count of leukocytes in blood was 8.81/nL ± 0.92. The mean ratios of granulocytes and monocytes out of leukocytes were 67.8% ± 3.79 and 6.8% ± 0.98, respectively in trauma patients and 43.4% ± 2.35 and 6.6% ± 0.36, respectively in healthy subjects. The data are summarized in Table 1.

Table 1. Patient cohort.

	Parameter	SEM
Age	38.2 years old	4.99
Gender	10 men/5 women	-
ISS	27.7	2.27
Hospital stay	29.0 days	7.32
ICU stay	15.5 days	4.15
Ventilation	8.4 days	2.97
Death	0	-
Leukocytes	8.81/nL *	0.92
Neutrophils	67.8% of leukocytes	3.79
Monocytes	6.8% of leukocytes	0.98
Pneumonia	1 patient	-
ARDS	0	-
Sepsis	0	-

* Normal range: 3.92–9.81/nL. ARDS, acute respiratory distress syndrome; ICU, intensive care unit; ISS, injury severity score; SEM, standard error of mean.

3.2. Severe Trauma Modulates the Distribution of CD16+ Neutrophil Subsets

As it is known that severe traumatic injury has modulating effects on the immune system, we investigated the distribution of three neutrophil subsets according their CD16 and CD62L expression. Circulatory neutrophils were stained ex vivo and evaluated by flow cytometry. The gating strategy as well as the representative figures of $CD16^{dim}CD62L^{bright}$ (immature), $CD16^{bright}CD62L^{bright}$ (mature) and $CD16^{bright}CD62L^{dim}$ ($CD62L^{dim}$) neutrophil subsets in healthy volunteers and trauma patients are shown in Figure 1A. The main population of neutrophils in healthy volunteers and trauma patients is formed by mature neutrophils (Figure 1B). Immature and $CD62L^{dim}$ neutrophil populations are significantly less present compared to mature neutrophils (Figure 1B, $p < 0.05$). Comparing healthy volunteers to severely injured patients, the numbers of immature neutrophils significantly increase following major injury (Figure 1B, $p < 0.05$), whereas the counts of mature neutrophils do not change, and a decreasing trend is shown in $CD62L^{dim}$ neutrophil subset (Figure 1B).

3.3. Severe Traumatic Injury Causes a Phenotypic Shift of CD14+ Monocytes

Similar to neutrophils, we evaluated the phenotypic redistribution of CD14+ monocytes following traumatic injury. The gating strategy as well as the representative figures of $CD16^-CD14^{bright}$ (classical), $CD16^+CD14^{bright}$ (intermediate) and $CD16^+CD14^{dim}$ (non-classical) monocyte subsets in healthy volunteers and trauma patients are shown in Figure 2A. In healthy volunteers, classical monocytes present the most abundant monocyte population, whereas intermediate and non-classical monocytes are significantly less present compared to this subset (Figure 2B, $p < 0.05$). The population of non-classical monocytes is also significantly smaller than the intermediate monocyte population (Figure 2B, $p < 0.05$). In trauma patients, intermediate subset presents the most abundant monocyte population and the classical monocyte counts have a decreasing trend compared to this subset (Figure 2B). Non-classical monocytes of trauma patients are significantly less present than classical and intermediate monocytes (Figure 2B, $p < 0.05$). Comparing healthy volunteers to trauma patients, classical monocyte population decreases in trauma patients, whereas intermediate monocyte population becomes significantly more abundant (Figure 2B, $p < 0.05$). The numbers of the non-classical monocytes significantly decrease in trauma patients (Figure 2B, $p < 0.05$).

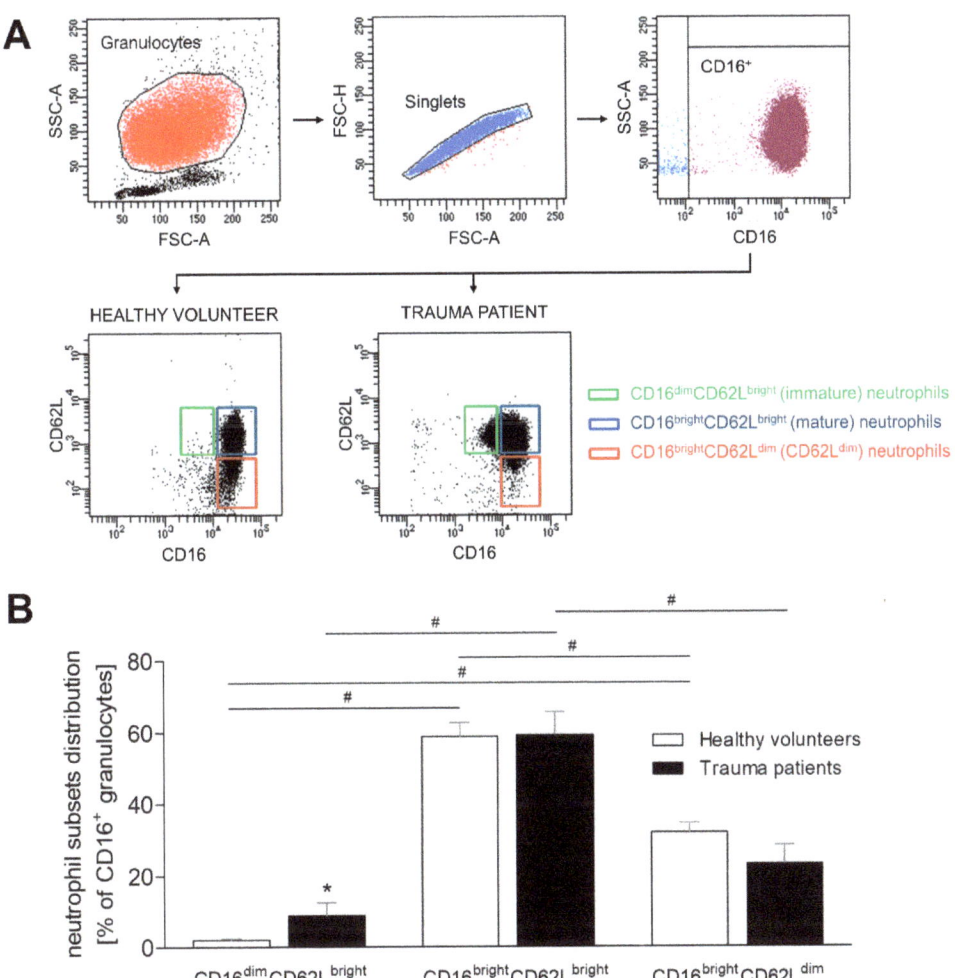

Figure 1. Impact of severe traumatic injury on neutrophil subset distribution. (**A**) Representative gating strategy for phenotyping human neutrophil subsets, including size discrimination, doublet exclusion, selection of $CD16^+$ cells, and separation according to expression of CD16 and CD62L. (**B**) The percentage distribution of $CD16^{dim}CD62L^{bright}$ (immature), $CD16^{bright}CD62L^{bright}$ (mature) and $CD16^{bright}CD62L^{dim}$ ($CD62L^{dim}$) neutrophils out of $CD16^+$ granulocytes was determined in healthy subjects (white bars) and severely injured patients (black bars) within 12 h postinjury. Data are presented as mean ± standard error of the mean. *: $p < 0.05$ vs. healthy volunteers; #: $p < 0.05$ vs. respective subset.

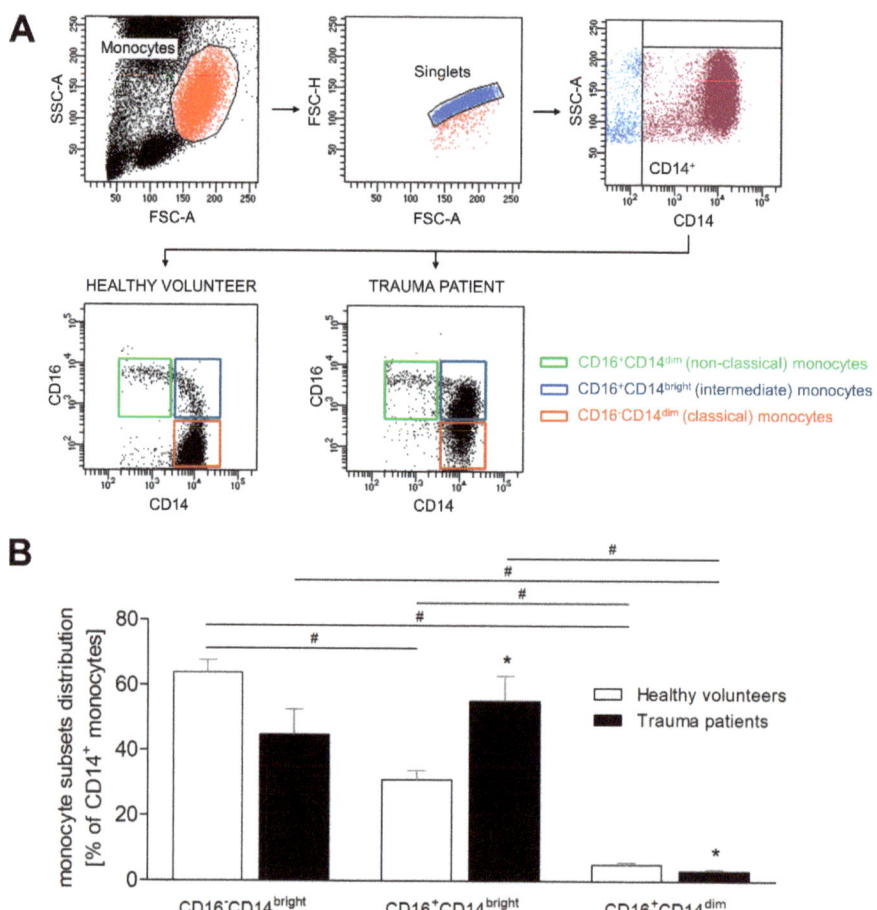

Figure 2. Impact of severe traumatic injury on monocyte subset distribution. (**A**) Representative gating strategy for phenotyping human monocyte subsets, including size discrimination, doublet exclusion, selection of CD14$^+$ cells, and separation according to expression of CD16 and CD14. (**B**) The percentage distribution of CD14^{bright}CD16$^-$ (classical), CD14^{bright}CD16$^+$ (intermediate) and CD14^{dim}CD16$^+$ (non-classical) monocytes out of CD14$^+$ monocytes was determined in healthy subjects (white bars) and severely injured patients (black bars) within 12 h postinjury. Data are presented as mean ± standard error of the mean. *: $p < 0.05$ vs. healthy volunteers; #: $p < 0.05$ vs. respective subset.

3.4. Severe Trauma Does Not Affect Phagocytic Capacity of Neutrophils at Early Time Point

Severely injured patients often develop secondary infectious complications, which may be caused by reduced phagocyting capacity [16]. Therefore, we evaluated the bacterial intake of neutrophils following traumatic injury. All three neutrophil populations obtained from healthy volunteers incorporate comparable numbers of FITC-labeled *E. coli* bioparticles, with slight increase in mature and CD62L^{dim} neutrophils, however, without significance (Figure 3A). Within the first 12 h after injury, the counts of phagocyting cells do not significantly change compared to respective subsets in healthy volunteers (Figure 3A).

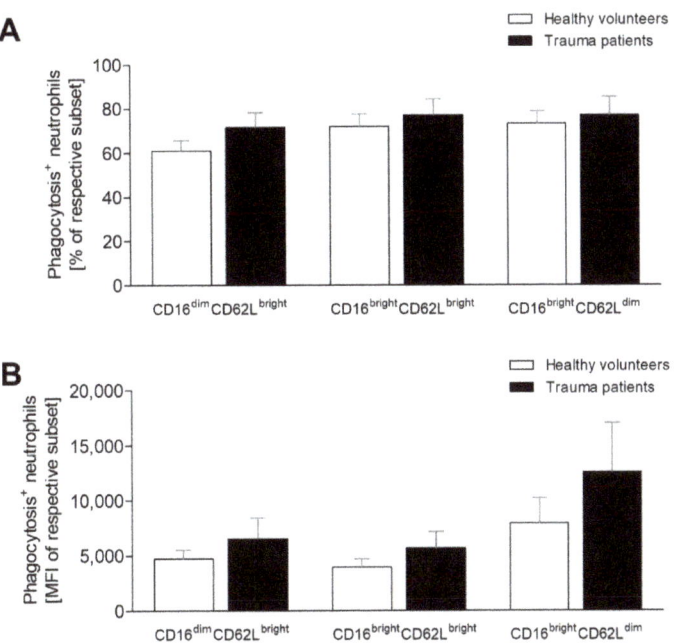

Figure 3. Impact of severe traumatic injury on phagocytic capacity of neutrophil subsets. The (**A**) percentage and (**B**) mean intensity of phagocytosis positive $CD16^{dim}CD62L^{bright}$ (immature), $CD16^{bright}CD62L^{bright}$ (mature) and $CD16^{bright}CD62L^{low}$ ($CD62L^{dim}$) neutrophils were determined in healthy subjects (white bars) and severely injured patients (black bars) within 12 h postinjury. Data are presented as mean ± standard error of the mean.

The mean bioparticle intake per cell is comparable in immature and mature neutrophils of healthy volunteers, whereas the $CD62L^{dim}$ neutrophils display higher phagocyting capacity compared to these two subsets (Figure 3B). Following traumatic injury, all three subsets exert increased mean phagocyting capacity without statistical significance compared to healthy volunteers (Figure 3B).

3.5. Severe Trauma Elevates the Production of Reactive Oxygen Species in Mature and $CD62L^{dim}$ Neutrophils

As it is known that enhanced ROS production contributes to endothelial dysfunction and tissue injury, we evaluated ROS levels in neutrophils. In healthy volunteers, significantly more immature neutrophils form ROS compared to mature and $CD62L^{dim}$ neutrophils (Figure 4A, $p < 0.05$), whereas in trauma patients the counts of ROS positive neutrophils are equal in all three subsets (Figure 4A). Following traumatic injury, the counts of ROS positive immature neutrophils are comparable with these in healthy volunteers (Figure 4A), whereas the mature and $CD62L^{dim}$ neutrophil subsets display significant increase of ROS positive neutrophils (Figure 4A, $p < 0.05$). Ex vivo stimulation of whole blood with fMLP does not affect the ratio of ROS positive neutrophils in the immature subset of healthy volunteers but significantly increases in the mature and $CD62L^{dim}$ subset (Figure 4A, $p < 0.05$). In trauma patients, the fLMP-induced generation of ROS tends to increase compared to unstimulated samples, however, without significance (Figure 4A).

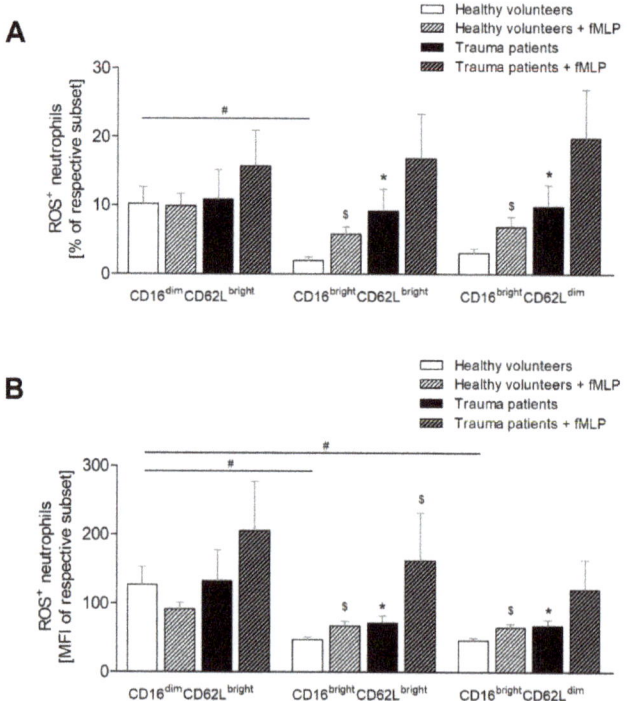

Figure 4. Impact of severe traumatic injury on generation of reactive oxygen species (ROS) by neutrophil subsets. The (**A**) percentage and (**B**) mean intensity of ROS positive $CD16^{dim}CD62L^{bright}$ (immature), $CD16^{bright}CD62L^{bright}$ (mature) and $CD16^{bright}CD62L^{low}$ ($CD62L^{dim}$) neutrophils were determined in healthy subjects (white bars) and severely injured patients (black bars) within 12 h postinjury. Whole blood was stimulated with PMA ex vivo (diagonally striped bars). Data are presented as mean ± standard error of the mean. *: $p < 0.05$ vs. healthy volunteers; #: $p < 0.05$ vs. respective subset; $: $p < 0.05$ vs. unstimulated corresponding subset.

Similarly, the mean ROS production intensity per cell is the highest in immature neutrophil subset in both, healthy volunteers and trauma patients (Figure 4B). Those levels are significantly lower in mature and $CD62L^{dim}$ neutrophils of trauma patients compared to immature neutrophils (Figure 4B, $p < 0.05$) and the levels in healthy volunteers are clearly lower as well, however, without statistical significance (Figure 4B). Comparing the ROS levels in trauma patients to healthy volunteers within the individual subsets, the mean ROS production of immature neutrophils does not change following traumatic injury (Figure 4B), whereas the levels in mature and $CD62L^{dim}$ neutrophil population significantly increase (Figure 4B, $p < 0.05$). Similar to ROS positive neutrophils, the mean ROS generation intensity per cell does not change in the immature neutrophils of healthy volunteers following ex vivo fMLP stimulation and is significantly higher in mature and CD62L subsets (Figure 4B, $p < 0.05$). fMLP stimulation of trauma patient's blood increases the mean generation of ROS compared to that of healthy subjects in the mature neutrophils, whereas the immature and $CD62L^{dim}$ subsets show only increasing tendency (Figure 4B, $p < 0.05$).

3.6. Severe Traumatic Injury Increases the Production of Reactive Oxygen Species in Monocytes

Similar to neutrophils, monocytes display subset specific differences in ROS production following traumatic injury. In healthy volunteers, the same ratio of classical and intermediate monocytes generates ROS, whereas non-classical monocyte population displays significantly higher number of ROS positive cells (Figure 5A, $p < 0.05$). The monocytes obtained from trauma patients have increasing ratios of ROS positive cell from classical over intermediate to non-classical monocytes, whereby the difference between classical and non-classical subset is significant (Figure 5A, $p < 0.05$). When comparing trauma patients with healthy volunteers, there is an increasing ratio of ROS positive monocytes in all subsets, with significance in the intermediate subset (Figure 5A, $p < 0.05$). Ex vivo stimulation of whole blood of both healthy and injured subjects with PMA significantly increases the ratio of ROS positive monocytes within all three subsets compared to the unstimulated samples (Figure 5A, $p < 0.05$). However, only the non-classical monocytes of injured patients generate significantly less ROS following PMA stimulation compared to the equivalent subsets in healthy subjects (Figure 5A, $p < 0.05$).

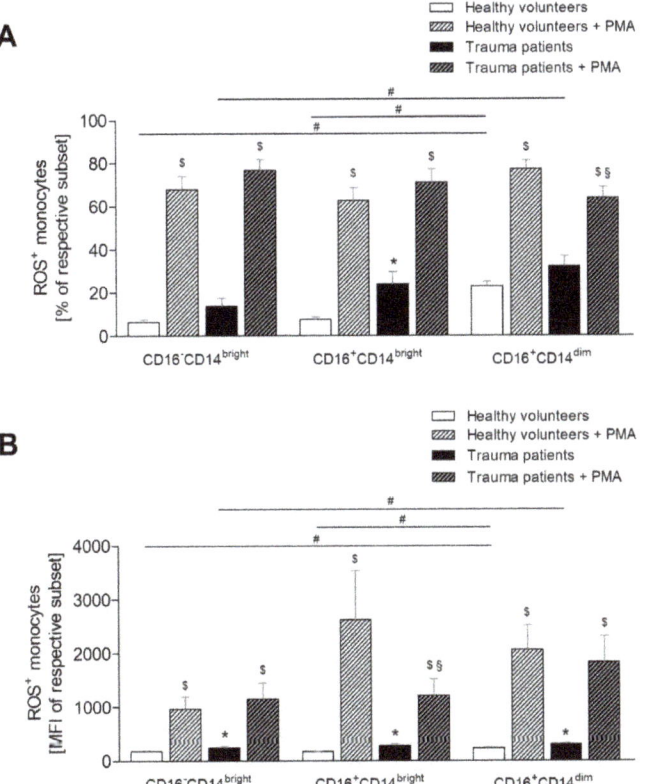

Figure 5. Impact of severe traumatic injury on generation of reactive oxygen species (ROS) by monocyte subsets. The (**A**) percentage and (**B**) mean intensity of ROS positive CD14brightCD16− (classical), CD14^{bright}CD16$^+$ (intermediate) and CD14^{dim}CD16$^+$ (non-classical) monocytes were determined in healthy subjects (white bars) and severely injured patients (black bars) within 12 h postinjury. Whole blood was stimulated with PMA ex vivo (diagonally striped bars). Data are presented as mean ± standard error of the mean. *: $p < 0.05$ vs. healthy volunteers; #: $p < 0.05$ vs. respective subset; $: $p < 0.05$ vs. unstimulated corresponding subset; §: $p < 0.05$ vs. healthy volunteers + PMA.

The mean ROS production per cell is the highest in the non-classical subset, whereas classical and intermediate monocyte population is significantly less positive for ROS compared to non-classical monocytes (Figure 5B, $p < 0.05$). In trauma patients, classical monocytes produce significantly less ROS than non-classical monocytes (Figure 5B,

$p < 0.05$), whereas the mean ROS production intensity of intermediate subset is comparable with that of non-classical monocyte population (Figure 5B). Comparing the respective subsets, all monocyte populations display significantly increased mean ROS production intensity following traumatic injury compared to healthy volunteers (Figure 5B, $p < 0.05$). Ex vivo stimulation with PMA leads similarly to the ratios of ROS positive monocytes, and also to a significant increase of mean ROS generation intensity in both healthy and injured subjects compared to untreated samples (Figure 5B, $p < 0.05$). This increase is significantly lower in the intermediate subset of severely injured patients compared to healthy subjects, whereas the mean intensity does not change in the classical and non-classical monocytes (Figure 5B, $p < 0.05$).

3.7. Fluorescence-Activated Cell Sorting Reveals an Exhaustion of Neutrophils and Monocytes and Aligns the Functional Differences between the Subsets

The individual neutrophil subsets of healthy volunteers were sorted by fluorescence-activated cell sorting (FACS) and subsequently analyzed for ROS production and phagocytic capacity. Nearly 100% of mature and CD62L^{dim} neutrophils were positive for ROS (Figure S1A) and the mean ROS production did not differ between the subsets as well (Figure S1B). Compared to whole blood analyses (see Figure 3), the production of ROS approximately increased 30-fold. The counts of phagocytosis positive neutrophils (Figure S1C) and the mean phagocytic capacity (Figure S1D) did not vary between the mature and CD62L^{dim} subsets. The bacterial intake is significantly impeded compared to whole blood analyses (see Figure 4). The immature neutrophil subset was not analyzed due to its low numbers and nearly absence in HV.

Similarly, nearly 100% of classical, intermediate, and non-classical monocytes were positive for ROS following FACS (Figure S2A). The mean production of ROS did not differ between the subsets (Figure S2B). Compared to whole blood analyses (see Figure 5), all monocyte subsets produce significantly higher amounts of ROS.

4. Discussion

Although the clinical treatment algorithms of severely injured trauma patients have improved over the last decades, leading to higher post-traumatic survival rates, those patients are still highly vulnerable to secondary infections during their clinical stay. The development of infectious complications has been associated with a dysregulated immune response, wherefore a mapping and characterization of immunological changes and intercellular interactions may predict post-traumatic vulnerability to secondary complications and potentially represent promising therapeutic targets in future [2–4]. Neutrophils and monocytes have been shown to initiate an immediate innate immune response with the aim to clear tissue damage and provide protection from invading pathogens [7–10]. Therefore, we investigated the phenotypical changes of different neutrophil and monocyte subsets in severely injured trauma patients as well as their functionality regarding the ROS generation and phagocytic capacity.

In this study, severely injured patients' leukocyte counts remain in the normal range, whereas the ratio of granulocytes significantly increases compared to healthy subjects. Emergency granulopoiesis, which has been extensively described following traumatic injury and microbial challenge [27,28], is a part of the first line of cellular defense that crucially modulate subsequent repair processes after tissue damage [29]. However, on the other hand, an exaggerated release of neutrophils leads to bone marrow exhaustion and in turn, can impair the innate immune response to secondary hit such as surgery or infection [21].

Subset-specifically, we observed that in both, healthy volunteers and severely injured patients mature neutrophils (CD16^{brigh}CD62L^{bright}) represent the most abundant neutrophil subset. Although it has been reported that only a homogenous population of mature neutrophils can be found in healthy individuals, we detected additionally the CD62L^{dim} population (CD16^{brigh}CD62L^{dim}). Comparing healthy volunteers with severely injured patients, the counts of CD16^{brigh}CD62L^{dim} neutrophils did not differ between those.

A significantly increased frequency and absolute cell numbers of $CD16^{brigh}CD62L^{dim}$ neutrophils in trauma patients is extensively described in the literature and thus, contradictory to our results [30]. $CD16^{brigh}CD62L^{dim}$ neutrophils occur within the first hour after the injury [30] and locally release hydrogen peroxide into the immunological synapse between the neutrophils and T cells in Mac-1-dependend manner, leading to the suppression of T cell activation [22]. This suggests that a neutrophil subset with dimmer CD62L expression exhibits immunosuppressive features. Although CD62L is rapidly shed from the cell surface upon neutrophil activation [31], also changes in osmotic pressure, pH value, or hemodynamic shear stress can cause CD62L shedding [32–34]. Thus, regarding our results, $CD16^{brigh}CD62L^{dim}$ population in healthy volunteers may not constitute of $CD62L^{dim}$ neutrophils but rather we might potentially detect the mature neutrophils that underwent CD62L shedding ex vivo caused by mechanical stress caused by the isolation and analysis methods. This, however, should be the case for both healthy donors and trauma patients.

Further, we observed a massive presence of immature ($CD16^{dim}CD62L^{bright}$) neutrophils in severely injured patients, whereas healthy individuals lack this population. It is assumed that immature neutrophils have impaired functional ability [21]. Moreover, Spijkerman et al. have shown that the ratio of immature neutrophils positively correlates with the severity of the injury and the development of infectious complication [28]. This indicates that immature neutrophils have an inadequate immune response towards traumatic stimuli depending on the injury severity and wherefore, the ratio of immature neutrophils may become a potent tool in the prediction of infectious complications following traumatic injury.

For a timely resolution of inflammation and recovery from injury, phagocytes such as neutrophils and monocytes recognize and eliminate microbes and cell debris [13,14]. Thus, if the phagocytes fail to engulf and clear their targets, the tissue inflammation is prolonged, causing tissue damage with subsequent infectious complications [10]. In the present study, we did not observe any significant differences between the severely injured patients and healthy individuals and the individual neutrophil subsets regarding the phagocytosis in the first twelve hours after trauma. Actually, the references about aberrated phagocytic capacity of neutrophils following traumatic injury are not consistent [17,35,36]. However, it must be considered that the most studies evaluate the intake of fluorochrome-conjugated bacteria or bacterial bioparticles by neutrophils and not directly their killing potential. That an accurate engulfment of bacteria does not necessarily mean that the pathogens are also adequate killed is underlined by the study by Leliefeld et al., analyzing the incorporation of bacteria and the capacity of killing the bacteria by neutrophils in human experimental endotoxemia model [37]. Interestingly, immature neutrophils exhibit a superior engulfment of bacteria and killing capacity. However, even though mature and $CD62L^{dim}$ subsets incorporate bacteria at comparable level to immature neutrophils, they are incapable to kill the bacteria, that has been associated with higher intraphagosomal pH, subsequent intracellular bacterial growth and escape of the pathogens from the neutrophils [37]. This indicates that the above-described positive correlation between the elevated ratio of immature neutrophils and the development of inflammatory complications does not depend on defective phagocytosis. Moreover, as severe traumatic injury leads to neutrophilia with subsequent bone marrow exhaustion and the $CD62L^{dim}$ subset appears within the first hour after the injury [21,27,28,30], this may together with the incapability of $CD62L^{dim}$ neutrophils to adequately kill the bacteria [37] contribute to the development of infectious complications in later time course, because the immune system might not adequate respond to the bacterial escape from the $CD62L^{dim}$ neutrophils.

The generation of ROS is an elemental mechanism to clear the pathogens within the phagosome, but it also acts as a chemoattractant for immune cells to clear and repair the tissue. However, an exaggerated release of free radicals can have detrimental consequences to the host such a loss of junctional integrity of vascular microvessels that contributes to the development of pulmonary edema and has been associated with the development of ARDS, systemic inflammatory response syndrome and multiorgan failure (MOF) [7,20,21,38–40].

Although the extent of the generation of ROS seems to be injury severity-dependent [17] and the contribution of neutrophil-induced exaggerated oxidative burst in the development of secondary complications after trauma is generally accepted, there is no evidence about neutrophil subset-specific generation of ROS.

We have shown that the oxidative burst significantly increases in mature and CD62L^{dim} neutrophils of severely injured patients, but its level remains stable in immature neutrophils compared to healthy individuals. However, immature neutrophils have the highest ratio of ROS compared to the other subsets. This supports the suggestion that immature neutrophils may be the key players in development of secondary post-traumatic complications. In line, the mean generation of ROS in the immature neutrophils noticeable increases in severely injured patients following ex vivo stimulation with N-formyl-methionyl-leucyl-phenylalanine (fMLP) compared to stimulated blood samples from healthy subjects. It has been shown that immature neutrophils are apoptosis resistant [41], whereas an exaggerated oxidative burst to secondary hit post-trauma has been associated with uncontrolled inflammatory response, resulting in endothelial permeability and tissue damage [42–44]. This along with our data indicates that the ROS-induced collateral tissue damage and subsequent infectious complications following traumatic injury could be primarily caused by immature neutrophil subset. Taken together, neutrophils undergo phenotypical and functional changes in severely injured patients dependently on the injury severity and contribute to the development of secondary complications. Therefore, a consequent monitoring of those during the whole period of hospital stay along with the incidence of infectious complications could provide data about the prediction of post-traumatic vulnerability to secondary infections.

Similar to neutrophils, monocytes have a multi-faced role in maintaining the tissue homeostasis and responding to inflammatory stimuli in order to clear the pathogens and cellular debris with subsequent restoration of tissue integrity [45]. However, the initial monocyte activation after trauma is rapidly followed by substantial paralysis of monocyte function, reflected by the decreased surface presentation of human leukocyte antigen (HLA)-DR [46,47]. Delayed recovery of HLA-DR expression and decreased release of pro-inflammatory mediators such as interleukin (IL)-1β, IL-6, IL-8 and tumor necrosis factor-α (TNF-α) have been associated with the development of secondary infections and MOF [46,47]. However, these studies focus mainly on aberrated monocyte functions from 24 h after trauma and there are no data about potential phenotypical changes of human monocytes following traumatic injury at early time point. Therefore, we analyzed the redistribution of monocyte subsets within the first twelve hours after severe trauma.

It is generally accepted that classical CD16$^-$CD14^{bright} monocytes, which is the main monocyte population in healthy individuals, are precursors for pro-inflammatory intermediate CD16$^+$CD14^{bright} monocytes that in turn differentiate into patrolling non-classical CD16$^+$CD14^{low} monocytes [48]. In trauma patients, the numbers of circulating intermediate monocytes significantly increase, whereas we have observed a decrease of classical and non-classical subsets, suggesting a phenotype switch toward the pro-inflammatory phenotype. Classical monocytes have anti-microbial features with superior phagocytic capacity and after entering the tissues, they differentiate into monocyte-derived macrophages or dendritic cells [24]. Thus, the initial decrease of circulating classical monocytes after severe trauma might be caused on the one hand by a differentiation into intermediate monocytes and on the other hand by their transmigration to injury site in order to shape and resolve the inflammation. Regarding the intermediate monocytes, such an exaggerated elevation has been shown in severely injured patients 48 h post-trauma [49] and under inflammatory conditions such as sepsis or bacterial and viral infections [9], paralleled by sequestration of high amounts of TNF-α, IL-1β, and IL-6 [50]. Such an exaggerated release of pro-inflammatory cytokines has been associated with a so-called cytokine storm, that in turn can lead to blood pressure collapse, coagulopathy, up to MOF and death [51]. Therefore, the extent of the intermediate subset may prospectively provide an information about secondary post-traumatic complications.

Although an excessive oxidative burst has been already shown in monocytes of severely injured patients [52,53], there is no evidence whether the monocyte subsets generate ROS in a different extent and thus, may differently contribute to the pathogen and tissue clearance. In the present study, all monocyte subsets have significantly increased mean capacity to produce ROS compared to healthy individuals, which is comparable between the subsets. The ratio of ROS positive monocytes was elevated also in all subsets; however, a significant increase has been observed only in the pro-inflammatory intermediate monocytes. This along with the significant increase of the intermediate monocyte numbers support the assumption that the very early post-traumatic phase is characterized by a pro-inflammatory immune response of monocytes. Interestingly, ex vivo stimulation of whole blood with phorbol 12-myristate 13-acetate (PMA) leads to significant increase of mean generation of ROS compared to unstimulated samples, but this increase is significantly lower in the intermediate subset of severely injured patients compared to healthy volunteers. Once a pathogen is phagocytized, ROS contribute to the elimination of ingested pathogen and in the case of their not sufficient intracellular level, pathogen can escape and survive [54]. Thus, this inadequate intracellular oxidative burst of intermediate monocyte subset upon secondary stimuli may contribute to the susceptibility to infectious complications.

Interestingly, intermediate monocytes display the highest expression of HLA-DR in human experimental endotoxemia model compared to another two subsets over the whole observation period of 24 h [9]. Considering the post-traumatic monocyte deactivation within the first 48 h [9], it would be reasonable to follow the redistribution of monocyte subsets of severely injured patients and the subset-specific HLA-DR expression and the generation of ROS over the entire intensive care unit stay. We assume that the extent and the timing of the initial pro-inflammatory phase followed by the immunosuppressive phase in combination with the monocyte subsets distribution might provide valuable insight into post-traumatic monocyte kinetics and prospectively also a potent tool for counteracting the secondary infections.

For the evaluation of the physiological role of the neutrophil and monocyte subsets, studies on isolated subsets are necessary. Thus, we isolated the subsets by FACS. Although we obtained viable and clearly defined populations verified by flow cytometry, the above discussed functional differences between the subsets were no longer visible. Whereas nearly 100% of the cells were positive for oxidative burst and the mean levels elevated extraordinary, the bacterial incorporation was significantly impaired compared to whole blood analyses. We used BD FACSCalibur flow cytometer (BD Biosciences, USA), which is the first multicolor benchtop flow cytometry system capable of analyzing and sorting cells of interest for further study. The cell sorting rate and consequently the velocity, in which we obtained the requested cell counts, were extremely low. As both neutrophils and monocytes respond overly sensitive to their environment, so prolonged isolation led to cell exhaustion and impaired functionality. Thus, we have not been successful in isolating the individual subsets and subsequent analyzing their physiological roles and further studies under optimum conditions are necessary.

5. Limitations

This study provides a solid fundament for understanding the early post-traumatic phenotypic shift of neutrophils and monocytes and their antimicrobial functions, however, it also has several limitations. First, we only included fifteen polytrauma patients. Although the results shown are conclusive, increasing the number of study participants would enable a more precise group allocation according to the trauma pattern, and also correlation analyses of the evaluated neutrophil and monocyte subsets with clinical parameters such as ISS, bacterial complications, or ARDS. Second, we evaluated the phenotypic and functional changes only at the early time point. As severely injured patients develop secondary inflammatory complications in later time course, it would be reasonable to follow-up on the changes during the entire stay at intensive care unit. Third, as we did not use counting beads during the flow cytometry measurements, we obtained only relative fractions of neutrophil and monocyte subsets. Additionally, the percentage of neutrophils and monocytes out of leukocytes was evaluated by flow cytometry and, thus, this is not so precise as the blood analysis by hospital laboratory would be. Therefore, for achieving the absolute numbers, counting beads must be included in the upcoming studies as well as the blood work performed by hospital laboratory for evaluation of the ratios between the different leukocyte subpopulations. Lastly, FITC-labeled *E. coli* BioParticles were used for the phagocytic assay. This is a proper assay for the evaluation of bacterial intake; however, it is not possible to make a statement regarding the bacterial killing. A combination of the assessment of the bacterial intake and killing by neutrophils and monocytes would provide an immerse improvement of understanding the post-traumatic antimicrobial kinetics of leukocytes.

6. Conclusions

Severe traumatic injury induces an immediate phenotype shift of neutrophils as well as monocytes accompanied by their alterations in ROS generation compared to healthy subjects. In the circulation of trauma patients, the ratio of immature neutrophils is immensely elevated, whereas numbers of mature and $CD62L^{dim}$ neutrophils do not change. All three subsets display an increasing tendency in phagocytic capacity and the mature and $CD62L^{dim}$ neutrophils produce significantly more free radicals than those in healthy individuals. Thereby, an ex vivo stimulation with fMLP increases mean generation of ROS by trauma patients' immature neutrophils compared to healthy subjects. Similarly, monocytes shift toward the pro-inflammatory intermediate phenotype and the classical and non-classical subsets becomes less abundant in trauma patients. All monocyte subsets generate high levels of ROS after severe traumatic injury. However, the intermediate and non-classical monocytes of severely injured patients generate significantly less ROS following ex vivo stimulation with PMA compared to healthy subjects. The here presented post-traumatic dynamic changes of those cells of innate immune system provide a solid fundament for functional studies of the individual subsets. The data following the ex vivo stimulation suggest that neutrophils may more contribute to the endothelial permeability and tissue damage, whereas monocytes seem to more contribute to higher susceptibility to secondary infections by their hyporesponsiveness to secondary hit. Future directions will include a larger cohort of severely injured patient and the analysis of trauma-induced phenotypical and functional changes of neutrophils and monocytes over an observation period of two weeks. We assume that the appearance and the antimicrobial functions of immature neutrophils and intermediate monocytes may be decisive for the development of secondary infectious complications in severely injured patients. The gained findings may improve the therapeutic approach or even contribute to a prevention of developing life-threatening infections.

Supplementary Materials: The following are available online at https://www.mdpi.com/article/10.3390/jcm10184139/s1, Figure S1: Generation of reactive oxygen species and phagocytic capacity in isolated neutrophil subsets obtained from healthy volunteers, Figure S2: Generation of reactive oxygen species in isolated monocyte subsets obtained from healthy volunteers.

Author Contributions: Conceptualization, B.R.; methodology, B.R., A.J. and N.B.; validation, A.J.; formal analysis, A.J.; investigation, A.J., N.B. and B.X.; resources, B.R.; data curation, A.J.; writing—original draft preparation, A.J.; writing—review and editing, B.R., M.S., L.N., N.W., A.J.M., J.B. and I.M.; visualization, A.J.; supervision, B.R.; funding acquisition, B.R. All authors have read and agreed to the published version of the manuscript.

Funding: This research was funded by Deutsche Forschungsgemeinschaft, grant number RE 3304/8-1.

Institutional Review Board Statement: The study was conducted according to the guidelines of the Declaration of Helsinki and following the Strengthening the Reporting of Observational studies in Epidemiology-guidelines [26]. The current study was approved by the institutional ethics committee of the University Hospital of the Goethe-University Frankfurt with the nr. 312/10.

Informed Consent Statement: Informed consent was obtained from all subjects involved in the study.

Data Availability Statement: All data generated or analyzed during this study are included in this published article.

Conflicts of Interest: The authors declare no conflict of interest. The funders had no role in the design of the study; in the collection, analyses, or interpretation of data; in the writing of the manuscript, or in the decision to publish the results.

Abbreviations

ARDS	acute respiratory distress syndrome
CD	cluster of differentiation
FACS	fluorescence-activated cell sorting
fMLP	N-formyl-methionyl-leucyl-phenylalanine
IL	interleukin
ISS	injury severity score
MOF	multi organ failure
PBS	phosphate-buffered saline
PBMCs	peripheral blood mononuclear cells
PMA	phorbol 12-myristate 13-acetate
ROS	reactive oxygen species

References

1. *Injuries and Violence: The Facts*; World Health Organization: Geneve, Switzerland, 2010.
2. Hellebrekers, P.; Leenen, L.P.; Hoekstra, M.; Hietbrink, F. Effect of a standardized treatment regime for infection after osteosynthesis. *J. Orthop. Surg. Res.* **2017**, *12*, 41. [CrossRef]
3. Horiguchi, H.; Loftus, T.J.; Hawkins, R.B.; Raymond, S.L.; Stortz, J.A.; Hollen, M.K.; Weiss, B.P.; Miller, E.S.; Bihorac, A.; Larson, S.D.; et al. Efron, Sepsis, and I. Critical Illness Research Center. Innate Immunity in the Persistent Inflammation, Immunosuppression, and Catabolism Syndrome and Its Implications for Therapy. *Front. Immunol.* **2018**, *9*, 595. [CrossRef]
4. Mira, J.C.; Brakenridge, S.C.; Moldawer, L.L.; Moore, F.A. Persistent Inflammation, Immunosuppression and Catabolism Syndrome. *Crit. Care Clin.* **2017**, *33*, 245–258. [CrossRef]
5. Stormann, P.; Lustenberger, T.; Relja, B.; Marzi, I.; Wutzler, S. Role of biomarkers in acute traumatic lung injury. *Injury* **2017**, *48*, 2400–2406. [CrossRef] [PubMed]
6. Villar, J.; Blanco, J.; Kacmarek, R.M. Current incidence and outcome of the acute respiratory distress syndrome. *Curr. Opin. Crit. Care* **2016**, *22*, 1–6. [CrossRef] [PubMed]
7. Kellner, M.; Noonepalle, S.; Lu, Q.; Srivastava, A.; Zemskov, E.; Black, S.M. ROS Signaling in the Pathogenesis of Acute Lung Injury (ALI) and Acute Respiratory Distress Syndrome (ARDS). *Adv. Exp. Med. Biol.* **2017**, *967*, 105–137. [PubMed]
8. Hesselink, L.; Spijkerman, R.; van Wessem, K.J.P.; Koenderman, L.; Leenen, L.P.H.; Huber-Lang, M.; Hietbrink, F. Neutrophil heterogeneity and its role in infectious complications after severe trauma. *World J. Emerg. Surg.* **2019**, *14*, 24. [CrossRef]
9. Tak, T.; van Groenendael, R.; Pickkers, P.; Koenderman, L. Monocyte Subsets Are Differentially Lost from the Circulation during Acute Inflammation Induced by Human Experimental Endotoxemia. *J. Innate. Immun.* **2017**, *9*, 464–474. [CrossRef] [PubMed]
10. Westman, J.; Grinstein, S.; Marques, P.E. Phagocytosis of Necrotic Debris at Sites of Injury and Inflammation. *Front. Immunol.* **2019**, *10*, 3030. [CrossRef]
11. Rani, M.; Nicholson, S.E.; Zhang, Q.; Schwacha, M.G. Damage-associated molecular patterns (DAMPs) released after burn are associated with inflammation and monocyte activation. *Burns* **2017**, *43*, 297–303. [CrossRef]
12. Amulic, B.; Cazalet, C.; Hayes, G.L.; Metzler, K.D.; Zychlinsky, A. Neutrophil function: From mechanisms to disease. *Annu. Rev. Immunol.* **2012**, *30*, 459–489. [CrossRef]
13. Filep, J.G.; Ariel, A. Neutrophil heterogeneity and fate in inflamed tissues: Implications for the resolution of inflammation. *Am. J. Physiol. Cell Physiol.* **2020**, *319*, C510–C532. [CrossRef]
14. Andrews, T.; Sullivan, K.E. Infections in patients with inherited defects in phagocytic function. *Clin. Microbiol. Rev.* **2003**, *16*, 597–621. [CrossRef]
15. Reine, J.; Rylance, J.; Ferreira, D.M.; Pennington, S.H.; Welters, I.D.; Parker, R.; Morton, B. The whole blood phagocytosis assay: A clinically relevant test of neutrophil function and dysfunction in community-acquired pneumonia. *BMC Res. Notes* **2020**, *13*, 203. [CrossRef]
16. Kanyilmaz, S.; Hepguler, S.; Atamaz, F.C.; Gokmen, N.M.; Ardeniz, O.; Sin, A. Phagocytic and oxidative burst activity of neutrophils in patients with spinal cord injury. *Arch. Phys. Med. Rehabil.* **2013**, *94*, 369–374. [CrossRef]
17. Liao, Y.; Liu, P.; Guo, F.; Zhang, Z.Y.; Zhang, Z. Oxidative burst of circulating neutrophils following traumatic brain injury in human. *PLoS ONE* **2013**, *8*, e68963.

18. Ritzel, R.M.; Doran, S.J.; Barrett, J.P.; Henry, R.J.; Ma, E.L.; Faden, A.I.; Loane, D.J. Chronic Alterations in Systemic Immune Function after Traumatic Brain Injury. *J. Neurotrauma* **2018**, *35*, 1419–1436. [CrossRef]
19. Hellebrekers, P.; Hietbrink, F.; Vrisekoop, N.; Leenen, L.P.H.; Koenderman, L. Neutrophil Functional Heterogeneity: Identification of Competitive Phagocytosis. *Front. Immunol.* **2017**, *8*, 1498. [CrossRef]
20. Santos, S.S.; Brunialti, M.K.; Rigato, O.; Machado, F.R.; Silva, E.; Salomao, R. Generation of nitric oxide and reactive oxygen species by neutrophils and monocytes from septic patients and association with outcomes. *Shock* **2012**, *38*, 18–23. [CrossRef]
21. Mulder, P.P.G.; Vlig, M.; Boekema, B.; Stoop, M.M.; Pijpe, A.; van Zuijlen, P.P.M.; de Jong, E.; van Cranenbroek, B.; Joosten, I.; Koenen, H. Persistent Systemic Inflammation in Patients With Severe Burn Injury Is Accompanied by Influx of Immature Neutrophils and Shifts in T Cell Subsets and Cytokine Profiles. *Front. Immunol.* **2020**, *11*, 621222. [CrossRef]
22. Pillay, J.; Kamp, V.M.; van Hoffen, E.; Visser, T.; Tak, T.; Lammers, J.W.; Ulfman, L.H.; Leenen, L.P.; Pickkers, P.; Koenderman, L. A subset of neutrophils in human systemic inflammation inhibits T cell responses through Mac-1. *J. Clin. Investig.* **2012**, *122*, 327–336. [CrossRef] [PubMed]
23. Greco, M.; Mazzei, A.; Palumbo, C.; Verri, T.; Lobreglio, G. Flow Cytometric Analysis of Monocytes Polarization and Reprogramming From Inflammatory to Immunosuppressive Phase During Sepsis. *EJIFCC* **2019**, *30*, 371–384. [PubMed]
24. Kapellos, T.S.; Bonaguro, L.; Gemund, I.; Reusch, N.; Saglam, A.; Hinkley, E.R.; Schultze, J.L. Human Monocyte Subsets and Phenotypes in Major Chronic Inflammatory Diseases. *Front. Immunol.* **2019**, *10*, 2035. [CrossRef]
25. Cros, J.; Cagnard, N.; Woollard, K.; Patey, N.; Zhang, S.Y.; Senechal, B.; Puel, A.; Biswas, S.K.; Moshous, D.; Picard, C.; et al. Human CD14dim monocytes patrol and sense nucleic acids and viruses via TLR7 and TLR8 receptors. *Immunity* **2010**, *33*, 375–386. [CrossRef]
26. von Elm, E.; Altman, D.G.; Egger, M.; Pocock, S.J.; Gotzsche, P.C.; Vandenbroucke, J.P.; Initiative, S. The Strengthening the Reporting of Observational Studies in Epidemiology (STROBE) statement: Guidelines for reporting observational studies. *J. Clin. Epidemiol.* **2008**, *61*, 344–349. [CrossRef]
27. Lawrence, S.M.; Corriden, R.; Nizet, V. The Ontogeny of a Neutrophil: Mechanisms of Granulopoiesis and Homeostasis. *Microbiol. Mol. Biol. Rev.* **2018**, *82*, e00057-17. [CrossRef]
28. Spijkerman, R.; Hesselink, L.; Bongers, S.; van Wessem, K.J.P.; Vrisekoop, N.; Hietbrink, F.; Koenderman, L.; Leenen, L.P.H. Point-of-Care Analysis of Neutrophil Phenotypes: A First Step Toward Immuno-Based Precision Medicine in the Trauma ICU. *Crit. Care Explor.* **2020**, *2*, e0158. [CrossRef]
29. Kovtun, A.; Messerer, D.A.C.; Scharffetter-Kochanek, K.; Huber-Lang, M.; Ignatius, A. Neutrophils in Tissue Trauma of the Skin, Bone, and Lung: Two Sides of the Same Coin. *J. Immunol. Res.* **2018**, *2018*, 8173983. [CrossRef]
30. Hazeldine, J.; Naumann, D.N.; Toman, E.; Davies, D.; Bishop, J.R.B.; Su, Z.; Hampson, P.; Dinsdale, R.J.; Crombie, N.; Duggal, N.A.; et al. Prehospital immune responses and development of multiple organ dysfunction syndrome following traumatic injury: A prospective cohort study. *PLoS Med.* **2017**, *14*, e1002338. [CrossRef]
31. Cappenberg, A.; Margraf, A.; Thomas, K.; Bardel, B.; McCreedy, D.A.; van Marck, V.; Mellmann, A.; Lowell, C.A.; Zarbock, A. L-selectin shedding affects bacterial clearance in the lung: A new regulatory pathway for integrin outside-in signaling. *Blood* **2019**, *134*, 1445–1457. [CrossRef]
32. Lee, D.; Schultz, J.B.; Knauf, P.A.; King, R.M. Mechanical shedding of L-selectin from the neutrophil surface during rolling on sialyl Lewis x under flow. *J. Biol. Chem.* **2007**, *282*, 4812–4820. [CrossRef]
33. Mitchell, M.J.; Lin, K.S.; King, M.R. Fluid shear stress increases neutrophil activation via platelet-activating factor. *Biophys. J.* **2014**, *106*, 2243–2253. [CrossRef] [PubMed]
34. Peng, S.; Chen, S.B.; Li, L.D.; Tong, C.F.; Li, N.; Lu, S.Q.; Long, M. Impact of real-time shedding on binding kinetics of membrane-remaining L-selectin to PSGL-1. *Am. J. Physiol. Cell Physiol.* **2019**, *316*, C678–C689. [CrossRef] [PubMed]
35. Pap, G.; Furesz, J.; Fennt, J.; Kovacs, G.C.; Nagy, L.; Hamar, J. Self-regulation of neutrophils during phagocytosis is modified after severe tissue injury. *Int. J. Mol. Med.* **2006**, *17*, 649–654. [CrossRef] [PubMed]
36. Sturm, R.; Heftrig, D.; Mors, K.; Wagner, N.; Kontradowitz, K.; Jurida, K.; Marzi, I.; Relja, B. Phagocytizing activity of PMN from severe trauma patients in different post-traumatic phases during the 10-days post-injury course. *Immunobiology* **2017**, *222*, 301–307. [CrossRef] [PubMed]
37. Leliefeld, P.H.C.; Pillay, J.; Vrisekoop, N.; Heeres, M.; Tak, T.; Kox, M.; Rooijakkers, S.H.M.; Kuijpers, T.W.; Pickkers, P.; Leenen, L.P.H.; et al. Differential antibacterial control by neutrophil subsets. *Blood Adv.* **2018**, *2*, 1344–1355. [CrossRef]
38. Mortaz, E.; Alipoor, S.D.; Adcock, I.M.; Mumby, S.; Koenderman, L. Update on Neutrophil Function in Severe Inflammation. *Front. Immunol.* **2018**, *9*, 2171. [CrossRef]
39. Partrick, D.A.; Moore, F.A.; Moore, E.E.; Barnett, C.C., Jr.; Silliman, C.C. Neutrophil priming and activation in the pathogenesis of postinjury multiple organ failure. *New Horiz.* **1996**, *4*, 194–210.
40. Swain, S.D.; Rohn, T.T.; Quinn, M.T. Neutrophil priming in host defense: Role of oxidants as priming agents. *Antioxid. Redox Signal.* **2002**, *4*, 69–83. [CrossRef]
41. Wang, L.; Ai, Z.; Khoyratty, T.; Zec, K.; Eames, H.L.; van Grinsven, E.; Hudak, A.; Morris, S.; Ahern, D.; Monaco, C.; et al. ROS-producing immature neutrophils in giant cell arteritis are linked to vascular pathologies. *JCI Insight* **2020**, *5*, e139163. [CrossRef]
42. Botha, A.J.; Moore, F.A.; Moore, E.E.; Kim, F.J.; Banerjee, A.; Peterson, V.M. Postinjury neutrophil priming and activation: An early vulnerable window. *Surgery* **1995**, *118*, 358–364, discussion 364–365. [CrossRef]

43. Mortaz, E.; Zadian, S.S.; Shahir, M.; Folkerts, G.; Garssen, J.; Mumby, S.; Adcock, I.M. Does Neutrophil Phenotype Predict the Survival of Trauma Patients? *Front. Immunol.* **2019**, *10*, 2122. [CrossRef]
44. Zhu, L.; Castranova, V.; He, P. fMLP-stimulated neutrophils increase endothelial [Ca^{2+}]i and microvessel permeability in the absence of adhesion: Role of reactive oxygen species. *Am. J. Physiol. Heart Circ. Physiol.* **2005**, *288*, H1331–H1338. [CrossRef]
45. Olingy, C.E.; Emeterio, C.L.S.; Ogle, M.E.; Krieger, J.R.; Bruce, A.C.; Pfau, D.D.; Jordan, B.T.; Peirce, S.M.; Botchwey, E.A. Non-classical monocytes are biased progenitors of wound healing macrophages during soft tissue injury. *Sci. Rep.* **2017**, *7*, 447. [CrossRef]
46. Flohe, S.; Flohe, S.B.; Schade, F.U.; Waydhas, C. Immune response of severely injured patients–influence of surgical intervention and therapeutic impact. *Langenbecks Arch. Surg.* **2007**, *392*, 639–648. [CrossRef]
47. Kirchhoff, C.; Biberthaler, P.; Mutschler, W.E.; Faist, E.; Jochum, M.; Zedler, S. Early down-regulation of the pro-inflammatory potential of monocytes is correlated to organ dysfunction in patients after severe multiple injury: A cohort study. *Crit. Care* **2009**, *13*, R88. [CrossRef]
48. Patel, A.A.; Zhang, Y.; Fullerton, J.N.; Boelen, L.; Rongvaux, A.; Maini, A.A.; Bigley, V.; Flavell, R.A.; Gilroy, D.W.; Asquith, B.; et al. The fate and lifespan of human monocyte subsets in steady state and systemic inflammation. *J. Exp. Med.* **2017**, *214*, 1913–1923. [CrossRef]
49. West, S.D.; Goldberg, D.; Ziegler, A.; Krencicki, M.; Clos, T.W.D.; Mold, C. Transforming growth factor-beta, macrophage colony-stimulating factor and C-reactive protein levels correlate with CD14(high)CD16+ monocyte induction and activation in trauma patients. *PLoS ONE* **2012**, *7*, e52406. [CrossRef]
50. Stansfield, B.K.; Ingram, D.A. Clinical significance of monocyte heterogeneity. *Clin. Transl. Med.* **2015**, *4*, 5. [CrossRef]
51. Hotchkiss, R.S.; Monneret, G.; Payen, D. Immunosuppression in sepsis: A novel understanding of the disorder and a new therapeutic approach. *Lancet Infect. Dis.* **2013**, *13*, 260–268. [CrossRef]
52. Bao, F.; Bailey, C.S.; Gurr, K.R.; Bailey, S.I.; Rosas-Arellano, M.P.; Dekaban, G.A.; Weaver, L.C. Increased oxidative activity in human blood neutrophils and monocytes after spinal cord injury. *Exp. Neurol.* **2009**, *215*, 308–316. [CrossRef] [PubMed]
53. Seshadri, A.; Brat, G.A.; Yorkgitis, B.K.; Keegan, J.; Dolan, J.; Salim, A.; Askari, R.; Lederer, J.A. Phenotyping the Immune Response to Trauma: A Multiparametric Systems Immunology Approach. *Crit. Care Med.* **2017**, *45*, 1523–1530. [CrossRef]
54. Paiva, C.N.; Bozza, M.T. Are reactive oxygen species always detrimental to pathogens? *Antioxid. Redox Signal.* **2014**, *20*, 1000–1037. [CrossRef] [PubMed]

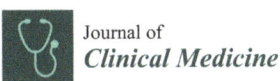

Article

I-FABP as a Potential Marker for Intestinal Barrier Loss in Porcine Polytrauma

Jan Tilmann Vollrath [1], Felix Klingebiel [1,2,3], Felix Bläsius [4], Johannes Greven [4], Eftychios Bolierakis [4], Aleksander J. Nowak [3], Marija Simic [3], Frank Hildebrand [4], Ingo Marzi [1] and Borna Relja [3,*]

[1] Department of Trauma, Hand and Reconstructive Surgery, Goethe University, 60596 Frankfurt, Germany
[2] Department of Trauma, University of Zurich, Universitätsspital Zurich, 8091 Zurich, Switzerland
[3] Experimental Radiology, Department of Radiology and Nuclear Medicine, Otto von Guericke University, 39120 Magdeburg, Germany
[4] Department of Trauma and Reconstructive Surgery, RWTH Aachen University, 52074 Aachen, Germany
* Correspondence: info@bornarelja.com

Abstract: Polytrauma and concomitant hemorrhagic shock can lead to intestinal damage and subsequent multiple organ dysfunction syndrome. The intestinal fatty acid-binding protein (I-FABP) is expressed in the intestine and appears quickly in the circulation after intestinal epithelial cell damage. This porcine animal study investigates the I-FABP dynamics in plasma and urine after polytrauma. Furthermore, it evaluates to what extent I-FABP can also act as a marker of intestinal damage in a porcine polytrauma model. Eight pigs (Sus scrofa) were subjected to polytrauma which consisted of lung contusion, tibial fracture, liver laceration, and hemorrhagic shock followed by blood and fluid resuscitation and fracture fixation with an external fixator. Eight sham animals were identically instrumented but not injured. Afterwards, intensive care treatment including mechanical ventilation for 72 h followed. I-FABP levels in blood and urine were determined by ELISA. In addition, immunohistological staining for I-FABP, active caspase-3 and myeloperoxidase were performed after 72 h. Plasma and urine I-FABP levels were significantly increased shortly after trauma. I-FABP expression in intestinal tissue showed significantly lower expression in polytraumatized animals vs. sham. Caspase-3 and myeloperoxidase expression in the immunohistological examination were significantly higher in the jejunum and ileum of polytraumatized animals compared to sham animals. This study confirms a loss of intestinal barrier after polytrauma which is indicated by increased I-FABP levels in plasma and urine as well as decreased I-FABP levels in immunohistological staining of the intestine.

Keywords: I-FABP; biomarker; intestinal damage; hemorrhagic shock; major trauma

Citation: Vollrath, J.T.; Klingebiel, F.; Bläsius, F.; Greven, J.; Bolierakis, E.; Nowak, A.J.; Simic, M.; Hildebrand, F.; Marzi, I.; Relja, B. I-FABP as a Potential Marker for Intestinal Barrier Loss in Porcine Polytrauma. *J. Clin. Med.* **2022**, *11*, 4599. https://doi.org/10.3390/jcm11154599

Academic Editors: Roman Pfeifer and Bernard Allaouchiche

Received: 31 March 2022
Accepted: 2 August 2022
Published: 7 August 2022

Publisher's Note: MDPI stays neutral with regard to jurisdictional claims in published maps and institutional affiliations.

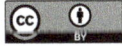

Copyright: © 2022 by the authors. Licensee MDPI, Basel, Switzerland. This article is an open access article distributed under the terms and conditions of the Creative Commons Attribution (CC BY) license (https://creativecommons.org/licenses/by/4.0/).

1. Introduction

Despite significant achievements that reduced injury-related morbidity and mortality in recent decades, the number of polytraumatized patients admitted to hospitals still remains high and worldwide approximately 4.8 million human deaths per year are caused by traumatic injuries [1]. After traumatized patients survive the first phase after injury, they are at high mortality risk from late-occurring complications such as multiple organ failure (MOF) and/or sepsis [2,3]. For several decades, the gut has been considered to play an important role in the development of systemic inflammation, sepsis and multiple organ dysfunction syndrome (MODS) after trauma, hemorrhagic shock and in critically ill patients in general [4,5]. The predominant theory in the 1980s associating the gut with MODS underlines the key role of bacterial translocation caused by an increased intestinal hyperpermeability allowing bacteria to enter the portal blood and cause downstream organ dysfunction [5,6]. In contrast, more recent studies emphasize the role of the mesenteric lymph as a carrier of gut-derived danger-associated molecular patterns (DAMPs) to the lung and the systemic circulation, leading to the "gut-lymph hypothesis" [6,7]. Furthermore, recent data suggest that gut luminal contents, including the mucus gel layer, pancreatic proteases and gut flora, as well as the luminal response to splanchnic ischemia, play an important role in modulating gut injury [4]. Regardless of the underlying mechanisms, early recognition of patients with intestinal injury and at risk of developing MODS or MOF is of enormous clinical relevance. D-lactate, glutathione S-transferase (GST) and intestinal fatty acid binding protein (I-FABP) have been proposed as novel biomarkers of intestinal ischemia, and plasma citrulline levels have been proposed as a novel quantitative biomarker of significantly reduced enterocyte mass and function [4,8]. FABPs are small proteins localized intracellularly or within the plasma membrane and are released in their soluble form into the extracellular space early after cell or tissue damage [9,10]. Therefore, FABPs can be used as urine and plasma markers for tissue-specific injuries [9,11]. I-FABP is present in enterocytes of the small intestine as well as partly in the colon and appears quickly in the circulation after intestinal epithelial cell damage [9,12]. Voth et al. investigated I-FABP levels in polytraumatized patients and confirmed I-FABP as a useful and promising early marker for the detection of abdominal injury [9,13]. Furthermore, even in the absence of an abdominal injury, I-FABP indicated intestinal damage by hemorrhagic shock [9]. In this study, we investigated I-FABP plasma and urine levels in a standardized porcine trauma model which consisted of lung contusion, tibial fracture, liver laceration, and hemorrhagic shock followed by fluid resuscitation and fracture fixation with an external fixator. Furthermore, this study provides insights into changes in I-FABP-, caspase-3- and myeloperoxidase levels in intestinal tissue after polytrauma which are not possible to be investigated in human clinical studies.

2. Materials and Methods

2.1. Ethics

All experiments were conducted in compliance with federal German law. Especially with regard to the protection of animals, institutional guidelines and the criteria in "Guide for the Care and Use of Laboratory Animals" (Eighth Edition The National Academies Press, 2011) [14]. All animals were continuously treated in consensus with the ARRIVE guidelines [15]. Experiments were authorized by the responsible government authority ("Landesamt für Natur-, Umwelt- und Verbraucherschutz": LANUV-NRW, Germany, AZ: 81.02.04.2018.A113). The in vivo experiments were performed at the Institute of Laboratory Animal Science & Experimental Surgery, RWTH Aachen University, Germany.

2.2. Animals

16 German landrace pigs (*Sus scrofa*, 30 ± 5 kg, male, three months old) from a disease-free barrier breeding facility were used for the experiment. Before the beginning of the experiment, the animals were fasted overnight but had free access to water ad libitum. The animals were held in rooms with air-conditioning and had the opportunity to acclimatize to the new environment for a minimum of seven days before the experiment started. Furthermore, animals were examined by a veterinarian ahead of the beginning of the experiment. The porcine polytrauma model is well established in our study group and has been reported in detail by Horst et al. [16]. The underlying study was part of a larger animal study containing polytraumatized animals and sham animals that were not injured.

2.3. Porcine Polytrauma Model

A total of eight pigs were attributed to a standardized polytrauma which consisted of a tibia fracture, a liver laceration, a unilateral blunt chest trauma and hemorrhagic shock (40 ± 5 mm Hg for 90 min). During the following, ATLS-phase animals were resuscitated and the fracture was fixated with the help of an external fixator. Eight sham animals underwent identical instrumentation but were not traumatized. In advance of the beginning of the experiment, all animals received an intramuscular application of 4 mg/kg azaperone (Stressnil™, Janssen, Neuss, Germany). Before surgery and every 24 h during the further experiment a prophylactic antibiotic treatment was administered (1.5 g cefuroxime i.v., Fresenius Kabi, Bad Homburg, Germany). In order to induce anesthesia, propofol was injected into the vein at a dosage of 3 mg/kg (Propofol Claris 2% MCT, Pharmore GmbH, Ibbenbüren, Germany). After that, pigs were intubated orotracheally with a 7.5 ch tube (Hi-Lo Lanz™, Medtronic, Meerbusch, Germany). In order to prevent awareness and pain during the further course of the experiment, general anesthesia was sustained with intravenous application of propofol, fentanyl (Rotexmedica, Trittau, Germany) and midazolam (Rotexmedica, Trittau, Germany). During the whole experiment, pigs were ventilated with lung protective ventilation (Draeger, Evita 4, Lübeck, Germany). The tidal volume was set to 6–8 mL/kg. Furthermore, positive end-expiratory pressure (PEEP) was set to 8 mm Hg (plateau pressure < 28 mm Hg) and arterial pCO_2 was aimed to be between 35 and 45 mm Hg which was regularly controlled with the help of blood gas analysis. To maintain anesthesia, and monitor central venous pressure and provide fluids, a sterile central venous catheter (4-Lumen Catheter, 8,5 Fr, Arrow Catheter, Teleflex Medical, Fellbach, Germany) was inserted into the right external jugular vein. Furthermore, a sterile two-lumen hemodialysis catheter (Arrow International, Teleflex Medical, Fellbach, Germany) was implemented into the left femoral vein to generate hemorrhagic shock adequately in the further experimental course. To monitor blood pressure and to generate arterial blood gas analysis an arterial catheter (PiCCO, Pulsion Medical Systems, Feldkirchen, Germany) was inserted into the right femoral artery. Moreover, a urinary catheter was inserted into the bladder (12.0 Fr, Cystofix, Braun, Melsungen, Germany). The first blood samples were taken shortly after the implementation of the central venous catheter. Before subjecting the pigs to polytrauma, an equilibration period of one hour was awaited. The porcine polytrauma was induced as previously described by Horst et al. but with slight modifications [16]. To represent the situation and condition during trauma more closely the fraction of inspired oxygen (FiO_2) was set to 21% before the initiation of trauma. Furthermore, fluid administration was restricted to a minimum of 10 mL/h. The endeavors to maintain normothermia with the help of forced-air warming systems were stopped and a drop in body temperature into hypothermia was not prevented anymore to imitate the preclinical situation. Animals were placed on the left side and the tibia was fractured with the help of a bolt gun (Blitz-Kerner, turbocut JOBB GmbH, Bad Neustadt an der Saale, Germany; Ammunition: 9 × 17 mm^2, RUAG Ammotec GmbH, Fürth, Germany). Then pigs were placed on the right side followed by induction of blunt thoracic trauma with the help of a bolt shot to the left dorsal lower thorax. After that, a midline-laparotomy was performed and the caudal lobe of the liver was incised (4.5 × 4.5 cm^2) leading to uncontrolled bleeding. Bleeding was stopped after 30 s by packing with five sterile gauze compresses (10 × 10 cm^2). To induce hemorrhagic shock, blood was withdrawn from the femoral venous catheter until a mean arterial blood pressure (MAP) of 40 ± 5 mm Hg. This state of hemorrhagic shock was maintained for 90 min. Resuscitation was performed by returning the withdrawn blood, adjusting the FiO_2 to baseline and infusion of crystalloid fluids (4 mL/kg body weight/h). To reach normothermia (38.7–39.8 °C) again, warm air was applied with the help of a forced-air warming system. The tibial fracture was fixated with the help of an external fixator. Further intensive care treatment, as well as the management of complications (e.g., pneumothorax), were performed according to the latest recommendations of the European Resuscitation Council and the Advanced Trauma Life Support (ATLS®) [17,18]. After 72 h pigs were euthanized with the help of potassium chloride. Figure 1 shows an overview of the experimental design.

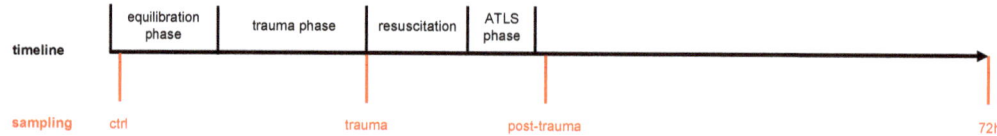

Figure 1. The experimental design is shown. Animals were subjected to polytrauma which consisted of lung contusion, tibial fracture, liver laceration and hemorrhagic shock. Polytrauma was followed by blood and fluid resuscitation as well as fracture fixation with an external fixator. Blood sampling was performed at the beginning shortly after implementation of the central venous catheter (ctrl), shortly after trauma (trauma) and in the further course after the Advanced Trauma Life Support (ATLS) phase (post-trauma).

2.4. Blood and Urine Sampling and Processing

Blood samples were obtained shortly after the implementation of the central venous catheter (ctrl), shortly after trauma (trauma) and in the further course after the ATLS phase (post-trauma) in prechilled ethylendiaminetetraacetic acid tubes (EDTA, S-Monovette®, Sarstedt, Nümbrecht, Germany) and kept on ice. Then, blood samples were centrifuged at $2000 \times g$ for 15 min at 4 °C and the supernatant was stored at −80 °C until further analysis. The same protocol was applied for urine samples.

2.5. ELISA Measurements

I-FABP ELISA measurements were performed with plasma and urine samples in accordance with the manufacturer's manuals (Porcine IFABP/FABP2 (Intestinal Fatty Acid Binding Protein) ELISA Kit, #MBS2501296, MyBioSource, Inc., San Diego, CA, USA). According to the manufacturer the used I-FABP ELISA Kit has a sensitivity is 46.88 pg/mL. Before ELISA blood and urine were centrifuged at $2000 \times g$ for 15 min at 4 °C and supernatant was stored at −80 °C until further analysis.

2.6. Immunohistochemical Staining of Intestine Tissue

Parts of jejunum and ileum (1×1 cm^2) were stored in 4% formalin for overnight fixation and kept in 70% ethanol until paraffin embedding and sectioning. Paraffin-embedded intestine samples were sectioned (3 µm), deparaffinized, rehydrated and stained with anti-FABP2 antibody (Cloud-Clone Corp., Houston, TX, USA), anti-Myeloperoxidase antibody (Abcam, Cambridge, UK) or anti-Caspase-3 antibody (Abcam, Cambridge, UK). Following deparaffinization, antigen retrieval was conducted under a steam atmosphere using an R-Universal epitope recovery buffer (Aptum, Kassel, Germany) for one hour (Retriever 2010, Prestige Medical). The endogenous tissue peroxidase activity was blocked with hydrogen peroxide according to the manufacturer's instructions (Peroxidase UltraVision Block, Dako, Hamburg, Germany). After washing with water and PBS, anti-FABP2 antibody (1:100, PAA559Po01), anti-Myeloperoxidase antibody (1:100, ab9535) or anti-Caspase-3 antibody (1:100, ab4051) was applied as a primary antibody. After the incubation at room temperature for one hour, and a subsequent washing procedure, a secondary anti-rabbit horseradish peroxidase-linked antibody (Nichirei Biosciences Inc., Tokyo, Japan) was applied to detect specific binding. As the substrate, 3-amino-9-ethylcarbazole (AEC, DCS Innovative Diagnostik-Systeme, Hamburg, Germany) was applied. Then, the sections were counterstained with hematoxylin. The relative staining intensity of the AEC substrate per slide was evaluated using the ImageJ software in a blinded manner by an independent examiner for anti-FABP2 staining. For MPO and caspase-3 15–20 high power fields per slide were quantified by counting positively stained cells.

2.7. Statistical Analyses

Statistical analyses were performed by using GraphPad Prism 6 (Graphpad Software Inc., San Diego, CA, USA). Data are presented as mean ± standard error of the mean.

Based on the D'Agostino–Pearson normality test differences between the groups were determined by the non-parametric Kruskal–Wallis test followed by Dunn's post hoc test for the correction of multiple comparisons. The comparison between polytrauma and sham groups was performed using the unpaired Mann–Whitney test. A p-value less than 0.05 was considered to be statistically significant.

3. Results
3.1. Data Decription
3.1.1. Plasma and Urine I-FABP Concentrations after Trauma

The time course of I-FABP concentration in the blood shows a significant increase shortly after trauma compared to the control before trauma ($p < 0.05$). In the further posttraumatic course, I-FABP concentration in the blood decreases again reaching the pre-trauma ctrl levels (Figure 2A). The time course of urine I-FABP-concentration shows a distinct and statistically significant increase shortly after trauma and in the further posttraumatic course compared with the ctrl ($p < 0.05$, Figure 2B).

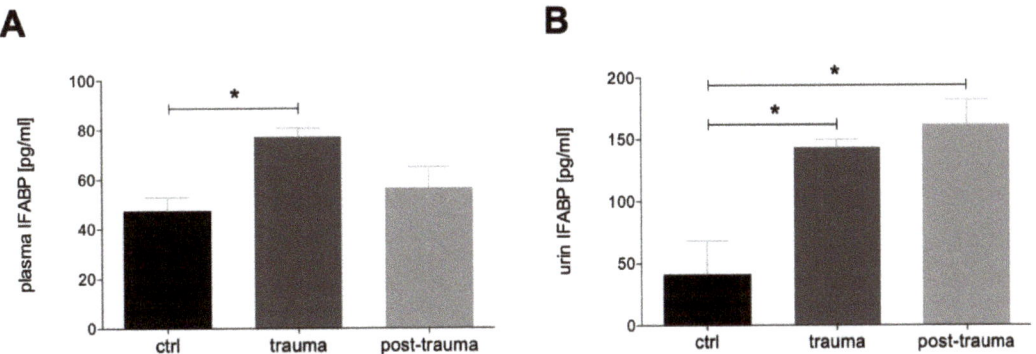

Figure 2. Intestinal fatty acid binding protein (I-FABP) levels in plasma and urine. Plasma (**A**) and urine (**B**) I-FABP levels shortly after implementation of the central venous catheter (ctrl), shortly after trauma (trauma, within 90 min during trauma and hemorrhagic shock) and in the further course after the Advanced Trauma Life Support (ATLS) phase (post-trauma, within 6 h after reperfusion and surgery) are shown. *: $p < 0.05$.

3.1.2. I-FABP Expression in Intestinal Tissue

A comparison of the I-FABP expression in the intestinal tissue of sham and polytraumatized animals shows significantly lower I-FABP expression in the jejunum of polytraumatized animals compared to sham animals ($p < 0.05$, Figure 3A). The same significantly decreased expression after polytrauma vs. sham can be observed in the ileum ($p < 0.05$, Figure 3B). Figure 3C shows exemplary histological I-FABP stainings from the jejunum and ileum in sham and polytraumatized animals.

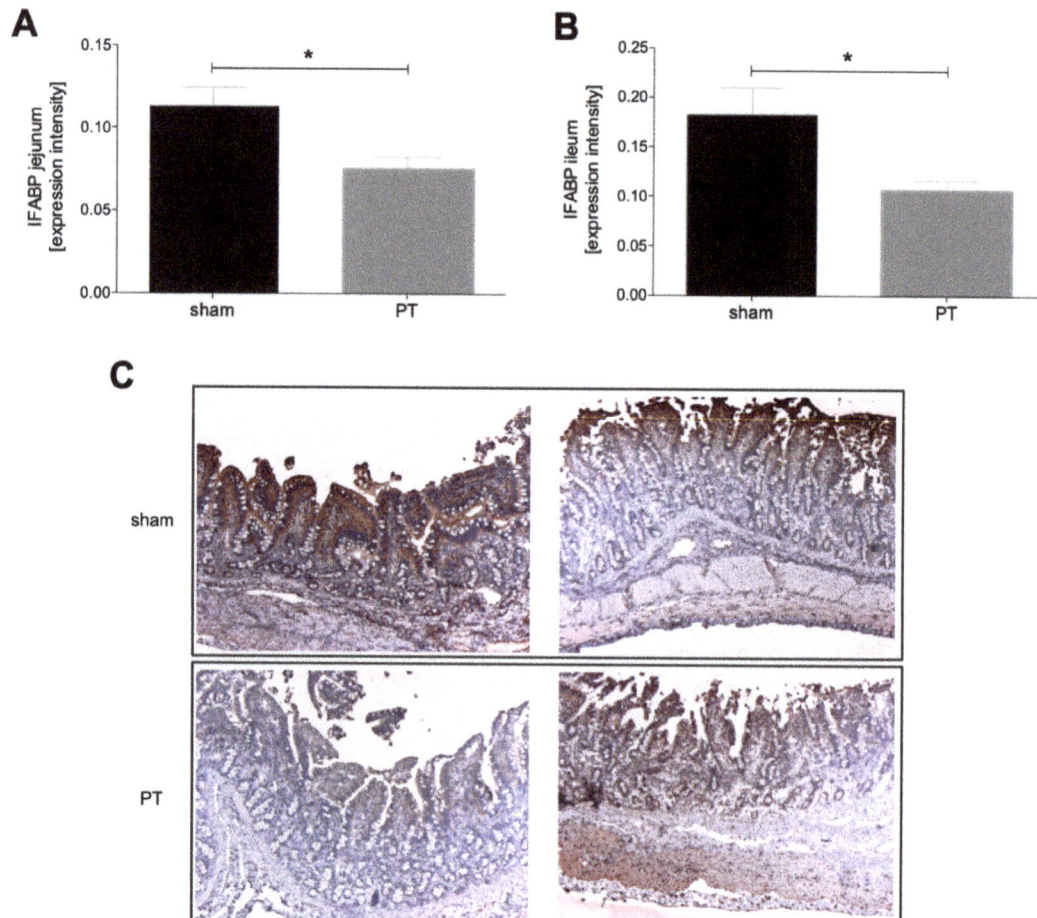

Figure 3. Expression intensity of intestinal fatty acid binding protein (I-FABP) in jejunum (**A**) and ileum (**B**) in polytraumatized (PT) and sham animals after 72 h is shown. (**C**) Exemplary images of immunohistological staining for I-FABP of ileum and jejunum from polytraumatized and sham animals. *: $p < 0.05$.

3.1.3. Caspase-3 Expression in Intestinal Tissue

A comparison of the active caspase-3 expression in intestinal tissue from sham and polytraumatized animals shows significantly higher expression in the jejunum of polytraumatized animals compared to sham animals ($p < 0.05$, Figure 4A). Significantly increased expression after polytrauma vs. sham can be observed in the ileum ($p < 0.05$, Figure 4B). Figure 4C shows exemplary histological caspase-3 stainings from the jejunum and ileum in sham and polytraumatized animals.

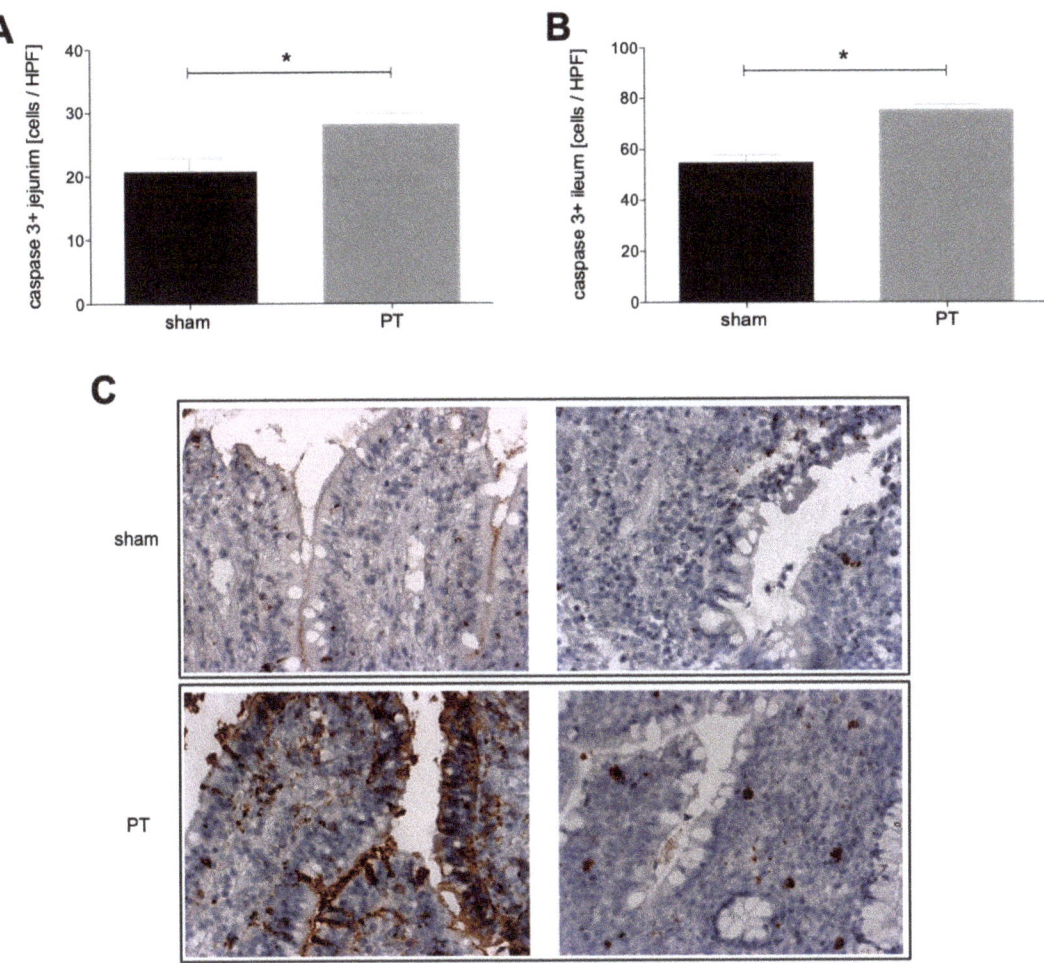

Figure 4. Number of caspase-3 positive cells per high power field (HPF) in jejunum (**A**) and ileum (**B**) of polytraumatized (PT) and sham animals after 72 h is shown. (**C**) Exemplary images of immunohistological staining for caspase-3 of ileum and jejunum from polytraumatized and sham animals. *: $p < 0.05$.

3.1.4. Myeloperoxidase Expression in Intestinal Tissue

A comparison of the myeloperoxidase expression in intestinal tissues from sham and polytraumatized animals shows significantly higher expression in both jejunum and ileum of polytraumatized animals compared to sham animals ($p < 0.05$, Figure 5A,B).

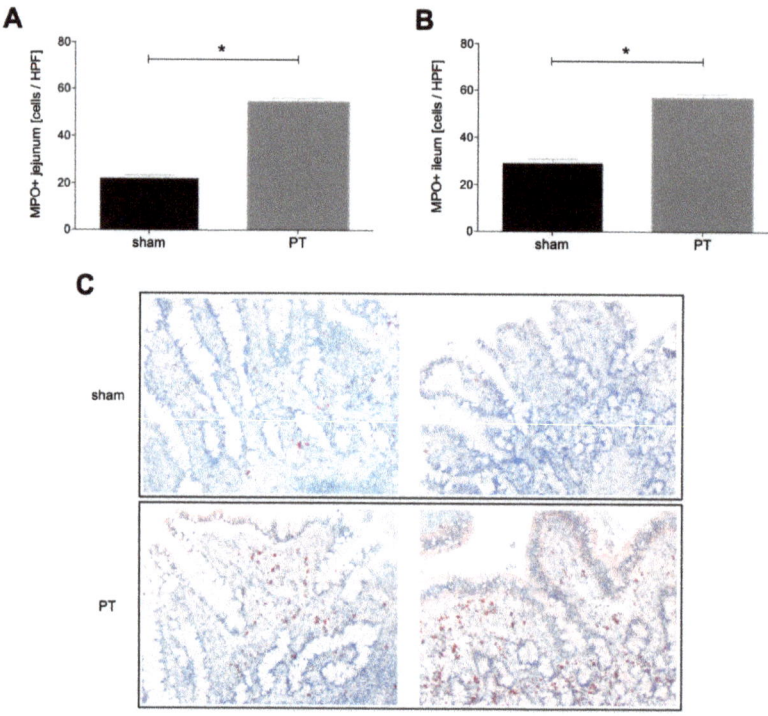

Figure 5. Number of myeloperoxidase positive cells (MPO$^+$) per high power field (HPF) in jejunum (**A**) and ileum (**B**) of polytraumatized (PT) and sham animals after 72 h is shown. (**C**) Exemplary images of immuno-histological staining for MPO of ileum and jejunum from polytraumatized and sham animals. *: $p < 0.05$.

4. Discussion

In the recent study, we investigated plasma and urine I-FAPB levels in a standardized porcine polytrauma model and observed significantly increased plasma I-FABP levels immediately after trauma while plasma I-FABP decreased in the further course. This is in line with studies by Voth et al. showing increased I-FABP levels already in the emergency room in polytraumatized patients with concomitant abdominal injury, as well as in polytraumatized patients with hemorrhagic shock [9,13]. Voth et al. observed I-FABP levels decreasing to control levels already on day one after trauma [9,13]. Khadaroo et al. investigated I-FABP as a biomarker for the early diagnosis of acute mesenteric ischemia in mice and observed significantly increased plasma I-FABP levels already after ischemia of 30 min resulting in a further increase with values continuing to rise clearly with increasing ischemia time [19]. Furthermore, a significant rise in plasma I-FABP concentrations could already be demonstrated 15–30 min after clamping of the mesenteric artery in a porcine ischemia model [20]. Several other studies report elevated serum I-FABP levels in patients with mesenteric ischemia [21–23]. In line with these studies which observed increased levels of I-FABP in the blood in the context of an undersupply of the intestine, we assume that in our polytrauma model an undersupply of the intestine with blood probably occurs in the context of the hemorrhagic shock phase. This theory is supported by the underlying data showing significantly more caspase-3 positive cells in the intestine of polytraumatized animals, which corresponds to an increased apoptosis rate. However, since our study does not have a separate group with hemorrhagic shock without further injuries, this can only be speculated. In line with our results, Hotchkiss et al. reported rapidly occurring apoptosis in lymphocyte and intestinal epithelial cells in patients with trauma and ischemia/reperfusion injury and concluded that their results support the theory that gut mucosal apoptosis may compromise bowel integrity and lead to translocation of bacteria and endotoxin into the systemic circulation [24].

In line with this, we observed decreased I-FABP expression in the small intestine and increased I-FABP plasma levels in animals that were exposed to multiple traumas, which could be an indication of possible damage to the intestinal barrier. Sturm et al. also observed a significant increase in I-FABP in serum following acute alcohol consumption and concluded that this might suggest possible damage to the intestinal barrier [25]. In line with the study by Khadaroo et al. showing increased serum I-FABP levels as well as increased MPO activity in the intestine after mesenteric ischemia [19], we also observed increased MPO activity in the intestine after polytrauma. Furthermore, Khadaroo et al. observed that intestinal ischemia resulted in lung injury in a time-dependent manner and that I-FABP also directly correlated with resultant lung injury [19]. The potential link between the gut and the lung might be the mesenteric lymph as shown by Lu et al. [26]. In an animal model the authors could demonstrate that trauma-hemorrhagic shock induces pulmonary endothelial cell apoptosis and that pulmonary endothelial and nonendothelial cell apoptosis occurs largely due to gut-derived factors carried in the mesenteric lymph [26]. Nowadays it is undisputed that intestinal barrier dysfunction and increased gut permeability are associated with the development of MODS [7]. While clinical data did not confirm the initial theory of bacterial translocation, the current pathogenetic aspects support the gut-lymph axis which is reviewed in detail elsewhere [7]. Anyway, the gut seems to be a pivotal proinflammatory organ promoting deleterious effects in even remote organs, through the release of DAMPs, without the need for systemic bacterial translocation [7]. However, what both theories have in common is the loss of the intestinal barrier, which was also shown in this study by lower I-FABP expressions in the immunohistological staining of the intestine as well as increased blood and urine I-FABP levels after trauma.

It must be mentioned and considered that this animal study has several limitations. First of all, and of utmost importance, is the limited sample size which is due to animals' welfare and the very high cost of large animal models. Moreover, due to the limited duration of the experiment, we cannot make a well-founded statement about whether the observed changes in the intestinal barrier will influence the outcome beyond the observational period of 72 h. Furthermore, we must be aware of the immunological variability among different species, when we transfer findings from animal experiments to humans [27]. Another limitation of the study is that it only indicates a loss of the intestinal barrier after polytrauma. It is purely observational, without investigating the pathogenesis and does not answer the question of which aspect of the traumatic injury (hemorrhagic shock, fracture, lung injury, etc.) leads to the disruption of the intestinal barrier. Furthermore, additional biochemical or observational markers of severity have not been associated with I-FABP levels. However, in this regard, we need to consider the original characterization study of the underlying model, where a descriptive assessment of inflammatory changes has been performed. Horst et al. have described an early systemic increase in inflammatory parameters with a decline during the time course after polytrauma [16]. In another study in polytraumatized patients, we have shown that I-FABP correlated with IL-6 und PCT levels. That study revealed the early presence of intestinal epithelial cell damage in trauma patients. The extent of intestinal damage was associated with the presence of shock and injury severity. Early intestinal damage preceded and was related to the subsequent developing inflammatory response [28]. In the underlying study, we measured IL-6 at 72 h after polytrauma in the samples that still were available. We found very low but still detectable levels of IL-6 by using a high-sensitivity ELISA kit. The levels of IL-6 were statistically significantly different between sham and polytrauma (1.685 ± 0.389 vs. 3.387 ± 0.532 pg/mL, $p = 0.030$) after 72 h. Taken together, according to that and the studies reported above, I-FABP increase appears associated with an increase in inflammatory parameters in the underlying model. Another limitation of the study is the administration of medications such as antibiotics, opiates, or the lack of enteral nutrition during the experiment which can lead to a distortion of the results. Furthermore, the quantification of I-FABP expression is a bit arbitrary, and in future studies, western blot analyses, as well as additional markers of enterocyte damage, should be implemented. Moreover, since we did not do other tissue-specific analyses of FABP, we cannot exclude that this array cross-reacts with FABP from origins other than the intestine. Another limitation is certainly I-FABP itself which is still arguably a biomarker without clinical applicability. Timmermans et al. investigated intestinal damage using I-FABP in trauma patients during the first days of their hospital admission and observed substantial differences in plasma I-FABP levels between patients with abdominal trauma and low Hb/MAP and patients with other trauma types and normal/high Hb/MAP [29]. Therefore, the authors concluded that targeted interventions, such as (more aggressive or more goal-directed) fluid resuscitation and/or hemodynamic support, may represent a viable treatment option in these subgroups of patients. Because the intestinal injury is suggested to be related to late complications, such as MODS or sepsis in trauma patients, strategies to prevent intestinal damage consequences or the persisting damage itself after trauma could be of benefit to these patients. Yet, clinicians can also make decisions on the amount of volume resuscitation or hemodynamic support based on other clinical or technical parameters as well. Measurement of I-FABP can only provide an additional read-out parameter. Voth et al. showed that I-FABP levels are significantly increased in patients with an intestinal injury compared to patients with abdominal injury but without intestinal damage and concluded that I-FABP might be a useful and promising early marker for the detection of an injury to the small or large intestine [13]. Thus, a threshold of the initial I-FABP level indicating the need for exploratory surgery would be of significant clinical importance. Thus, it is of utmost clinical importance to elaborate on whether I-FABP allows early diagnosis of specific intestinal injuries that cannot be seen on CT scan and therefore may be overlooked.

5. Conclusions

In conclusion, our study indicates a loss of intestinal barrier after polytrauma which is demonstrated by increased I-FABP levels in plasma and urine, as well as decreased I-FABP levels in immunohistological staining of the intestine. Future studies in larger cohorts need to investigate the pathogenesis, the underlying molecular pathways and possible treatment options.

Author Contributions: Conceptualization, B.R.; methodology, J.T.V., F.K., F.B., J.G., E.B. and B.R.; validation, J.T.V.; formal analysis, B.R. and J.T.V.; investigation, J.T.V., F.B., J.G. and E.B.; data curation, J.T.V.; writing—original draft preparation, J.T.V.; writing—review and editing, J.T.V., F.K., F.B., J.G., E.B., A.J.N., M.S., F.H., I.M. and B.R.; visualization, J.T.V. and B.R.; supervision, B.R.; project administration, J.T.V., F.B. and B.R.; funding acquisition, B.R. and F.H. All authors have read and agreed to the published version of the manuscript.

Funding: The work was supported by grants from the DFG HI 820/5-1, DFG WU 820/2-1 and RE 3304/8-1.

Institutional Review Board Statement: All experiments were performed in compliance with the federal German law with regards to the protection of animals, institutional guidelines and the criteria in "Guide for the Care and Use of Laboratory Animals" (Eighth Edition The National Academies Press, 2011). During the study duration animals were consistently handled in accordance with the ARRIVE guidelines and experiments were authorized by the responsible government authority ("Landesamt für Natur-, Umwelt- und Verbraucherschutz": LANUV-NRW, Germany, AZ: 81.02.04.2018.A113). All Animal experiments were performed at the Institute of Laboratory Animal Science & Experimental Surgery, RWTH Aachen University, Germany.

Data Availability Statement: The data are available upon a reasonable request from the corresponding author.

Acknowledgments: We thank Katrin Jurida, Kerstin Kontradowitz and Alexander Schaible for outstanding technical assistance.

Conflicts of Interest: The authors declare no conflict of interest. The funders had no role in the design of the study; in the collection, analyses, or interpretation of data; in the writing of the manuscript, or in the decision to publish the results.

References

1. Haagsma, J.A.; Graetz, N.; Bolliger, I.; Naghavi, M.; Higashi, H.; Mullany, E.C.; Abera, S.F.; Abraham, J.P.; Adofo, K.; Al-sharif, U.; et al. The global burden of injury: Incidence, mortality, disability-adjusted life years and time trends from the Global Burden of Disease study 2013. *Inj. Prev. J. Int. Soc. Child. Adolesc. Inj. Prev.* **2016**, *22*, 3–18. [CrossRef] [PubMed]
2. Nast-Kolb, D.; Aufmkolk, M.; Rucholtz, S.; Obertacke, U.; Waydhas, C. Multiple organ failure still a major cause of morbidity but not mortality in blunt multiple trauma. *J. Trauma* **2001**, *51*, 835–841; discussion 841–842. [CrossRef] [PubMed]
3. Relja, B.; Mörs, K.; Marzi, I. Danger signals in trauma. *Eur. J. Trauma Emerg. Surg. Off. Publ. Eur. Trauma Soc.* **2018**, *44*, 301–316. [CrossRef] [PubMed]
4. Sertaridou, E.; Papaioannou, V.; Kolios, G.; Pneumatikos, I. Gut failure in critical care: Old school versus new school. *Ann. Gastroenterol.* **2015**, *28*, 309–322.
5. Mittal, R.; Coopersmith, C.M. Redefining the gut as the motor of critical illness. *Trends Mol. Med.* **2014**, *20*, 214–223. [CrossRef]
6. Patel, J.J.; Rosenthal, M.D.; Miller, K.R.; Martindale, R.G. The gut in trauma. *Curr. Opin. Crit. Care* **2016**, *22*, 339–346. [CrossRef]
7. Assimakopoulos, S.F.; Triantos, C.; Thomopoulos, K.; Fligou, F.; Maroulis, I.; Marangos, M.; Gogos, C.A. Gut-origin sepsis in the critically ill patient: Pathophysiology and treatment. *Infection* **2018**, *46*, 751–760. [CrossRef]
8. Evennett, N.J.; Petrov, M.S.; Mittal, A.; Windsor, J.A. Systematic review and pooled estimates for the diagnostic accuracy of serological markers for intestinal ischemia. *World J. Surg.* **2009**, *33*, 1374–1383. [CrossRef]
9. Voth, M.; Lustenberger, T.; Relja, B.; Marzi, I. Is I-FABP not only a marker for the detection abdominal injury but also of hemorrhagic shock in severely injured trauma patients? *World J. Emerg. Surg. WJES* **2019**, *14*, 49. [CrossRef]
10. Glatz, J.F.; van der Vusse, G.J. Cellular fatty acid-binding proteins: Their function and physiological significance. *Prog. Lipid Res.* **1996**, *35*, 243–282. [CrossRef]
11. Pelsers, M.M.A.L.; Hermens, W.T.; Glatz, J.F.C. Fatty acid-binding proteins as plasma markers of tissue injury. *Clin. Chim. Acta Int. J. Clin. Chem.* **2005**, *352*, 15–35. [CrossRef]
12. Pelsers, M.M.A.L.; Namiot, Z.; Kisielewski, W.; Namiot, A.; Januszkiewicz, M.; Hermens, W.T.; Glatz, J.F.C. Intestinal-type and liver-type fatty acid-binding protein in the intestine. Tissue distribution and clinical utility. *Clin. Biochem.* **2003**, *36*, 529–535. [CrossRef]
13. Voth, M.; Duchene, M.; Auner, B.; Lustenberger, T.; Relja, B.; Marzi, I. I-FABP is a Novel Marker for the Detection of Intestinal Injury in Severely Injured Trauma Patients. *World J. Surg.* **2017**, *41*, 3120–3127. [CrossRef]
14. National Research Council (US) Committee for the Update of the Guide for the Care and Use of Laboratory Animals. *Guide for the Care and Use of Laboratory Animals*, 8th ed.; The National Academies Collection: Reports funded by National Institutes of Health; National Academies Press: Washington, DC, USA, 2011. Available online: http://www.ncbi.nlm.nih.gov/books/NBK54050/ (accessed on 1 April 2022).
15. Kilkenny, C.; Browne, W.J.; Cuthi, I.; Emerson, M.; Altman, D.G. Improving bioscience research reporting: The ARRIVE guidelines for reporting animal research. *Vet. Clin. Pathol.* **2012**, *41*, 27–31. [CrossRef]
16. Horst, K.; Simon, T.P.; Pfeifer, R.; Teuben, M.; AlMahmoud, K.; Zhi, Q.; Santos, S.A.; Wembers, C.C.; Leonhardt, S.; Heussen, N.; et al. Characterization of blunt chest trauma in a long-term porcine model of severe multiple trauma. *Sci. Rep.* **2016**, *6*, 39659. [CrossRef]
17. ATLS Subcommittee; American College of Surgeons' Committee on Trauma; International ATLS Working Group. Advanced trauma life support (ATLS®): The ninth edition. *J. Trauma Acute Care Surg.* **2013**, *74*, 1363–1366.
18. Nikolaou, N.I.; Welsford, M.; Beygui, F.; Bossaert, L.; Ghaemmaghami, C.; Nonogi, H.; O'Connor, R.E.; Pichel, D.R.; Scott, T.; Walters, D.L.; et al. Part 5: Acute coronary syndromes: 2015 International Consensus on Cardiopulmonary Resuscitation and Emergency Cardiovascular Care Science with Treatment Recommendations. *Circulation* **2015**, *132*, S146–S176.
19. Khadaroo, R.G.; Fortis, S.; Salim, S.Y.; Streutker, C.; Churchill, T.A.; Zhang, H. I-FABP as biomarker for the early diagnosis of acute mesenteric ischemia and resultant lung injury. *PLoS ONE* **2014**, *9*, e115242. [CrossRef]
20. Niewold, T.A.; Meinen, M.; van der Meulen, J. Plasma intestinal fatty acid binding protein (I-FABP) concentrations increase following intestinal ischemia in pigs. *Res. Vet. Sci.* **2004**, *77*, 89–91. [CrossRef]
21. Uzun, O.; Turkmen, S.; Eryigit, U.; Mentese, A.; Turkyilmaz, S.; Turedi, S.; Karahan, S.C.; Gunduz, A. Can Intestinal Fatty Acid Binding Protein (I-FABP) Be a Marker in the Diagnosis of Abdominal Pathology? *Turk. J. Emerg. Med.* **2014**, *14*, 99–103. [CrossRef]
22. Kanda, T.; Tsukahara, A.; Ueki, K.; Sakai, Y.; Tani, T.; Nishimura, A.; Yamazaki, T.; Tamiya, Y.; Tada, T.; Hirota, M.; et al. Diagnosis of ischemic small bowel disease by measurement of serum intestinal fatty acid-binding protein in patients with acute abdomen: A multicenter, observer-blinded validation study. *J. Gastroenterol.* **2011**, *46*, 492–500. [CrossRef] [PubMed]
23. Sun, D.L.; Cen, Y.Y.; Li, S.M.; Li, W.M.; Lu, Q.P.; Xu, P.Y. Accuracy of the serum intestinal fatty-acid-binding protein for diagnosis of acute intestinal ischemia: A meta-analysis. *Sci. Rep.* **2016**, *6*, 34371. [CrossRef] [PubMed]
24. Hotchkiss, R.S.; Schmieg, R.E.; Swanson, P.E.; Freeman, B.D.; Tinsley, K.W.; Cobb, J.P.; Karl, I.E.; Buchman, T. Rapid onset of intestinal epithelial and lymphocyte apoptotic cell death in patients with trauma and shock. *Crit. Care Med.* **2000**, *28*, 3207–3217. [CrossRef] [PubMed]

25. Sturm, R.; Haag, F.; Janicova, A.; Xu, B.; Vollrath, J.T.; Bundkirchen, K.; Dunay, I.R.; Neunaber, C.; Marzi, I.; Relja, B. Acute alcohol consumption increases systemic endotoxin bioactivity for days in healthy volunteers-with reduced intestinal barrier loss in female. *Eur. J. Trauma Emerg. Surg. Off. Publ. Eur. Trauma Soc.* **2022**, *48*, 1569–1577. [CrossRef] [PubMed]
26. Lu, Q.; Xu, D.Z.; Davidson, M.T.; Haskó, G.; Deitch, E.A. Hemorrhagic shock induces endothelial cell apoptosis, which is mediated by factors contained in mesenteric lymph. *Crit. Care Med.* **2004**, *32*, 2464–2470. [CrossRef]
27. Matute-Bello, G.; Frevert, C.W.; Martin, T.R. Animal models of acute lung injury. *Am. J. Physiol. Lung Cell Mol. Physiol.* **2008**, *295*, L379–L399. [CrossRef] [PubMed]
28. de Haan, J.J.; Lubbers, T.; Derikx, J.P.; Relja, B.; Henrich, D.; Greve, J.W.; Marzi, I.; Buurman, W.A. Rapid development of intestinal cell damage following severe trauma: A prospective observational cohort study. *Crit. Care* **2009**, *13*, R86. [CrossRef]
29. Timmermans, K.; Özcan, S.; Kox, M.; Vaneker, M.; De Jong, C.; Gerretsen, J.; Edwards, M.; Scheffer, G.J.; Pickkers, P. Circulating iFABP Levels as a marker of intestinal damage in trauma patients. *Shock* **2015**, *43*, 117–120. [CrossRef]

Article

Correlation between Platelet Count and Lung Dysfunction in Multiple Trauma Patients—A Retrospective Cohort Analysis

Frederik Greve [1,*], Olivia Mair [1], Ina Aulbach [1,2], Peter Biberthaler [1] and Marc Hanschen [1]

[1] Department of Trauma Surgery, Klinikum Rechts der Isar, Technical University of Munich, 81675 Munich, Germany; oliviaanna.mair@mri.tum.de (O.M.); ina.aulbach@charite.de (I.A.); peter.biberthaler@mri.tum.de (P.B.); marc.hanschen@mri.tum.de (M.H.)
[2] Department of Traumatology and Reconstructive Surgery, Charité-Universitätsmedizin Berlin, 12203 Berlin, Germany
* Correspondence: frederik.greve@mri.tum.de; Tel.: +49-89-4140-2126

Abstract: (1) Background: Current findings emphasize the potential contribution of platelets to the immunological response after severe trauma. As clinical relevance remains unclear, this study aims to analyze the correlation between platelets and lung dysfunction in severely injured patients. (2) Methods: We retrospectively enrolled all multiple trauma patients presenting to our level 1 trauma center from 2015 to 2016 with an Injury-Severity Score (ISS) $\geq$ 16. Apart from demographic data, platelet counts and PaO_2/FiO_2 as an approximate indicator for lung physiology were analyzed and correlated on subsequent days after admission. (3) Results: 83 patients with a median ISS of 22 (IQR 18–36) were included. Compared to day 1, platelet counts were decreased on day 3 ($p \leq 0.001$). Platelet counts were significantly lower on day 3 in patients with an ISS $\geq$ 35 ($p = 0.011$). There were no differences regarding PaO_2/FiO_2 index. Correlation analysis revealed a positive link between increased platelet counts and PaO_2/FiO_2 index on day 1 only in severely injured patients ($p = 0.007$). (4) Conclusions: This work supports the concept of platelets modulating the posttraumatic immune response by affecting lung dysfunction in the early phase after multiple trauma in dependence of injury severity. Our findings contribute to the understanding of the impact of platelets on systemic processes in multiple trauma patients.

Keywords: platelets; trauma; immune system; posttraumatic organ failure; posttraumatic lung dysfunction; posttraumatic hyperinflammation

1. Introduction

Trauma-induced injury is the leading cause of death among people until 44 years of age in the United States as well as one of the leading global causes of death and disability [1,2]. Late posttraumatic mortality is caused by systemic hyperinflammation, leading to multiple organ failure (MOF) with high lethality rates up to 50% [3–6].

Multifactorial pathophysiological mechanisms contribute to increased sensitivity and risk of MOF in the early stages of multiple trauma. The primary components are the pro-inflammatory systemic inflammatory response syndrome (SIRS) and compensatory anti-inflammatory response syndrome (CARS). High intensity and disbalance of these conflicting trauma-induced inflammatory responses trigger the progress of inflammation and development of organ dysfunction and MOF [7–12].

Lung injury is frequently observed after multiple trauma and is either caused directly (e.g., thoracic trauma) or indirectly in the context of posttraumatic hyperinflammation or sepsis [13–15]. Triggered by SIRS, activated leukocytes migrate into the pulmonary interstitium. Complex intercellular pathways and various cytokines lead to increased endothelial permeability with consecutive alveolar edema and impaired gas exchange. This is followed by a local inflammation, which further contributes to cytokine release and promotes systemic inflammation leading to MOF [16–18]. Lung injury clinically manifests as acute respiratory distress syndrome (ARDS), which, according to the latest definition, consists of acute hypoxemia, conspicuous radiological investigations, and exclusion of hydrostatic edema due to cardiac failure [19].

Recently, the impact of platelets on the posttraumatic immune disturbance gained increasing interest. It is well known that platelets serve as immunological mediators besides their distinctive function during hemostasis [20–26].

Several findings from animal studies indicate that especially in the pathophysiology of lung injury, platelet–neutrophil interactions seem to play a crucial role [27–31]. Driven by pro-inflammatory mediators, platelets adhere to lung capillary endothelial cells, become activated, and release chemokines and lipid mediators [27,28,32,33]. This is followed by activation of attached neutrophils, additional capturing of circulating leukocytes from the blood flow, and further release of pro-inflammatory mediators by endothelial cells [32,34]. Currently, our understanding of the pro- and anti-inflammatory impact of platelets is limited and the subject of ongoing studies.

Several registry studies focused on risk factors for the development of either MOF or ARDS after multiple trauma [35–39]. However, studies reflecting the direct clinical influence of platelets on injury-induced lung impairment are limited. Thus, the present work investigates the correlation between platelet count and lung dysfunction in multiple injury patients. As recent findings revealed a demographic influence on posttraumatic platelet counts [37,40] as well as on MOF and ARDS [35,39,41], we hypothesized that a potential correlation between platelet count and PaO_2/FiO_2 index would differ in varying subgroups of gender, age, and injury severity. We aim for a transfer of gaining molecular understanding of platelet interaction to a clinical setting to improve the overall understanding of the immunoinflammatory impact of platelets during posttraumatic hyperinflammation.

2. Materials and Methods

The key objective of this study is the clinical investigation of the influence of posttraumatic platelet counts on PaO_2/FiO_2 index as approximate measure of pulmonary end-organ failure in multiple trauma patients. For comprehensive evaluation, the posttraumatic dynamics of platelet counts and PaO_2/FiO_2 index were additionally analyzed.

We included all multiple trauma patients from our level 1 trauma center in this retrospective analysis from 2015 to 2016. Inclusion was prompted by an injury-severity score (ISS) of 16 or above. The study protocol was approved by the ethics committee of the Technical University of Munich (vote No. 129/17 S). The study was registered in the German Clinical Trial Registry (www.drks.de (accessed on 1 December 2021), trial number: DRKS00027235) and linked to the international Clinical Trials Registry Platform of the World Health Organization (https://trialsearch.who.int (accessed on 1 December 2021)).

2.1. Descriptive Analysis

Patient data were analyzed for demographic information (gender, age), cause of injury (blunt vs. penetrating), injury patterns, platelet count (G/l), PaO_2/FiO_2 index (mmHg), ICU stay, and outcome (survival vs. non-survival). For assessment of trauma severity, the ISS was calculated as per definition using the Abbreviated Injury Scale (AIS) [42]. This anatomical grading method provides an overall score for patients suffering from multiple injuries. Several body regions are scored from 0–6 (no injury up to non-survivable injury). The top three severity scores are squared and added. The range of the ISS is given from 0–75 [43]. Platelet count and PaO_2/FiO_2 index (also called Horovitz quotient or oxygenation index) as approximate measure of posttraumatic lung dysfunction were assessed in the early posttraumatic phase on day 1 and day 3 after admission to our trauma bay. For assessment of dynamic changes, platelet counts and PaO_2/FiO_2 index on day 3 were compared to base values on day 1. Statistical testing was performed by use of paired t-test after testing for normal distribution (D'Agostino and Pearson test). Testing for differences within the subgroups was performed by t-test and Mann–Whitney U test. Descriptive analysis was performed by use of mean and standard deviation in case of normal distribution or median and interquartile range in case of non-normally distributed parameters.

2.2. Correlation Analysis

As descriptive analysis only allows for interpretation of the kinetics and comparison between the respective subgroups, additional correlation analysis was performed to investigate a potential relationship between platelet count and PaO_2/FiO_2 index.

Correlation between PaO_2/FiO_2 index and platelet count for the entire study population and for patients in dependence of thoracic trauma—assessed for each day—was performed by use of Pearson (in case of normal distribution and linear relationship) or Spearman's correlation coefficient. The identic correlation as named above was performed after dividing the study population into three subgroups (gender: male/female; ISS: $<35/\geq35$; age: <60 years/≥60 years). Correlation coefficients of PaO_2/FiO_2 index and platelet count of the respective subgroups were compared. A Z-test was performed to compare correlation coefficients from independent samples. For application of the Z-test, Fisher's Z-transformation was considered.

The level of significance was set as $p < 0.05$. Statistical testing was performed by use of GraphPad PRISM Software (San Diego, CA, USA).

3. Results

3.1. Descriptive Data

For this study, data from 189 patients hospitalized to our trauma center were screened. With an ISS higher than 16 and full datasets for the measurement of PaO_2/FiO_2 index and platelet count on subsequent days, 83 individuals were found to be appropriate for inclusion in this research.

The leading cause of injury was a blunt trauma mechanism. The largest proportion was diagnosed with head/neck or extremities/pelvic trauma. Almost half of the patients presented thoracic trauma. The majority suffered a severe trauma expressed by a median ISS of 22 (IQR 18–36). The majority of the patients were admitted to ICU with an average stay of 8 days. Lethal outcome was observed in 10% of the cases. For further details, please see Table 1.

Table 1. Demographic patient data of the study population.

Demography	Number n (%)	Median (IQR Q_{25}–Q_{75})/Mean ± SD
Included patients	83 (100%)	-
Age		Median 51 years (34–64 years)
<60 years	57 (68.7%)	Median 43 years (29–51 years)
≥60 years	26 (31.3%)	Median 73 years (66–76 years)
Gender		
Male	62 (74.7%)	-
Female	21 (25.3%)	-
Mechanisms of injury		
Blunt trauma	76 (91.6%)	-
Penetrating trauma	7 (8.4%)	-
AIS		
Head/neck	59 (71.1%)	Median 3 (0–4)
Face	28 (33.7%)	Median 0 (0–2)
Thorax	45 (54.2%)	Median 2 (0–3)
Abdomen	28 (33.7%)	Median 0 (0–3)
Extremities/pelvis	62 (74.7%)	Median 3 (0–4)
Other	25 (30.1%)	Median 0 (0–1)
ISS	-	Median 22 (18–36)
<35	62 (74.7%)	Median 19 (17–25)
≥35	21 (25.3%)	Median 41 (38–57)
ICU stay		
Days on ICU	1–56 days	Mean 8.3 ± 13.0 days
Patients without ICU stay	16 (19%)	Mean 15.1 ± 5.8 days
Patients with ICU stay	67 (81%)	Mean 10.1 ± 13.7 days
Mortality		
Deaths	10 (12%)	-
Survivors	73 (88%)	-

SD, standard deviation; IQR, interquartile range; AIS, abbreviated injury scale; ISS, injury-severity score; ICU, intensive care unit.

3.2. Dynamics of Platelet Counts and PaO_2/FiO_2 Index

Platelet counts were gathered in the early phase after admission and analyzed for differences between day 1 and day 3 after trauma (Table 2, Figure 1).

Table 2. Platelet counts and PaO_2/FiO_2 on day (D) 1 and 3 of the entire study population.

	Platelet Count (G/L) (Mean ± SD)	p	PaO_2/FiO_2 (mmHg) (Mean ± SD)	p
D1	185.5 ± 69.6	-	325 ± 181.6	
D3	139.9 ± 53.5	≤0.001 ***	336.8 ± 172.8	0.755

Testing for statistical significance was performed between D3 and D1 as base value during admission in the trauma bay. SD, standard deviation; *** = $p \leq 0.001$; level of significance was set as $p < 0.05$.

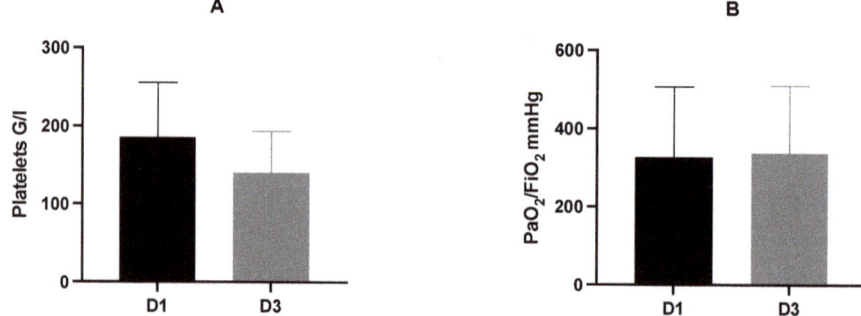

Figure 1. Mean and standard deviation of platelet count (**A**) and PaO2/FiO2 index (**B**) on D1 and D3 after trauma. Mean platelet count on D3 was significantly decreased compared to D1 (D1: mean 185.5 ± 69.7 G/l vs. D3: mean 139.9 ± 53.5 G/l; $p \leq 0.001$). There was no significant difference of the PaO_2/FiO_2 index between D1 and D3 (D1: mean 325 ± 181.6 mmHg vs. D3: mean 336.8 ± 172.8 mmHg; $p = 0.755$). D, day.

In relation to day 1 as base value, platelet counts decreased significantly on day 3 (D1: mean 185.5 G/l ± 69.6 G/l vs. D3: mean 139.9 G/l ± 53.5 G/l; $p \leq 0.001$).

Platelet counts were also analyzed within subgroups in dependence of age, gender, and injury severity (Table 3, Figure 2). Age and gender did not affect platelet counts on day 1 and day 3 after trauma. No significant differences between patients younger/older than 60 years and male/female patients were detected on day 1 and day 3 after admission for multiple trauma. In severely injured patients (ISS ≥ 35), platelet counts were significantly decreased on day 1 (ISS < 35: mean 197.7 ± 65.5 G/l vs. ISS ≥ 35: mean 150.6 ± 70.9 G/l; $p = 0.012$ *) and day 3 (ISS < 35: mean 149.0 ± 52.2 G/l vs. ISS ≥ 35: mean 113.2 ± 49.4 G/l; $p = 0.011$ *).

Table 3. Platelet counts on day (D) 1 and 3 in dependence of age, gender and injury severity.

Platelet Count (G/l)	<60 Years (Mean ± SD)	≥60 Years (Mean ± SD)	p
D1	189.4 ± 71.7	176.7 ± 65.3	0.437
D3	140.5 ± 50.5	138.7 ± 60.2	0.895
	Female	**Male**	**p**
D1	176.4 ± 76.0	188.6 ± 67.7	0.518
D3	129.8 ± 63.6	143.3 ± 49.8	0.408
	ISS < 35	**ISS ≥ 35**	**p**
D1	197.7 ± 65.5	150.6 ± 70.9	0.012 *
D3	149.0 ± 52.2	113.2 ± 49.4	0.011 *

SD, standard deviation; ISS, injury-severity score; * = $p < 0.05$; level of significance was set as $p < 0.05$.

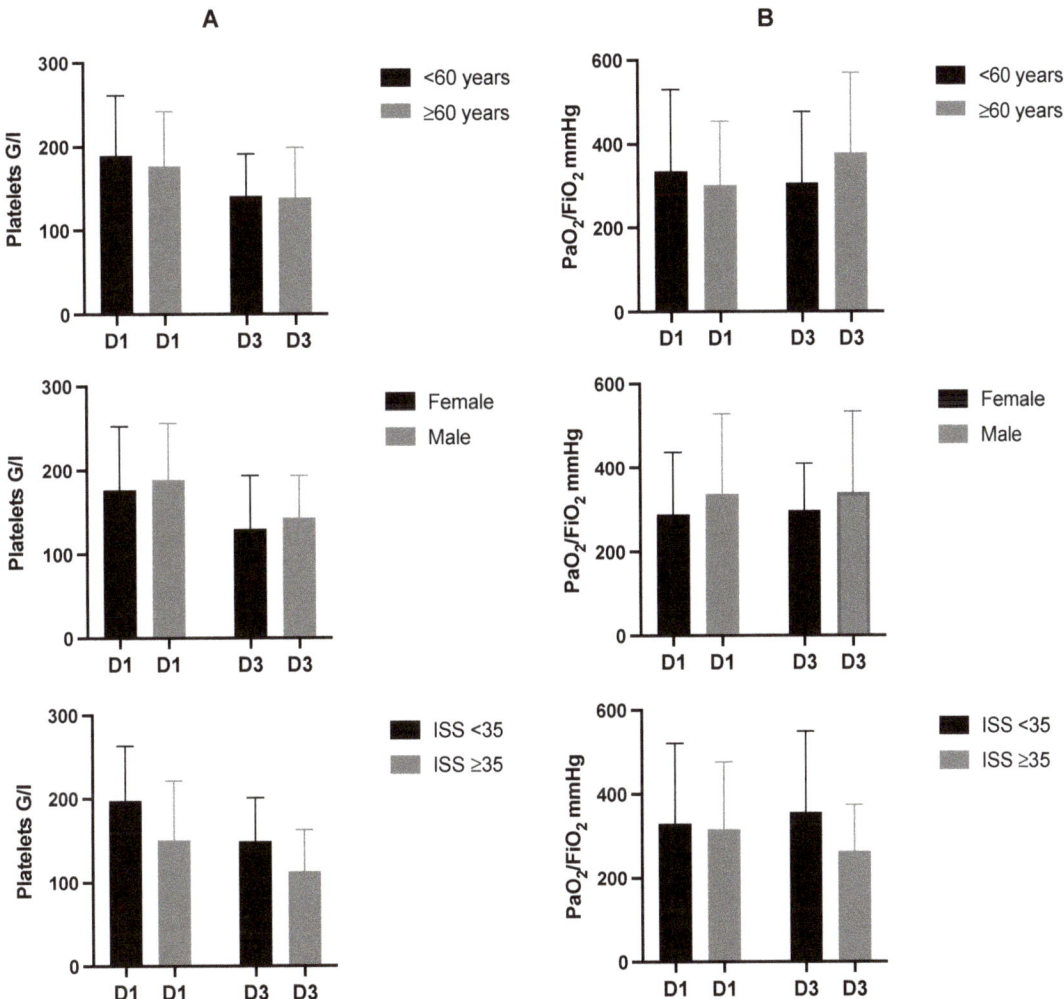

Figure 2. Descriptive subgroup analysis according to age, gender, and injury severity. Mean and standard deviation of platelet count (**A**) and PaO$_2$/FiO$_2$ index (**B**) on D1 and D3 after trauma. Comparison of platelet count and PaO$_2$/FiO$_2$, index in dependence of age and gender did not show any significant difference. Platelet count was significantly increased in patients with less severe injury (ISS < 35) compared to severely injured patients (ISS ≥ 35) on D1 (ISS < 35: mean 197.7 ± 65.5 G/l vs. ISS ≥ 35: mean 150.6 ± 70.9 G/l; p = 0.012) and D3 (ISS < 35: mean 149.0 ± 52.2 G/l vs. ISS ≥ 35: mean 113.2 ± 49.4 G/l; p = 0.011). There was no significant difference regarding PaO$_2$/FiO$_2$ index. D, day.

In analogy to platelet counts, PaO$_2$/FiO$_2$ index was determined on day 1 and day 3 after admission (Table 2, Figure 1) and additionally analyzed within the subgroups (Table 4, Figure 2). There were no significant differences.

Table 4. PaO$_2$/FiO$_2$ index on day (D) 1 and 3 in dependence of age, gender, and injury severity.

PaO$_2$/FiO$_2$ Index (mmHg)	<60 Years (Mean ± SD)	≥60 Years (Mean ± SD)	p
D1	353.3 ± 194.6	302.8 ± 151.3	0.672
D3	307.3 ± 169.1	378.5 ± 190.7	0.236
	Female	Male	p
D1	288.4 ± 148.8	337.4 ± 191.1	0.411
D3	297.9 ± 114.4	340.2 ± 193.9	0.881
	ISS < 35	ISS ≥ 35	p
D1	328.9 ± 190.7	315.5 ± 160.7	>0.999
D3	355.8 ± 192.9	263.8 ± 109.8	0.117

SD, standard deviation; ISS, injury-severity score; level of significance was set as $p < 0.05$.

3.3. Correlation Analysis

In a first step, correlation analysis of the entire study population was performed on day 1 and day 3 after multiple trauma (Figure 3). Correlation coefficients revealed a trend that increased platelet counts tend to be associated with increased PaO$_2$/FiO$_2$ index without reaching level of significance (D1: r = 0.23, p = 0.068; D3: r = 0.149, p = 0.306). To account for the potential impact of thoracic trauma, we performed correlation analysis after dividing the study population in dependence of diagnosed thoracic trauma. There was no significant correlation in patients with or without thoracic trauma between platelet count and PaO$_2$/FiO$_2$ index on day 1 (thoracic trauma: r = 0.19, p = 0.258; no thoracic trauma: r = 0.32, p = 0.109) and day 3 (thoracic trauma: r = 0.07, p = 0.723; no thoracic trauma: r = 0.287, p = 0.248).

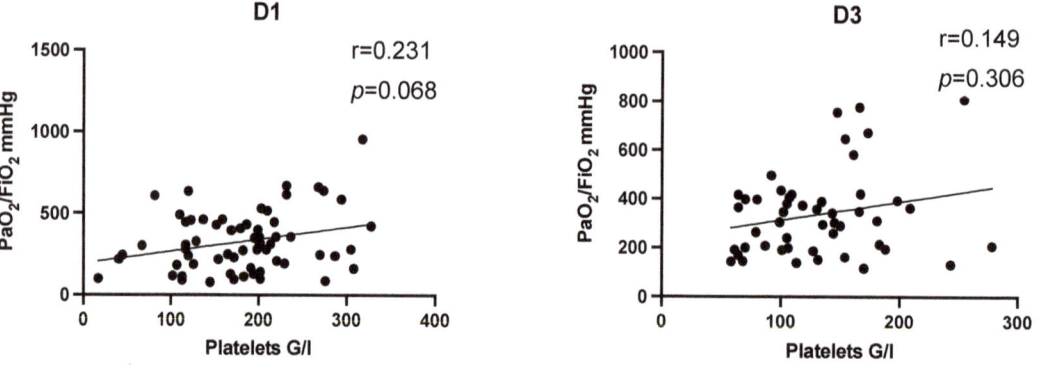

Figure 3. Correlation analysis of the entire study population on D1 and D3 after multiple trauma. Correlation analysis showed a slight positive correlation of platelet count and PaO$_2$/FiO$_2$ without reaching level of significance. The effect tends to be more pronounced on D1 (r = 0.231, p = 0.068). D, day; r, Spearman/Pearson correlation coefficient; p, level of significance.

The same analysis was performed in the respective subgroups to account for a potential influence of age, gender, and injury severity.

In patients younger than 60 years, a trend was detected that increased platelet counts seem to correlate with high PaO$_2$/FiO$_2$ index on day 1 after multiple trauma (r = 0.263, p = 0.092) (Figure 4, D1). The observations did not reach level of significance.

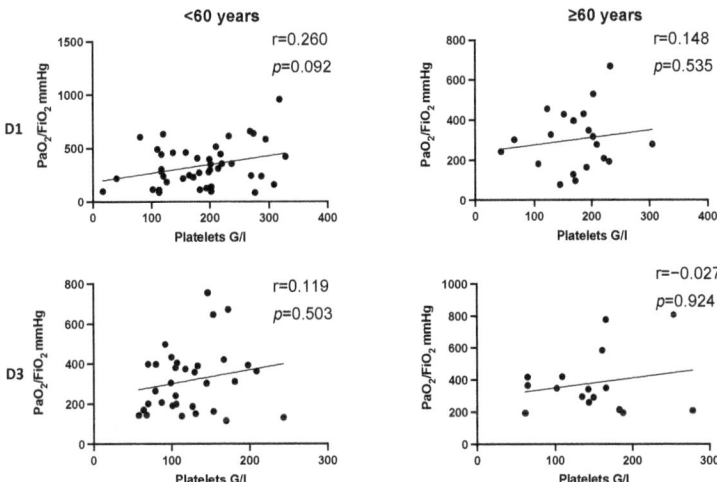

Figure 4. Correlation between platelet count and PaO_2/FiO_2 index following injury in dependence of age. There is no significant correlation between platelet count and PaO_2/FiO_2 index on D1 and D3 in dependence of age after trauma. Correlation coefficients show a slight positive correlation of platelet counts and PaO_2/FiO_2 index in younger and older patients. In younger patients, the effect seems to be more pronounced (D1: $r = 0.26$, $p = 0.092$; D3: $r = 0.119$, $p = 0.503$). D, day; r, Spearman/Pearson correlation coefficient; p, level of significance.

In dependence of gender, there also was a pronounced positive correlation in male patients on day 1 after multiple trauma (D1: $r = 0.249$, $p = 0.091$) (Figure 5, D1). However, a significant correlation was not observed.

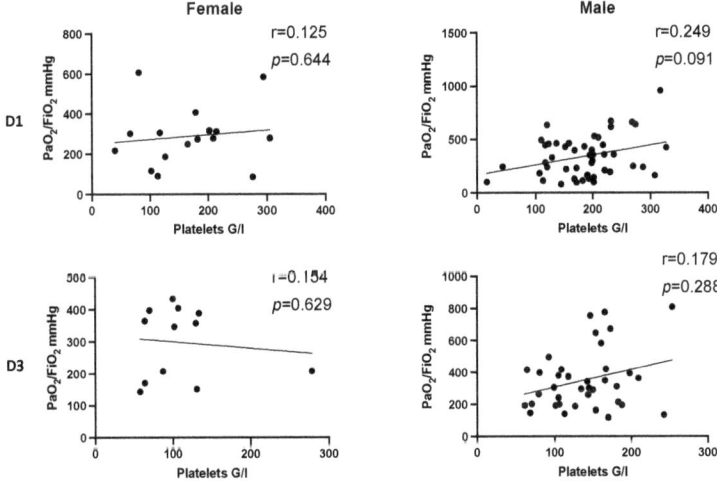

Figure 5. Correlation between platelet count and PaO_2/FiO_2 index following injury in dependence of gender. There is no significant correlation between platelet count and PaO_2/FiO_2 index on D1 and D3 in dependence of gender after trauma. Correlation coefficients in male patients on D1 ($r = 0.249$, $p = 0.091$) and D3 ($r = 0.179$, $p = 0.288$) indicate a pronounced effect that increased platelet counts tend to be associated with higher values of PaO_2/FiO_2 index. D, day; r, Spearman/Pearson correlation coefficient; p, level of significance.

In severely injured patients presenting an ISS ≥ 35, we detected a significant positive correlation indicating that increased platelet counts might correlate with increased PaO_2/FiO_2 index on day 1 after multiple trauma (D1: r = 0.609, p = 0.007 **). The effect was neither present in less severely injured patients (ISS < 35 D1: r = 0.096, p = 0.531; D3: r = 0.13, p = 0.457), nor did it last until day 3 (r = 0.293, p = 0.307) (Figure 6).

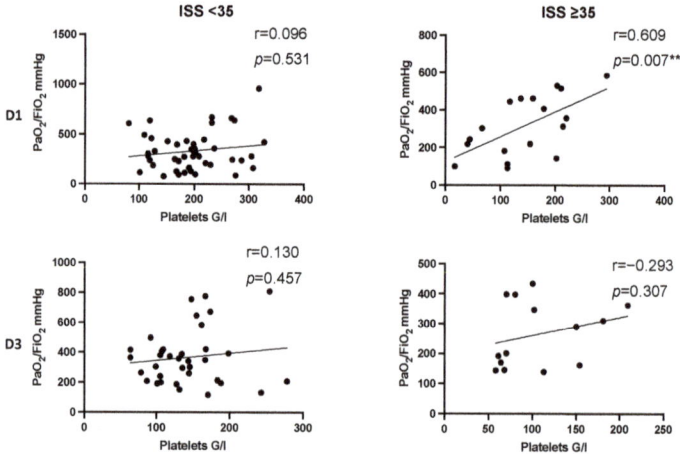

Figure 6. Correlation between platelet count and PaO_2/FiO_2 index following injury in dependence of injury severity (ISS). Correlation coefficients reveal a significantly positive correlation on D1 in severely injured patients (r = 0.609, p = 0.007). Increased platelet count seems to be associated with higher values of PaO_2/FiO_2 index. On D3, there is a pronounced positive correlation in severely injured patients without reaching level of significance. (r = 0.293, p = 0.307). D, day; r, Spearman/Pearson correlation coefficient; p, level of significance.

Subgroup analysis, which took into account the effects of age, gender, and injury severity, revealed various association patterns as shown in Figures 2–6. The level of significance was calculated as part of the statistical workup as shown in the legends of Figures 2–6. Table 5 allows for direct comparison of the given correlations, including the detailed indication of the patients included for each subgroup. For statistical comparison of the correlation coefficients, the Z-test was utilized.

Table 5. Correlation coefficients between platelet count and PaO_2/FiO_2 index in dependence of age, gender, and injury severity and comparison between correlation coefficients (Z-test).

Age	<60				≥60			Comparison of Correlation Coefficients	
	r	p		n	r	p	n	Z-test	p
D1	0.260	0.092	ns	43	0.148	0.535	20	0.404	0.686
D3	0.119	0.503	ns	33	−0.027	0.924	16	0.441	0.658
Gender	Female				Male			Comparison of Correlation Coefficients	
	r	p		n	r	p	n	Z-test	p
D1	0.125	0.644	ns	16	0.249	0.091	ns 47	−0.408	0.684
D3	0.154	0.629	ns	12	0.179	0.288	ns 37	−0.069	0.946
ISS	<35				≥35			Comparison of Correlation Coefficients	
	r	p		n	r	p	n	Z-test	p
D1	0.096	0.531	ns	45	0.609	0.007	** 18	−2.031	0.042 *
D3	0.130	0.457	ns	35	−0.293	0.307	ns 14	1.238	0.216

r, Spearman/Pearson correlation coefficient; p, level of significance; n, number of correlated pairs; ns, not significant; * p < 0.05; ** p < 0.01; level of significance was set as p < 0.05.

4. Discussion

In the setting of posttraumatic hyperinflammation, activated leukocytes migrate into the pulmonary microcirculation, leading to endothelial permeability and tissue edema formation with consecutive impaired gas exchange in the pulmonary alveoli [16–18]. Release of inflammatory mediators from the injured lung further contributes to additional end organ damage. Therefore, lung injury is an obligate early step and pacemaker in the development of MOF [38].

The assumption that platelets merely are a key player in hemostasis is outdated. Platelets contribute to inflammation as they release granules with pro-inflammatory cytokines, interact with neutrophils, and amplify endothelial-mediated inflammation and tissue injury [34,44].

In this study, our aim was to transfer increasing molecular understanding to a clinical setting. We performed a descriptive and correlation analysis of 83 multiple trauma patients (median ISS 22, IQR 18–36) to investigate the direct influence of platelet counts on PaO_2/FiO_2 index as a parameter for lung dysfunction.

4.1. Descriptive Analysis

Dynamics of Platelet Counts and PaO_2/FiO_2 Index after Multiple Trauma

Facing the entire study population, we detected a significant decrease of platelets on day 3 compared to day 1. There was no difference of PaO_2/FiO_2 index within the first days after trauma (Figure 1, Table 2). Subgroup analysis revealed significantly decreased platelet counts on day 1 in severely injured patients compared to less severely injured patients. There were no differences regarding PaO_2/FiO_2 index in dependence of age, gender, and injury severity (Figure 2, Tables 3 and 4).

Thrombocytopenia in the initial phase after trauma was also detected by Nydam and coworkers. In line with our results, low platelet counts were associated with increased injury severity. In addition, they were able to identify low post-injury platelet counts as a major independent risk factor for MOF and death, whereas higher platelet counts showed a protective effect several days after trauma [37]. Hefele and coworkers investigated post-injury dynamics of platelet counts and described low concentrations in the early phase and a recovery around ten days after multiple trauma with impaired function in thrombelastometry. Analogous to our findings, they detected decreased platelet counts in severely injured patients [40].

Thrombocytopenia in the early critical phase might be caused by dilution effects due to high-volume substitution in heavily injured patients. Furthermore, thrombocytopenia is associated with platelet sequestration in damaged pulmonary tissue by interactions with neutrophils promoted by adhesion molecule P-selectin [27,30,45,46]. We were surprised not to detect any differences in dynamics of PaO_2/FiO_2 index within the first 72 h after trauma. Several studies identified the lung to be the first affected organ in the cascade of MOF [13–15,38]. The large pulmonary capillary system filters the entire cardiac output, which is loaded with cytokines and inflammatory cells, such as neutrophils and macrophages. Ciesla and coworkers investigated a large multiple trauma collective for characterization of the onset of respective organ system impairment in the development of MOF. They detected lung dysfunction with decreased PaO_2/FiO_2 index to occur 1.6 days after trauma, followed by heart, liver, and kidney failure. The severity of lung dysfunction correlated with the extent of damage to other organ systems [38]. According to Sauaia and coworkers, almost every severe multiple trauma patient develops lung dysfunction, with the lowest influence on mortality. Mortality is believed to be highest for cardiovascular dysfunction, followed by acute kidney failure, liver injury, and lung dysfunction [7,47]. As several studies describe that age, gender, and injury severity influence MOF and lung dysfunction, we would have expected differences in the respected subgroups regarding PaO_2/FiO_2 index [7,35,36].

4.2. Correlation between Platelet Count and PaO$_2$/FiO$_2$ Index

We did not detect a significant correlation between platelet count and PaO$_2$/FiO$_2$ index facing the entire study population after multiple trauma (Figure 3). Correlation analysis within the subgroups showed no effect for age and gender (Figures 4 and 5, Table 5), but we detected a significantly positive correlation for severely injured patients on day 1 after multiple trauma. On day 3, there still is a tendency without reaching level of significance (Figure 6, Table 5). This indicates that decreased platelet count could be associated with decreased PaO$_2$/FiO$_2$ index as a parameter for impaired lung physiology within 48 h after severe multiple trauma (ISS $\geq$ 35).

We hypothesize that low platelet counts are caused by sequestration into the lungs as mentioned above [30]. This is followed by local inflammation leading to epithelial damage and fluid infiltration, which reduces alveolar integrity with dysfunctional gas exchange as a consequence [48–50]. High platelet counts might predict a less severe posttraumatic course.

Platelets are involved in the pathophysiology of acute lung injury merely by recruitment of neutrophils [34]. After activation, platelets release the content of their granules (procoagulant and fibrinolytic factors, pyrophosphate, calcium, and adhesion molecules) undergo change of shape and upregulate the expression of adhesion molecules (P-selectin, PECAM-1, Glycoprotein IIb/IIIa, fibronectin, and thrombospondin) [34,44,51]. Platelet attachment to pulmonary capillary endothelium is mainly mediated by P-selectin [28]. Subsequent attachment of neutrophils then leads to platelet–neutrophil interactions inducing local tissue injury [34]. Blockade of P-selectin in a rodent animal model for acute lung injury showed superior outcomes due to reduced platelet–neutrophil aggregates making this a potential therapeutic target [27].

Kasotakis and coworkers investigated the effect of platelet transfusions in multiple trauma patients. According to their results, high-volume platelet transfusions are associated with the development of ARDS [52]. This supports the theory of a detrimental effect of platelets on lung physiology. In contradiction to their findings, we detected that increasing platelet counts (without supplementation) are associated with improved lung function. The impact of transfused platelet units could potentially be amplified by HLA antibodies responsible for transfusion-related acute lung injury (TRALI) [52].

Several studies additionally reported that prehospital antiplatelet therapy was associated with lower incidence of lung dysfunction [53,54]. However, a large prospective, randomized, placebo-controlled clinical trial investigating the effect of aspirin on the development of ARDS in patients at risk ruled out a potential benefit [55]. Recent results from a multiple trauma animal model showed promising therapeutic results by use of tranexamic acid as an additional example of potential involvement of the coagulation system in lung dysfunction development. After administration of tranexamic acid, Wu and coworkers detected a decreased pulmonary platelet–neutrophil infiltration with reduced edema formation by increased integrity of epithelial barrier function [56].

In summary, our findings are in line with the existing literature and contribute to the understanding that platelets are involved in the pathophysiology of posttraumatic lung dysfunction. Precise pathways are still not understood and remain to be elucidated.

4.3. Limitations

The study's design, data processing, and data interpretation imply limitations that must be taken into account. The retrospective character of the study limits the control of data quality and data completeness although all efforts were made to ensure for best possible accuracy.

PaO$_2$/FiO$_2$ index is frequently used to sufficiently describe hypoxemia and lung dysfunction [37,38,52]. However, the current definition of ARDS additionally requires chest radiographs and assessment of right heart function, which are not routinely assessed in our clinic [19].

In addition, injury patterns (e.g., severity of thoracic trauma) and individual therapy (e.g., platelet transfusions) of multiple trauma patients vary significantly. Therefore, the heterogeneity of the patient population has the potential to bias the results. We are aware that direct thoracic trauma in severely injured individuals might have an impact on early PaO_2/FiO_2 index and potentially influences our results. However, there was no difference for the entire study population in dependence of thoracic trauma. Due to the rather small sample size, we waived additional subgroup analysis in dependence of thoracic trauma. Unfortunately, we were unable to assess platelet transfusions in patients' medical records, which could further bias our results due to the association with ARDS in multiple trauma patients [52]. We further point out that a study population of 83 individuals is underpowered to derive clear clinical conclusions yet sufficient enough for findings as basis for future studies with larger data sets (e.g., registry studies including the impact of direct thoracic trauma).

Finally, all attempts have been made to discuss the results of the present study with the highest degree of caution. Strong correlation, even reaching level of significance, does not imply causation. Therefore, further studies are needed to support our results.

5. Conclusions

In conclusion, the present retrospective clinical study is the first to investigate the clinical relevance of posttraumatic platelet count, highlighting the correlation between platelets and injury-induced respiratory organ failure.

We were able to present alterations in the dynamics of posttraumatic platelet counts. Severity of injury seems to have a pronounced impact within the first 72 h after trauma, whereas gender and age did not present a modulating influence. Dynamics of PaO_2/FiO_2 index as a parameter for lung injury remained stable without being influenced by gender, age, or trauma severity. Correlation analysis revealed that low platelet counts tend to be associated with impaired lung physiology only in severely injured patients. Being aware that correlation does not imply causation, our data resonate with previous findings supporting the theory that platelets tend to contribute to the development of posttraumatic lung dysfunction. Our clinical data cannot determine the exact mechanisms but can add further knowledge to the overall understanding of the complex posttraumatic immunological processes and build a basis for future studies.

Author Contributions: M.H. designed the research; F.G., O.M. and I.A. performed the research; F.G. and M.H. performed statistical analysis; F.G., I.A., O.M., P.B. and M.H. analyzed and interpreted data; F.G. and M.H. wrote the manuscript. All authors have read and agreed to the published version of the manuscript.

Funding: This research received no external funding.

Institutional Review Board Statement: The study protocol was approved by the local ethics committee "Ethics Committee Technical University of Munich, Ismaninger Strasse 22, 81675 Munich" (vote No. 129/17 S). Date of approval: 4 April 2017. The study was registered in the German Clinical Trial Register (www.drks.de (accessed on 1 December 2021), trial number: DRKS00025982). The study was carried out in accordance with the World Medical Declaration of Helsinki of 1975, revised in 2013.

Informed Consent Statement: Due to the retrospective character of this study and the use of only routinely assessed parameters, the above mentioned Ethics Committee approved that informed consent is not necessary for this study.

Data Availability Statement: The data presented in this study are available on request from the corresponding author. The data are not publicly available due to retrospective data collection without the necessity for informed consent (see above).

Acknowledgments: The authors thank Fritz Seidl for language editing.

Conflicts of Interest: The authors declare no conflict of interest.

References

1. Heron, M. Deaths: Leading Causes for 2019. *Natl. Vital Stat. Rep.* **2021**, *70*, 1–114. [PubMed]
2. World Health Organization. The Top 10 Causes of Death. Available online: https://www.who.int/news-room/fact-sheets/detail/the-top-10-causes-of-death (accessed on 1 April 2020).
3. Demetriades, D.; Kimbrell, B.; Salim, A.; Velmahos, G.; Rhee, P.; Preston, C.; Gruzinski, G.; Chan, L. Trauma Deaths in a Mature Urban Trauma System: Is "Trimodal" Distribution a Valid Concept? *J. Am. Coll. Surg.* **2005**, *201*, 343–348. [CrossRef] [PubMed]
4. Ciesla, D.J.; Moore, E.E.; Johnson, J.L.; Burch, J.M.; Cothren, C.C.; Sauaia, A. A 12-Year Prospective Study of Postinjury Multiple Organ Failure. *Arch. Surg.* **2005**, *140*, 432–440. [CrossRef] [PubMed]
5. Cohen, J. The immunopathogenesis of sepsis. *Nature* **2002**, *420*, 885–891. [CrossRef] [PubMed]
6. Brun-Buisson, C. The epidemiology of the systemic inflammatory response. *Intensive Care Med.* **2000**, *26*, S064–S074. [CrossRef]
7. Sauaia, A.; Moore, F.A.; Moore, E.E. Postinjury Inflammation and Organ Dysfunction. *Crit. Care Clin.* **2017**, *33*, 167–191. [CrossRef]
8. Zedler, S.; Faist, E. The impact of endogenous triggers on trauma-associated inflammation. *Curr. Opin. Crit. Care* **2006**, *12*, 595–601. [CrossRef]
9. Hirsiger, S.; Simmen, H.-P.; Werner, C.M.L.; Wanner, G.A.; Rittirsch, D. Danger Signals Activating the Immune Response after Trauma. *Mediat. Inflamm.* **2012**, *2012*, 315941. [CrossRef]
10. Bergmann, C.B.; Beckmann, N.; Salyer, C.E.; Hanschen, M.; Crisologo, P.A.; Caldwell, C.C. Potential Targets to Mitigate Trauma- or Sepsis-Induced Immune Suppression. *Front. Immunol.* **2021**, *12*, 622601. [CrossRef]
11. Gentile, L.F.; Cuenca, A.G.; Efron, P.A.; Ang, D.; Bihorac, A.; McKinley, B.A.; Moldawer, L.L.; Moore, F.A. Persistent inflammation and immunosuppression. *J. Trauma Acute Care Surg.* **2012**, *72*, 1491–1501. [CrossRef]
12. Moore, F.A.; Moore, E.E. The Evolving Rationale for Early Enteral Nutrition Based on Paradigms of Multiple Organ Failure: A Personal Journey. *Nutr. Clin. Pract.* **2009**, *24*, 297–304. [CrossRef] [PubMed]
13. Fry, D.E.; Pearlstein, L.; Fulton, R.L.; Polk, H.C. Multiple System Organ Failure. *Arch. Surg.* **1980**, *115*, 136–140. [CrossRef] [PubMed]
14. Faist, E.; Baue, A.E.; Dittmer, H.; Heberer, G. Multiple Organ Failure in Polytrauma Patients. *J. Trauma Inj. Infect. Crit. Care* **1983**, *23*, 775–787. [CrossRef]
15. Regel, G.; Grotz, M.; Weltner, T.; Sturm, J.A.; Tscherne, H. Pattern of Organ Failure following Severe Trauma. *World J. Surg.* **1996**, *20*, 422–429. [CrossRef] [PubMed]
16. Weinacker, A.B.; Vaszar, L.T. Acute Respiratory Distress Syndrome: Physiology and New Management Strategies. *Annu. Rev. Med.* **2001**, *52*, 221–237. [CrossRef]
17. Tasaka, S.; Hasegawa, N.; Ishizaka, A. Pharmacology of Acute Lung Injury. *Pulm. Pharmacol. Ther.* **2002**, *15*, 83–95. [CrossRef]
18. Bhatia, M.; Moochhala, S. Role of inflammatory mediators in the pathophysiology of acute respiratory distress syndrome. *J. Pathol.* **2004**, *202*, 145–156. [CrossRef]
19. ARDS Definition of Task Force; Ranieri, V.M.; Rubenfeld, G.D.; Thompson, B.T.; Ferguson, N.D.; Caldwell, E.; Fan, E.; Camporota, L.; Slutsky, A.S. Acute Respiratory Distress Syndrome: The Berlin Definition. *JAMA* **2012**, *307*, 2526–2533. [CrossRef]
20. Elzey, B.D.; Sprague, D.L.; Ratliff, T.L. The emerging role of platelets in adaptive immunity. *Cell. Immunol.* **2005**, *238*, 1–9. [CrossRef]
21. Clark, S.R.; Ma, A.C.; Tavener, S.A.; McDonald, B.; Goodarzi, Z.; Kelly, M.M.; Patel, K.D.; Chakrabarti, S.; McAvoy, E.; Sinclair, G.D.; et al. Platelet TLR4 activates neutrophil extracellular traps to ensnare bacteria in septic blood. *Nat. Med.* **2007**, *13*, 463–469. [CrossRef]
22. Henn, V.; Slupsky, J.R.; Gräfe, M.; Anagnostopoulos, I.; Forster, R.; Müller-Berghaus, G.; Kroczek, R.A. CD40 ligand on activated platelets triggers an inflammatory reaction of endothelial cells. *Nature* **1998**, *391*, 591–594. [CrossRef] [PubMed]
23. Danese, S.; De La Motte, C.; Reyes, B.M.R.; Sans, M.; Levine, A.D.; Fiocchi, C. Cutting Edge: T Cells Trigger CD40-Dependent Platelet Activation and Granular RANTES Release: A Novel Pathway for Immune Response Amplification. *J. Immunol.* **2004**, *172*, 2011–2015. [CrossRef] [PubMed]
24. Hilf, N.; Singh-Jasuja, H.; Schwarzmaier, P.; Gouttefangeas, C.; Rammensee, H.-G.; Schild, H. Human platelets express heat shock protein receptors and regulate dendritic cell maturation. *Blood* **2002**, *99*, 3676–3682. [CrossRef] [PubMed]
25. Klinger, M.H.; Jelkmann, W. Review: Role of Blood Platelets in Infection and Inflammation. *J. Interf. Cytokine Res.* **2002**, *22*, 913–922. [CrossRef]
26. Engelmann, B.; Massberg, S. Thrombosis as an intravascular effector of innate immunity. *Nat. Rev. Immunol.* **2013**, *13*, 34–45. [CrossRef]
27. Zarbock, A.; Singbartl, K.; Ley, K. Complete reversal of acid-induced acute lung injury by blocking of platelet-neutrophil aggregation. *J. Clin. Investig.* **2006**, *116*, 3211–3219. [CrossRef]
28. Kiefmann, R.; Heckel, K.; Schenkat, S.; Dörger, M.; Wesierska-Gądek, J.; Goetz, A.E. Platelet-endothelial cell interaction in pulmonary microcirculation: The role of PARS. *Thromb. Haemost.* **2004**, *91*, 761–770. [CrossRef]
29. Asaduzzaman, M.; Lavasani, S.; Rahman, M.; Zhang, S.; Braun, O.Ö.; Jeppsson, B.; Thorlacius, H. Platelets support pulmonary recruitment of neutrophils in abdominal sepsis. *Crit. Care Med.* **2009**, *37*, 1389–1396. [CrossRef]
30. Looney, M.R.; Nguyen, J.X.; Hu, Y.; van Ziffle, J.A.; Lowell, C.A.; Matthay, M.A. Platelet depletion and aspirin treatment protect mice in a two-event model of transfusion-related acute lung injury. *J. Clin. Investig.* **2009**, *119*, 3450–3461. [CrossRef]
31. Rahman, M.; Zhang, S.; Chew, M.; Ersson, A.; Jeppsson, B.; Thorlacius, H. Platelet-Derived CD40L (CD154) Mediates Neutrophil Upregulation of Mac-1 and Recruitment in Septic Lung Injury. *Ann. Surg.* **2009**, *250*, 783–790. [CrossRef]

32. Schulz, C.; Schäfer, A.; Stolla, M.; Kerstan, S.; Lorenz, M.; Von Brühl, M.-L.; Schiemann, M.; Bauersachs, J.; Gloe, T.; Busch, D.H.; et al. Chemokine Fractalkine Mediates Leukocyte Recruitment to Inflammatory Endothelial Cells in Flowing Whole Blood. *Circulation* **2007**, *116*, 764–773. [CrossRef] [PubMed]
33. Zhu, J.; Carman, C.V.; Kim, M.; Shimaoka, M.; Springer, T.A.; Luo, B.-H. Requirement of α and β subunit transmembrane helix separation for integrin outside-in signaling. *Blood* **2007**, *110*, 2475–2483. [CrossRef] [PubMed]
34. Zarbock, A. The role of platelets in acute lung injury (ALI). *Front. Biosci.* **2009**, *14*, 150–158. [CrossRef] [PubMed]
35. Sauaia, A.; Moore, E.E.; Johnson, J.L.; Chin, T.L.; Banerjee, A.; Sperry, J.L.; Maier, R.V.; Burlew, C.C. Temporal trends of postinjury multiple-organ failure. *J. Trauma Acute Care Surg.* **2014**, *76*, 582–593. [CrossRef]
36. Howard, B.M.; Kornblith, L.Z.; Hendrickson, C.M.; Redick, B.J.; Conroy, A.S.; Nelson, M.F.; Callcut, A.R.; Calfee, C.S.; Cohen, M.J. Differences in degree, differences in kind. *J. Trauma Acute Care Surg.* **2015**, *78*, 735–741. [CrossRef]
37. Nydam, T.L.; Kashuk, J.L.; Moore, E.E.; Johnson, J.L.; Burlew, C.C.; Biffl, W.L.; Barnett, C.C.; Sauaia, A. Refractory Postinjury Thrombocytopenia Is Associated With Multiple Organ Failure and Adverse Outcomes. *J. Trauma Inj. Infect. Crit. Care* **2011**, *70*, 401–407. [CrossRef]
38. Ciesla, D.J.; Moore, E.E.; Johnson, J.L.; Burch, J.M.; Cothren, C.C.; Sauaia, A. The role of the lung in postinjury multiple organ failure. *Surgery* **2005**, *138*, 749–758. [CrossRef]
39. Fröhlich, M.; Lefering, R.; Probst, C.; Paffrath, T.; Schneider, M.M.; Maegele, M.; Sakka, S.G.; Bouillon, B.; Wafaisade, A. Epidemiology and risk factors of multiple-organ failure after multiple trauma. *J. Trauma Acute Care Surg.* **2014**, *76*, 921–928. [CrossRef]
40. Hefele, F.; Ditsch, A.; Krysiak, N.; Caldwell, C.C.; Biberthaler, P.; van Griensven, M.; Huber-Wagner, S.; Hanschen, M. Trauma Induces Interleukin-17A Expression on Th17 Cells and CD4+ Regulatory T Cells as Well as Platelet Dysfunction. *Front. Immunol.* **2019**, *10*, 2389. [CrossRef]
41. Sauaia, A.; Moore, F.A.; Moore, E.E.; Haenel, J.B.; Read, R.A.; Lezotte, D.C. Early Predictors of Postinjury Multiple Organ Failure. *Arch. Surg.* **1994**, *129*, 39–45. [CrossRef]
42. Gennarelli, T.A.; Woodzin, E. *Abbreviated Injury Scale 2005: Update 2008*; Association for the Advancement of Automotive Medicine: Chicago, IL, USA, 2016.
43. Baker, S.P.; O'Neill, B.; Haddon, W., Jr.; Long, W.B. The injury severity score: A method for describing patients with multiple injuries and evaluating emergency care. *J. Trauma* **1974**, *14*, 187–196. [CrossRef] [PubMed]
44. Zarbock, A.; Polanowska-Grabowska, R.; Ley, K. Platelet-neutrophil-interactions: Linking hemostasis and inflammation. *Blood Rev.* **2007**, *21*, 99–111. [CrossRef] [PubMed]
45. Botha, A.J.; Moore, A.F.; Moore, E.E.; Kim, F.J.; Banerjee, A.; Peterson, V.M. Postinjury neutrophil priming and activation: An early vulnerable window. *Surgery* **1995**, *118*, 358–365. [CrossRef]
46. Laschke, M.W.; Dold, S.; Menger, M.D.; Jeppsson, B.; Thorlacius, H. Platelet-dependent accumulation of leukocytes in sinusoids mediates hepatocellular damage in bile duct ligation-induced cholestasis. *J. Cereb. Blood Flow Metab.* **2008**, *153*, 148–156. [CrossRef] [PubMed]
47. Ciesla, D.J.; Moore, E.E.; Johnson, J.L.; Cothren, C.C.; Banerjee, A.; Burch, J.M.; Sauaia, A. Decreased progression of postinjury lung dysfunction to the acute respiratory distress syndrome and multiple organ failure. *Surgery* **2006**, *140*, 640–648. [CrossRef]
48. Pugin, J.; Verghese, G.; Widmer, M.-C.; Matthay, M.A. The alveolar space is the site of intense inflammatory and profibrotic reactions in the early phase of acute respiratory distress syndrome. *Crit. Care Med.* **1999**, *27*, 304–312. [CrossRef]
49. Ware, L.B.; Matthay, M.A. The Acute Respiratory Distress Syndrome. *N. Engl. J. Med.* **2000**, *342*, 1334–1349. [CrossRef]
50. Wiener-Kronish, J.P.; Albertine, K.H.; Matthay, A.M. Differential responses of the endothelial and epithelial barriers of the lung in sheep to Escherichia coli endotoxin. *J. Clin. Investig.* **1991**, *88*, 864–875. [CrossRef]
51. Rendu, F.; Brohard-Bohn, B. The platelet release reaction: Granules' constituents, secretion and functions. *Platelets* **2001**, *12*, 261–273. [CrossRef]
52. Kasotakis, G.; The Inflammation and Host Response to Injury Investigators; Starr, N.; Nelson, E.; Sarkar, B.; Burke, P.A.; Remick, D.G.; Tompkins, R.G. Platelet transfusion increases risk for acute respiratory distress syndrome in non-massively transfused blunt trauma patients. *Eur. J. Trauma Emerg. Surg.* **2019**, *45*, 671–679. [CrossRef]
53. Chen, W.; Janz, D.R.; Bastarache, J.A.; May, A.K.; O'Neal, H.R.; Bernard, G.R.; Ware, L.B. Prehospital Aspirin Use Is Associated With Reduced Risk of Acute Respiratory Distress Syndrome in Critically Ill Patients. *Crit. Care Med.* **2015**, *43*, 801–807. [CrossRef] [PubMed]
54. Harr, J.; Moore, E.E.; Johnson, A.J.; Chin, T.L.; Wohlauer, M.V.; Maier, R.V.; Cuschieri, J.; Sperry, J.L.; Banerjee, A.; Silliman, C.C.; et al. Antiplatelet Therapy Is Associated with Decreased Transfusion-Associated Risk of Lung Dysfunction, Multiple Organ Failure, and Mortality in Trauma Patients. *Crit. Care Med.* **2013**, *41*, 399–404. [CrossRef] [PubMed]
55. Kor, D.J.; Carter, R.E.; Park, P.K.; Festic, E.; Banner-Goodspeed, V.; Hinds, R.; Talmor, D.; Gajic, O.; Ware, L.B.; Gong, M.N.; et al. Effect of Aspirin on Development of ARDS in At-Risk Patients Presenting to the Emergency Department. *JAMA* **2016**, *315*, 2406–2414. [CrossRef] [PubMed]
56. Wu, X.; Dubick, M.A.; Schwacha, M.G.; Cap, A.P.; Darlington, D.N. Tranexamic Acid Attenuates The Loss of Lung Barrier Function in a Rat Model of Polytrauma and Hemorrhage with Resuscitation. *Shock* **2017**, *47*, 500–505. [CrossRef]

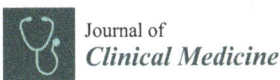

Article

Nutrition and Vitamin Deficiencies Are Common in Orthopaedic Trauma Patients

Jordan E. Handcox [1], Jose M. Gutierrez-Naranjo [1], Luis M. Salazar [2], Travis S. Bullock [1], Leah P. Griffin [3] and Boris A. Zelle [1,*]

[1] Department of Orthopaedics, UT Health San Antonio, 7703 Floyd Curl Dr., San Antonio, TX 78229, USA; handcox@uthscsa.edu (J.E.H.); gutierreznar@uthscsa.edu (J.M.G.-N.); bullockt@uthscsa.edu (T.S.B.)
[2] Long School of Medicine, UT Health San Antonio, 7703 Floyd Curl Dr., San Antonio, TX 78229, USA; salazarlm@livemail.uthscsa.edu
[3] Medical Solutions Division, 3M Health Care, San Antonio, TX 78249, USA; lpgriffin@mmm.com
* Correspondence: zelle@uthscsa.edu; Tel.: +1-210-743-4102

Citation: Handcox, J.E.; Gutierrez-Naranjo, J.M.; Salazar, L.M.; Bullock, T.S.; Griffin, L.P.; Zelle, B.A. Nutrition and Vitamin Deficiencies Are Common in Orthopaedic Trauma Patients. *J. Clin. Med.* **2021**, *10*, 5012. https://doi.org/10.3390/jcm10215012

Academic Editor: Roman Pfeifer

Received: 5 October 2021
Accepted: 26 October 2021
Published: 28 October 2021

Publisher's Note: MDPI stays neutral with regard to jurisdictional claims in published maps and institutional affiliations.

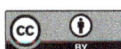

Copyright: © 2021 by the authors. Licensee MDPI, Basel, Switzerland. This article is an open access article distributed under the terms and conditions of the Creative Commons Attribution (CC BY) license (https://creativecommons.org/licenses/by/4.0/).

Abstract: Macro- and micronutrients play important roles in the biological wound-healing pathway. Although deficiencies may potentially affect orthopaedic trauma patient outcomes, data on nutritional deficiencies in orthopaedic trauma patients remain limited in the literature. The purpose of this study was to (1) evaluate the prevalence of macro- and micronutrient deficiencies in orthopaedic trauma patients with lower extremity fractures and (2) evaluate the impact of such deficiencies on surgical site complications. This retrospective study identified 867 patients with lower extremity fractures treated with surgical fixation from 2019 to 2020. Data recorded included albumin, prealbumin, protein, vitamins A/C/D, magnesium, phosphorus, transferrin and zinc, as well as wound complications. Nutritional deficiencies were found for prealbumin, albumin and transferrin at 50.5%, 23.4% and 48.5%, respectively. Furthermore, a high prevalence of micronutrient deficiencies (vitamin A, 35.4%; vitamin C, 54.4%; vitamin D, 75.4%; and zinc, 56.5%) was observed. We also recorded a statistically significant difference in wound complications in patients who were deficient in prealbumin (21.6% vs. 6.6%, $p = 0.0142$) and vitamin C (56.8% vs. 28.6%, $p = 0.0236$). Our study outlines the prevalence of nutritional deficiencies in an orthopaedic trauma population and identifies areas for possible targeted supplementation to decrease wound complications.

Keywords: orthopaedic trauma; nutritional deficiencies; vitamins; lower extremity; wound complications; nutrition wound healing

1. Introduction

The important role of nutrition in wound healing has been well documented in the literature, with macro- and micronutrients considered vital at every step of the wound healing pathway [1–3]. Unfortunately, malnutrition is common worldwide [4] and can be from a variety of causes, including advanced age, disease-related, food-insecurity/hunger or a mismatch between caloric intake and quality of nutrients consumed [5]. Malnutrition is a known contributor to poor clinical outcomes, from increased morbidity and mortality to wound and surgical complications [6,7]. As such, there is much interest in evaluating the role of nutrition in orthopaedic trauma patients, a vulnerable population sensitive to the effects of malnutrition.

Previous literature has demonstrated that malnutrition, as defined by hypoalbuminemia, is common in the orthopaedic trauma population [8]. Moreover, these authors recorded hypoalbuminemia and obesity as predictors of wound complications. Additionally, albumin deficiencies have been shown to correlate with wound complications in patients undergoing joint replacement surgery [9] and readmission rates for patients undergoing elective spine surgeries [10]. However, prior research has mostly focused on the geriatric populations, elective orthopaedic surgeries, and albumin and prealbumin as serum markers for malnutrition [11–14].

Even fewer studies have looked at the prevalence of micronutrient deficiencies in orthopaedic trauma patients. Among elderly hospitalized patients, vitamins C and D are commonly deficient [15,16]; however, there is limited data on its prevalence among a younger trauma population. Severe micronutrient deficiencies have well-known consequences, such as severe vitamin D deficiency leading to rickets and osteoporosis. Subtle deficiencies below the reference range may lead to wound-healing complications and other lesser-known sequela [5], and the orthopaedic literature has just started to explore the relationship between micronutrient deficiencies and negative clinical outcomes. For example, it has been shown that zinc deficiencies may lead to wound-healing complications in patients undergoing hemiarthroplasty [17]. Also, vitamin D has been shown to impact fracture healing rates in orthopaedic trauma patients [18]. Yet, data on micronutrient deficiencies in the orthopaedic trauma population remain limited in the literature.

The purpose of this study is to (1) evaluate the prevalence of macro- and micronutrient deficiencies in orthopaedic trauma patients with lower extremity fractures and (2) evaluate the impact of such deficiencies on surgical site complications in patients with high-risk lower extremity fractures. Our hypothesis is that deficiencies are common in the orthopaedic trauma population, and these deficiencies may be associated with an increase in surgical site complications in high-risk lower extremity fractures.

2. Materials and Methods

This study is a retrospective database analysis of orthopaedic trauma patients undergoing surgical fixation of their lower extremity fractures treated at a university-based level 1 trauma center between the years of 2019 and 2020. The study protocol was approved by our Institutional Review Board, and data collection, methods and analysis were performed in accordance with their rules and regulations. Inclusion criteria were patients over 18 years old with a minimum of 3 months follow-up and lower extremity fractures, identified through our electronic medical record system using the coding database. Patients were identified using the OTA classification system to include femur, tibia, tibia/fibula, fibula, talus, calcaneus and foot fractures. Subjects were excluded if they were under 18 years old, mentally or cognitively impaired, prisoners, or if they presented with a pathologic fracture, as well as those with less than 3 months follow-up.

Demographic data included age, gender, race/ethnicity, BMI, and the American Society of Anesthesiologists scale [19], as well as mechanism of injury and closed versus open injury. As our primary outcome measure, we recorded the available laboratory data on patients, including both macro- and micronutrient data: albumin (3.2–5.0 g/dL), prealbumin (17.0–37.1 mg/dL), protein total serum (6.2–8.1 g/dL), albumin/globulin ratio (1.06–1.61), transferrin (206–382 mg/dL), vitamin A (0.30–1.20 mg/L), vitamin C (23–114 mmol/L), vitamin D (30–80 ng/mL), vitamin K (0.22–4.88 nmol/L), magnesium (1.6–2.2 mg/dL), phosphorus (2.4/4.6 mg/dL), zinc (60.0–120 µg/dL), selenium (23–190 µg/L), TSH (0.350–5.500 µIU/mL) and PTH (19–88 pg/mL). An expanded panel of micronutrient data was obtained for patients who were deemed high risk by their treating orthopaedic surgeon; this expanded lab draw was at the discretion of the surgeon.

Secondary clinical outcome measures were tracked through a review of inpatient and outpatient charts and included data on wound complications (surgical site infections, wound dehiscence, hematoma) and surgical complications (malunion, nonunion, symptomatic hardware).

The statistical analysis was performed using SAS software version 9.4 (SAS Institute Inc., Cary, NC, USA). Categorical variables are summarized as count and percent. Chi-squared and Fisher's exact test were used to calculate differences for categorical variables. All tests were conducted at the alpha level of 0.05.

3. Results

3.1. Patient-Level Demographic Data

We identified 867 patients who met the inclusion criteria. Of these patients, 28.7% were age 65 or older. There were slightly more male patients (56.9%) compared to female patients. A majority of patients identified as White (95.6%) or Hispanic/Latino (62.1%). Finally, nearly 40% of patients were obese, as defined by BMI $\geq$ 30 (Table 1).

Table 1. Demographic and clinical data.

Number of Patients	n = 867
Age $\geq$ 65	249 (28.7%)
Ethnicity—Hispanic	538 (62.1%)
Race—White	829 (95.6%)
Gender (% Male)	493 (56.9%)
BMI $\geq$ 30	343 (39.6%)
Fracture location	n = 1008
Proximal Femur	195 (19.4%)
Femoral Shaft	107 (10.6%)
Distal Femur	34 (3.4%)
Proximal Tibia	98 (9.7%)
Tibial Shaft	84 (8.3%)
Ankle/Pilon	352 (34.9%)
Talus	20 (2.0%)
Calcaneus	51 (5.1%)
Foot	17 (1.7%)
Infection, Non-traumatic	38 (3.8%)
Others	12 (1.2%)

3.2. Nutritional Deficiencies

Albumin was measured for 745 patients, and of these, 23.4% were malnourished, as defined by albumin < 3.5 g/dL. Approximately half of the patients were deficient in prealbumin (50.5%). Finally, nearly half of the patients (48.5%) were deficient in transferrin.

Of those patients who had micronutrient data measured, 35.4% were deficient in vitamin A, 54.4% were deficient in vitamin C, and 75% were deficient in vitamin D. Over half of the patients were deficient in zinc (56.5% of patients). We did not observe significant deficiencies in magnesium, selenium or vitamin K (Table 2).

Table 2. Nutritional deficiencies by macro- or micronutrient.

Nutritional Markers	N	Deficient
Prealbumin	99	50 (50.5%)
Albumin	745	174 (23.4%)
Protein total serum	735	62 (8.4%)
Albumin/globulin ratio	734	512 (69.8%)
Transferrin	68	33 (48.5%)
Vitamin A	82	29 (35.4%)
Vitamin C	57	31 (54.4%)
Vitamin D	215	162 (75.4%)
Vitamin K	42	1 (2.4%)
Magnesium	619	21 (3.4%)
Phosphorus	609	100 (16.4%)
Zinc	92	52 (56.5%)
Selenium	63	0 (0%)
Thyroid-stimulating hormone	154	9 (5.8%)
Parathyroid hormone	97	2 (2.1%)

3.3. Nutritional Deficiencies by Demographic Group

There were significant differences in nutritional deficiencies between demographic groups. Of the patients 65 and older, 83.3% were deficient in prealbumin, compared to only 46.0% of patients younger than 65 years old ($p = 0.0153$). A similar trend was recorded with age and albumin, where 37% of patients over 65 years old were deficient, compared to 17.7% of patients under 65 years old ($p < 0.0001$). Compared to younger patients, patients over 65 years old were also at increased risk of deficiency in serum protein (11.7% deficient versus 7.1%, $p = 0.0396$) and transferrin (81.8% deficient versus 42.1%, $p = 0.0158$). With regards to age-related differences in micronutrients, patients over 65 years old were not at increased risk of deficiency in vitamins A, C, or zinc. Additionally, advanced age was protective against vitamin D deficiency, as 84.7% of younger patients had vitamin D deficiency, compared to 59.0% of patients over 65 ($p < 0.0001$).

Females were more likely to be deficient in albumin (29.2%) compared to males (19.2%, $p = 0.0015$). Micronutrient data showed that Hispanic patients were more likely to be vitamin D deficient than non-Hispanic patients (82.4% versus 65.6%, $p = 0.0047$). We did not observe statistically significant differences between these demographic groups in the remaining serum markers.

3.4. Complications by Nutritional Deficiency

To measure the rate of wound complications, we assessed the data at the fracture level, identifying 1008 individual lower extremity fractures, 181 (18.0%) of which had a wound complication. Low prealbumin was associated with a statistically significant difference in wound complications. We found that 21.6% of fractures with a prealbumin deficiency had a wound complication, compared to 6.6% of those with normal prealbumin levels ($p = 0.0142$). Vitamin C deficiency was also associated with wound complications; where 56.8% sustained a wound complication, compared to only 28.6% with normal vitamin C levels ($p = 0.0236$).

4. Discussion

Identifying macro- and micronutrient deficiencies in our orthopaedic trauma population is important, as it allows us to (1) understand the prevalence of this issue and (2) perform targeted interventions, which may lead to improvement in outcomes. Our data suggest that nutritional deficiencies have a high prevalence in orthopaedic trauma patients. Furthermore, macro- and micronutrient deficiencies may be associated with wound complications, most notably prealbumin and vitamin C deficiency.

There were some limitations to our study. One limitation was its retrospective design; this resulted in limited data for some of the studied micronutrients. Also, expanded micronutrient data collection was at the discretion of the treating surgeon at the time of hospital presentation. This led to variability in which nutritional markers were drawn for each patient. This may have contributed to the underrepresentation of certain micronutrients and difficulties in identifying other surgical complications, such as malunion/nonunion. Also, these data are from our local orthopaedic trauma population, which may lead to geographic variation in deficiency patterns.

Previous studies demonstrated improved outcomes with nutritional supplements in the geriatric population [14,20] and enhanced callus formation with zinc supplementation in young adult trauma patients with lower extremity fractures [21]. To our knowledge, there have not been any data reported on nutritional deficiencies using multiple serum markers in orthopaedic trauma patients with injuries at high risk for infection.

We have demonstrated profound malnutrition rates, including a hypoalbuminemia rate of 23.4%, which is slightly lower than previously found in this population (39.4%, Egbert et al.). Over half of our patients were deficient in prealbumin, which more closely correlates with perioperative nutritional deficiency, given its shorter half-life [22]. Prealbumin deficiency has previously been shown to correlate with surgical site infections in patients undergoing spinal surgery [23], and we did confirm a statistically significant difference in wound complications among those who were prealbumin deficient in our population. Almost half of the patients (48.5%) were deficient in transferrin, which also indicates significant malnutrition [24] and has been implicated in wound complications in arthroplasty [25]. Regarding micronutrient deficiencies, we found substantial deficiencies in vitamins A, C, D, and zinc, which is in line with the data available in the geriatric population [11,14]. In addition, Hispanic patients were also much more likely to be vitamin D deficient. Finally, we demonstrated that vitamin C deficiency is common, as is consistent with the existing literature [15] and found that deficiency in vitamin C may lead to wound complications.

Our study reinforces prior literature on the prevalence and impact of hypoalbuminemia in an orthopaedic trauma population [8,26] and confirms that malnutrition is a risk factor for wound complications [27,28]. Our study also confirms prior research demonstrating significant vitamin D deficiency in a diverse trauma population [12]. Our novel data on micronutrient deficiencies in the orthopaedic trauma population provides preliminary evidence for vitamin/nutritional supplementation in the perioperative period for a younger orthopaedic trauma population in order to improve clinical outcomes.

5. Conclusions

In summary, our study demonstrates a high prevalence of macro- and micronutrient deficiencies in an orthopaedic trauma patient population with lower extremity fractures. Deficiencies in prealbumin, and vitamins C, D and zinc were common, with over half of patients in our study group proving to be deficient. We also identified demographic risk factors for malnutrition, such as age, sex and ethnicity. Finally, we demonstrated that prealbumin and vitamin C may be associated with wound complications. This study lays the groundwork for identifying targeted supplement and nutritional interventions that may reduce the risk of surgical site complications. The reversal of these deficiencies in the perioperative period has the potential to improve patient outcomes and reduce hospital costs.

Author Contributions: Conceptualization, J.E.H., J.M.G.-N., L.M.S., T.S.B., L.P.G. and B.A.Z.; data curation, J.M.G.-N., L.M.S. and T.S.B.; formal analysis, L.P.G.; funding acquisition, L.P.G. and B.A.Z.; investigation, J.M.G.-N., L.M.S. and T.S.B.; methodology, J.E.H., J.M.G.-N., L.M.S., T.S.B., L.P.G. and B.A.Z.; project administration, J.E.H. and B.A.Z.; resources, B.A.Z.; software, L.P.G.; supervision, B.A.Z.; validation, L.P.G.; visualization, J.E.H.; writing—original draft, J.E.H., J.M.G.-N., L.M.S., T.S.B., L.P.G. and B.A.Z.; writing—review and editing, J.E.H., J.M.G.-N., L.M.S., T.S.B., L.P.G. and B.A.Z. All authors have read and agreed to the published version of the manuscript.

Funding: This research was partially funded by 3M KCI Inc.

Institutional Review Board Statement: The study was conducted according to the guidelines of the Declaration of Helsinki and approved by the Institutional Review Board of the University of Texas Health Science Center at San Antonio (project ID 165197).

Informed Consent Statement: Patient consent was waived by the IRB of our institution, as our study does not include any specific interventions or patient contact.

Data Availability Statement: The data are not publicly available online.

Conflicts of Interest: The authors declare no conflict of interest.

References

1. Palmieri, B.; Vadalà, M.; Laurino, C. Nutrition in wound healing: Investigation of the molecular mechanisms, a narrative review. *J. Wound Care* **2019**, *28*, 683–693. [CrossRef]
2. Stechmiller, J.K. Understanding the Role of Nutrition and Wound Healing. *Nutr. Clin. Pract.* **2010**, *25*, 61–68. [CrossRef]
3. Wild, T.; Rahbarnia, A.; Kellner, M.; Sobotka, L.; Eberlein, T. Basics in nutrition and wound healing. *Nutrition* **2010**, *26*, 862–866. [CrossRef] [PubMed]
4. World Health Organization. Malnutrition. Available online: https://www.who.int/news-room/fact-sheets/detail/malnutrition (accessed on 18 October 2021).

5. Cederholm, T.; Barazzoni, R.; Austin, P.; Ballmer, P.; Biolo, G.; Bischoff, S.C.; Compher, C.; Correia, I.; Higashiguchi, T.; Holst, M.; et al. ESPEN guidelines on definitions and terminology of clinical nutrition. *Clin. Nutr.* **2017**, *36*, 49–64. [CrossRef]
6. Reber, E.; Gomes, F.; Vasiloglou, M.F.; Schuetz, P.; Stanga, Z. Nutritional Risk Screening and Assessment. *J. Clin. Med.* **2019**, *8*, 1065. [CrossRef] [PubMed]
7. Tulchinsky, T.H. Micronutrient deficiency conditions: Global health issues. *Public Health Rev.* **2010**, *32*, 243–255. [CrossRef]
8. Egbert, R.C.; Bouck, T.T.; Gupte, N.N.; Pena, M.M.; Dang, K.H.; Ornell, S.S.; Zelle, B.A. Hypoalbuminemia and Obesity in Orthopaedic Trauma Patients: Body Mass Index a Significant Predictor of Surgical Site Complications. *Sci. Rep.* **2020**, *10*, 1953. [CrossRef]
9. Gu, A.; Malahias, M.; Strigelli, V.; Nocon, A.A.; Sculco, T.P.; Sculco, P.K. Preoperative Malnutrition Negatively Correlates with Postoperative Wound Complications and Infection After Total Joint Arthroplasty: A Systematic Review and Meta-Analysis. *J. Arthroplast.* **2019**, *34*, 1013–1024. [CrossRef] [PubMed]
10. Adogwa, O.; Elsamadicy, A.A.; Mehta, A.; Cheng, J.; Bagley, C.A.; Karikari, I.O. Preoperative Nutritional Status Is an Independent Predictor of 30-Day Hospital Readmission after Elective Spine Surgery. *Spine* **2016**, *16*, S271. [CrossRef] [PubMed]
11. Ernst, A.; Wilson, J.M.; Ahn, J.; Shapiro, M.; Schenker, M.L. Malnutrition and the Orthopaedic Trauma Patient: A Systematic Review of the Literature. *J. Orthop. Trauma* **2018**, *32*, 491–499. [CrossRef] [PubMed]
12. Zellner, B.; Dawson, J.; Reichel, L.; Schaefer, K.; Britt, J.; Hillin, C.; Reitman, C. Prospective Nutritional Analysis of a Diverse Trauma Population Demonstrates Substantial Hypovitaminosis D. *J. Orthop. Trauma* **2014**, *28*, e210–e215. [CrossRef]
13. Bohl, D.; Shen, M.; Hannon, C.; Fillingham, Y.; Darrith, B.; Della Valle, C. Serum Albumin Predicts Survival and Postoperative Course Following Surgery for Geriatric Hip Fracture. *J. Bone Jt. Surg. Am.* **2017**, *99*, 2110–2118. [CrossRef]
14. Roberts, J.L.; Drissi, H. Advances and Promises of Nutritional Influences on Natural Bone Repair. *J. Orthop. Res.* **2020**, *38*, 695–707. [CrossRef] [PubMed]
15. Teixeira, A.; Carrié, A.S.; Généreau, T.; Herson, S.; Cherin, P. Vitamin C deficiency in elderly hospitalized patients. *Am. J. Med.* **2001**, *111*, 502. [CrossRef]
16. Boettger, S.F.; Angersbach, B.; Klimek, C.N.; Wanderley, A.L.M.; Shaibekov, A.; Sieske, L.; Wang, B.; Zuchowski, M.; Wirth, R.; Pourhassan, M. Prevalence and predictors of vitamin D-deficiency in frail older hospitalized patients. *BMC Geriatr.* **2018**, *18*, 219. [CrossRef]
17. Zorrilla, P.; Salido, J.A.; Lopez-Alonso, A.; Silva, A. Serum Zinc as a Prognostic Tool for Wound Healing in Hip Hemiarthroplasty. *Clin. Orthop. Relat. Res.* **2004**, *420*, 304–308. [CrossRef] [PubMed]
18. Pourfeizi, H.H.; Tabriz, A.; Elmi, A.; Aslani, H. Prevalence of vitamin D deficiency and secondary hyperparathyroidism in nonunion of traumatic fractures. *Acta Med. Iran.* **2013**, *51*, 705–710. [PubMed]
19. Daabiss, M. American Society of Anaesthesiologists physical status classification. *Indian J. Anaesth.* **2011**, *55*, 111–115. [CrossRef] [PubMed]
20. He, Y.; Xiao, J.; Shi, Z.; He, J.; Li, T. Supplementation of enteral nutritional powder decreases surgical site infection, prosthetic joint infection, and readmission after hip arthroplasty in geriatric femoral neck fracture with hypoalbuminemia. *J. Orthop. Surg. Res.* **2019**, *14*, 292. [CrossRef]
21. Sadighi, A.; Roshan, M.M.; Moradi, A.; Ostadrahimi, A. The effects of zinc supplementation on serum zinc, alkaline phosphatase activity and fracture healing of bones. *Saudi Med. J.* **2008**, *29*, 1276–1279.
22. Keller, U. Nutritional Laboratory Markers in Malnutrition. *J. Clin. Med.* **2019**, *8*, 775. [CrossRef]
23. Tempel, Z.; Grandhi, R.; Maserati, M.; Panczykowski, D.; Ochoa, J.; Russavage, J.; Okonkwo, D. Prealbumin as a serum biomarker of impaired perioperative nutritional status and risk for surgical site infection after spine surgery. *J. Neurol. Surg. Part A Cent. Eur. Neurosurg.* **2015**, *76*, 139–143.
24. Gariballa, S.; Forster, S. Effects of acute-phase response on nutritional status and clinical outcome of hospitalized patients. *Nutrition* **2006**, *22*, 750–757. [CrossRef]
25. Roche, M.; Law, T.Y.; Kurowicki, J.; Sodhi, N.; Rosas, S.; Elson, L.; Summers, S.; Sabeh, K.; Mont, M.A. Albumin, Prealbumin, and Transferrin May Be Predictive of Wound Complications following Total Knee Arthroplasty. *J. Knee Surg.* **2018**, *31*, 946–951. [CrossRef]
26. Wilson, J.; Lunati, M.; Grabel, Z.; Staley, C.; Schwartz, A.; Schenker, M. Hypoalbuminemia Is an Independent Risk Factor for 30-Day Mortality, Postoperative Complications, Readmission, and Reoperation in the Operative Lower Extremity Orthopaedic Trauma Patient. *J. Orthop. Trauma* **2019**, *33*, 284–291. [CrossRef] [PubMed]
27. He, Z.; Zhou, K.; Tang, K.; Quan, Z.; Liu, S.; Su, B. Perioperative hypoalbuminemia is a risk factor for wound complications following posterior lumbar interbody fusion. *J. Orthop. Surg. Res.* **2020**, *15*, 538. [CrossRef] [PubMed]
28. Cross, M.; Yi, P.; Thomas, C.; Garcia, J.; Della Valle, C. Evaluation of Malnutrition in Orthopaedic Surgery. *JAAOS* **2014**, *22*, 193–199. [CrossRef] [PubMed]

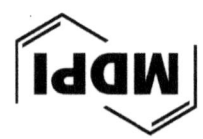

MDPI
St. Alban-Anlage 66
4052 Basel
Switzerland
Tel. +41 61 683 77 34
Fax +41 61 302 89 18
www.mdpi.com

Journal of Clinical Medicine Editorial Office
E-mail: jcm@mdpi.com
www.mdpi.com/journal/jcm

www.ingramcontent.com/pod-product-compliance
Lightning Source LLC
LaVergne TN
LVHW070618100526
838202LV00012B/680